Clinical Management of Heart Failure

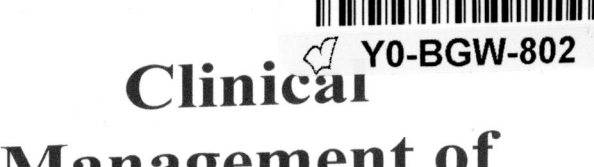

Third Edition

Javed Butler, MD, MPH
Professor of Medicine
Director, Division of Cardiovascular Medicine
Co-Director, Heart Institute
Stony Brook University School of Medicine

Roger M. Mills, MD, FACP, FACC
Cardiologist
Dexter, MI

James B. Young, MD
Professor of Medicine and Executive Dean
Cleveland Clinic Lerner College of Medicine
of Case Western University

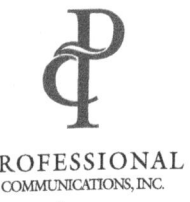

PROFESSIONAL
COMMUNICATIONS, INC.

Copyright 2017
Javed Butler, MD, MPH
Roger M. Mills, MD
James B. Young, MD

Professional Communications, Inc.

A Medical Publishing & Communications Company

400 Center Bay Drive
West Islip, NY 11795
(t) 631/661-2852
(f) 631/661-2167

1223 W. Main St, #1427
Durant, OK 74702-1427
(t) 580/745-9838
(f) 580/745-9837

All rights reserved. No part of this publication may be reproduced or transmitted in any form or by any means, electronic or mechanical, including photocopy, recording, or any other information storage and retrieval system, without the prior agreement and written permission of the publisher.

For orders only, please call
1-800-337-9838
or visit our Web site at
www.pcibooks.com

ISBN: 978-1-932610-36-9
Printed in the United States of America

DISCLAIMER

The opinions expressed in this publication reflect those of the authors. However, the authors make no warranty regarding the contents of the publication. The protocols described herein are general and may not apply to a specific patient. Any product mentioned in this publication should be taken in accordance with the prescribing information provided by the manufacturer.

This text is printed on recycled paper.

TABLE OF CONTENTS

1. Diagnosis of Heart Failure
2. Clinical Syndromes and Staging of Heart Failure
3. Pathophysiology of Heart Failure
4. Nonpharmacologic Management of Chronic Heart Failure: Diet, Activity, and Environment
5. Pharmacologic Management of Chronic Heart Failure
6. Cardiovascular Implantable Electrophysiologic Devices in the Management of Heart Failure
7. Heart Failure With Major Comorbidities
8. Interventions for Heart Failure
9. Acute Heart Failure
10. Psychosocial Issues in Heart Failure Management
11. Resources for Patients
12. Abbreviations/Acronyms
13. Index

TABLES

Table 1	ACC/AHA Recommendation System: Applying Class of Recommendation and Level of Evidence to Clinical Strategies, Interventions, Treatments, or Diagnostic Testing in Patient Care (Updated August 2015)	xvi
Table 1.1	Heart Failure Patients May Present With Any Possible Combination of Variables From These Categories	22
Table 1.2	The Evaluation of Salt and Water Retention, Exercise Intolerance, and Dyspnea	22
Table 1.3	Cardiovascular History	23
Table 1.4	Cardiovascular Physical Examination	24
Table 1.5.	Routine Laboratory Studies in the Evaluation of Suspected HF Patients	25
Table 1.6	Common Findings on the Resting 12-Lead ECG in Heart Failure Patients	26
Table 1.7	Important Findings on Routine Chest X-ray	27
Table 1.8	Important Data from 2D and Doppler Echocardiography	28
Table 1.9	Specialized Cardiac Imaging Studies	29
Table 1.10	Functional Cardiopulmonary Testing	30
Table 1.11	Outcomes of the Heart Failure Evaluation	32
Table 2.1	Demographics of Heart Failure	36
Table 2.2	Hemodynamic Patterns in Heart Failure	39
Table 2.3	The NYHA Classification	41
Table 2.4	ACC/AHA Stages of Heart Failure	41
Table 2.5	Examples of the Context Provided by Detailed Classification and Staging Systems	44
Table 3.1	Categories of Cardio-Renal Syndrome	55
Table 3.2	Suggested Mechanisms of Renal Impairment in Heart Failure	56
Table 3.3	Possible Mechanisms of Peripheral Muscle Abnormality in Heart Failure	60

Table 3.4	Cardiac Changes in HF-pEF	68
Table 3.5	Skeletal Muscle Impairment in HF-pEF	68
Table 4.1	Useful Conversion Factors for Prescribing Sodium Limitations	72
Table 4.2	Summary of Dietary Recommendations for Heart Failure Patients	74
Table 5.1	Classes of Pharmacologic Agents Available for Heart Failure Treatment	84
Table 5.2	Adverse Effects of ACE Inhibitors and ARBs	86
Table 5.3	ACE Inhibitors and ARB Contraindications and Cautions	86
Table 5.4	Summary of β-Blocker Comparisons	98
Table 5.5	Dosing Recommendations for MRAs	104
Table 5.6	Observed Laboratory Testing of Potassium and Creatinine Levels Among Patients Initiating Mineralocorticoid Receptor Antagonist Therapy for Heart Failure	110
Table 5.7	Comparison of PK and PD for Hydrochlorothiazide and Chlorthalidone	114
Table 5.8	Torsemide vs Furosemide Studies: Hospitalizations and Mortality	122
Table 5.9	Potential Benefits of Torsemide Compared With Furosemide	125
Table 5.10	Currently Available Agents for Pulmonary Hypertension	132
Table 6.1	Cardiac Effects of Right-Ventricular Pacing	150
Table 7.1	Ten Most Common Co-occurring Chronic Conditions Among Medicare Beneficiaries With HF, 2011	160
Table 7.2	Comorbidities in Patients With Acute Heart Failure From Three Large Registries	162
Table 7.3	Classes of Drugs Approved for T2D	165
Table 7.4	Currently Ongoing Cardiovascular Outcomes Trials With SGLT2 Inhibitors	178
Table 7.5	β-Blockers for HF and Their Effects on Lung Function and Symptoms in COPD Patients	181

Table 7.6	Baseline Characteristics of SHIFT Subjects With and Without COPD.....................182
Table 7.7	Prevalence of CKD in the General Population and in HF-rEF Patients.....................187
Table 7.8	Key Management Principles for Patients With Coexisting HF and CKD.....................194
Table 7.9	Systemic Anticancer Drugs With Important Cardiovascular Effects.....................206
Table 7.10	Frequency, Mechanism, and Reversibility of Important Anticancer Agents.....................208
Table 7.11	Cardiotoxicity Related to Anti-HER2 and VEGF: Frequency, Mechanism, and Reversibility of Important Anticancer Agents.....................210
Table 7.12	Assessment, Monitoring, and Management Recommendations for Patients at Risk of Cardiotoxicity (Stage A).....................212
Table 8.1	Complications of the MitraClip Procedure..........228
Table 8.2	INTERMACS (Interagency Registry for Mechanically Assisted Circulatory Support) Stages for Classifying Patients With Advanced Heart Failure.....................244
Table 8.3	Terms Describing Various Indications for Mechanical Circulatory Support.....................250
Table 8.4	Patients Potentially Eligible for Implantation of a Left Ventricular Assist Device.....................251
Table 9.1	Clinical Presentations of Acute Heart Failure.....256
Table 9.2	Initial Evaluation of the ADHF Patient...............258
Table 9.3	Common Precipitating Factors for ADHF..........259
Table 9.4	Adjusted Outcomes in Patients With and Without Hypotension.....................265
Table 9.5	Intravenous Inotropic Agents Used in Management of HF.....................267
Table 9.6	OPTIME: Adverse Effects in the Placebo and Milrinone Groups.....................268
Table 10.1	2016 ESC Guideline Recommendations on Frailty.....................280

Table 10.2	2016 ESC Guidelines Recommendations on Cognitive Dysfunction and Depression 281
Table 10.3	Clinical Indications for End-of-Life Planning 288
Table 10.4	Suggestions for Communication With Patients About HF Prognosis and Care Planning 290

FIGURES

Figure 2.1	Classification of Heart Failure Based on Timing of Symptoms...34
Figure 2.2	Hospital Discharges for Heart Failure, 1979-2006 34
Figure 2.3	Classification of Adults with Heart Failure on the Basis of Anatomy and Function 38
Figure 2.4	NYHA Classification and Peak Oxygen Uptake in Heart Failure Patients...40
Figure 2.5	The ACC/AHA Classification and the NYHA Classification..42
Figure 2.6	Phenotypes ("Clusters") in the HF-ACTION Study..46
Figure 3.1	Primary Negative Feedback Cycle in HF-rEF 50
Figure 3.2	RAAS Activation and the Natriuretic Peptides.....51
Figure 3.3	Relationship of Cardiac Performance and End Diastolic Volume...52
Figure 3.4	Pathophysiology of Renal Congestion and Renal Dysfunction...58
Figure 3.5	Physiology of HF-pEF 62
Figure 3.6	Pathophysiology of HF-pEF 64
Figure 3.7	PV Loops and Pressure vs Time Relationship in HF-pEF...64
Figure 3.8	Interplay Between HF-pEF and Comorbidities.....66
Figure 4.1	Canadian Hypertension Alcohol Intake Recommended Limits for Healthy Adults.............75
Figure 5.1	The Renin-Angiotensin Cascade...........................85

Figure 5.2	Molecular Structure of Entresto (Sacubitril and Valsartan) 90
Figure 5.3	Hazard Ratios for the Composite Endpoint and Components for LCZ vs Enalapril Displayed by Ejection Fraction (≤28%, >28%-33%, and ≥33%) 92
Figure 5.4	Algorithm for Choosing Dosing for Sacubitril/Valsartan Based on Current Treatment 94
Figure 5.5	Decline in High-Sensitivity Troponin T Over 36 Weeks With LCZ696 and With Valsartan in the PARAMOUNT Trial 96
Figure 5.6	SHIFT: Kaplan-Meir Plots for the Composite Endpoint, Cardiovascular Death, and Hospitalization, and Each Component Separately 100
Figure 5.7	TOPCAT Results by Region 108
Figure 5.8	Kaplan-Meier Survival Curves from A-HeFT 112
Figure 5.9	Potential Effects of Torsemide on the RAAS 118
Figure 5.10	Potential Effects of Torsemide on Myocardial Fibrosis 120
Figure 5.11	All-Cause Mortality Rates by Serum Digoxin Concentration Groups 126
Figure 5.12	Prevalence of Atrial Fibrillation in 6286 Patients Age 45 and Older in the General Population by Age and Sex 128
Figure 6.1	Incidence of Sudden Cardiac Death 142
Figure 6.2	Impact of ICD vs Conventional Therapy on Mortality in Trials in Patients With HF-rEF by Etiology 144
Figure 6.3	Relationship of QRS Duration and LV Dysfunction 146
Figure 6.4	Kaplan-Meier Curves Showing Survival in Patients with QRS <120 ms vs ≥120 ms 146
Figure 6.5	Effect of CRT vs Control on All-Cause Mortality and All-Cause Mortality Plus Hospitalization 148

Figure 6.6	Relationship of LVEF and Extent of Dyssynchrony with RV Pacing...........................150
Figure 6.7	AV Nodal Ablation vs Medical Rate Control for AF Patients Undergoing CRT........................151
Figure 6.8	Mortality With and Without Anticoagulation in Patients With HF, AF, and an IEPD 153
Figure 6.9	Recommended Management of Cardiac Implantable Device Infection...............................154
Figure 7.1	Long-Term Endpoints From STICHES: All-Cause Death, Cardiovascular Death, and All-Cause Death or Cardiovascular Hospitalization 164
Figure 7.2	Association Between Treatment With Incretin-Based Drugs and the Risk of Hospitalization for Heart Failure Among Patients With and Without a History of Heart Failure...167
Figure 7.3	Mechanism of Action of SGLT2 Inhibitors..........168
Figure 7.4	Efficacy Data, Systematic Review, and Network Meta-analysis 170
Figure 7.5	CV Outcomes and Death in the EMPA-REG OUTCOME Trial 174
Figure 7.6	Adverse Effects of SGLT2 Inhibitors...................176
Figure 7.7	Evaluation of Heart Failure During COPD Exacerbation Using B-Type Natriuretic Peptide Levels 179
Figure 7.8	Use of 2D and Doppler Echo and Radionuclide Ventriculography in the Cardiac Evaluation of Patients With Stable COPD...180
Figure 7.9	Ivabradine vs Placebo: K-M Curves for the Occurrence of the Primary Composite Endpoint in SHIFT for Patients With and Without COPD 185
Figure 7.10	K-M Plots for Cardiovascular Death or Admission for Chronic Heart Failure and All-Cause Mortality, Stratified by Albuminuria Status from CHARM 188

Figure 7.11 Multiple Processes Contribute to Negative Feedback Cycles in Patients With Both HF and CKD 189

Figure 7.12 Prevalence and Severity of Renal Dysfunction in Over 118,000 Hospital Admissions for Heart Failure...190

Figure 7.13 Kaplan-Meier Plot of All-Cause Mortality in a Propensity-Matched Analysis of the DIG Trial 191

Figure 7.14 Kaplan-Meier Plots Illustrating the Impact of Renal Dysfunction on the Incidence of Cardiovascular Death or Heart Failure Hospitalization for the Study Populations With HF-rEF and HF-pEF, Stratified by Renal Function 192

Figure 7.15 6-Minute Walk Test: Fatigue and Quality of Life Score Over Time 196

Figure 7.16 Algorithm for Diagnosis of Iron Deficiency in HF-rEF 201

Figure 7.17 Treatment Algorithm for Iron Deficiency in HF-rEF 202

Figure 7.18 Schematic Representation of the Main Mechanisms by Which Cardiomyocytes Are Damaged by the Most Cardiotoxic Anticancer Agents Among Those Currently in Use 204

Figure 8.1 Survival Rates After Heart Failure Hospitalization in Medically Managed Medicare Patients with Aortic Stenosis...............218

Figure 8.2 Changes in NYHA Class After TAVR, After SAVR, and with Conservative Treatment...220

Figure 8.3 Decision Making in Patients Referred for TAVR...224

Figure 8.4 MitraClip Implantation...225

Figure 8.5 Meta-analysis of 1 Year Events for MitraClip vs Surgery..227

Figure 8.6 The Watchman Left Atrial Appendage Closure Device...230

Figure 8.7	Kaplan-Meier Curves of Incidence of Endpoints 232
Figure 8.8	Kaplan Meier Curves for Freedom From Major Bleeding 234
Figure 8.9	Management Algorithm for the Active Treatment Arm in CHAMPION 238
Figure 8.10	Changes in Medication Overall and by Class of Agent in Active vs Control Groups in CHAMPION 240
Figure 8.11	Increases and Decreases in Medication Dose in the Active and Control Groups in CHAMPION 241
Figure 8.12	The HeartMate II LVAD 243
Figure 8.13	LVAD and Medical Management in Ambulatory HF: Treatmetn Algorithm to Guide Decisions on Noninotrope-Dependent Patients With Advanced HF 248
Figure 9.1	Hazard Ratio for Mortality Based on Number of HF Hospitalizations 254
Figure 9.2	A Scheme for Integrating Signs and Symptoms of ADHF Into an Overall Circulatory Assessment 258
Figure 9.3	60-Day Kaplan-Meier Curves for the Clinical Composite End Point of Death, Rehospitalization, or Emergency Department Visit in DOSE 261
Figure 9.4	EVEREST: K-M Curves for All-Cause Mortality and Cardiovascular Mortality/Heart Failure Hospitalization for Tolvaptan vs Placebo 263
Figure 9.5	ROSE Trial: Differences in Urine Volumes With Nesiritide and Dopamine as Compared With Placebo 270
Figure 10.1	Results of Cognitive Function Evaluation 284
Figure 10.2	Kaplan-Meier Curves Indicate the Composite End Point of Death or Hospitalization Because of Cardiovascular Disease 286
Figure 10.3	An Integrative Model for Palliative Care in Heart Failure 289

Introduction

Slightly more than a decade has passed since the previous (second) edition of this book. During that time, the movement toward practice guidelines promulgated by expert panels from the major cardiovascular societies has grown progressively stronger. At every level of experience, physicians are encouraged to follow guideline directed, evidence-based medical practice. So, why do we need another edition of this book? Why not simply say, "Read the guidelines and do what they say"?

First, the evidence base created from clinical trials has several important limitations. Most recent heart failure trials require that new drugs are tested "on top of" guideline-directed therapy rather than against placebo alone. In addition, trials have extensive inclusion and exclusion criteria. Finally, the practice of requiring "statistically significant" efficacy based on P values alone is suspect on multiple grounds, both practical and theoretical. These limitations may lead us to abandon development or use of drugs that have important benefits for smaller or unique populations.

Translating the evidence from clinical trials into practice is challenging. The problem that clinicians face is that patients do not come in neat packages with single problems. Rather, they come as themselves, as complex human beings with multiple comorbidities. Their caregivers face the issue of prioritizing the patients' problems, working out the most effective management strategies, and increasingly trying to limit the number and the cost of the drugs that they prescribe.

What we all must realize is that the more guidelines we have, the more messy spaces we will find in between the guidelines where professional judgement is required. That judgement must be based on an understanding of the evidence behind the guidelines, and a sense of priorities for the available options.

How can we, as authors, help? Our answer is largely expressed in our approach to the text, references, and format of this volume. We have made every effort to keep the text concise. We have attempted to base as much of the discussion of heart failure management on pathophysiologic principles as possible. We have provided references, whenever possible, to review articles and sound meta-analyses rather than primary data so that readers have access to the overall weight of evidence on a question. Technical abbreviations are listed with definitions in Chapter 12.

The format we have employed emphasizes the graphic display of information: Kaplan-Meir plots of mortality and re-hospitalization data, Forrest plots to show subgroup analyses, and tables to summarize lists. For any given patient, prognosis may vary widely based on demographics and comorbidities; we have emphasized the importance of careful, complete evaluation and management. In addition, clinicians should exercise the option for consultation with an experienced heart transplant/mechanical cardiac support device center early in the heart failure management process.

We hope that this volume will be a useful adjunct to health care professionals in practice, particularly those in the early stages of their careers. Our intent is for it to be handy, to be available, and to be easy to use.

— **JB, JBY, RMM**

Guidelines Update

When we wrote the second edition of *Clinical Management of Heart Failure,* publications and protocols often referred to "optimal medical management," or "evidence-based medicine." Today, authors use the phrase, "guideline-directed medical therapy" to describe best practices. This change indicates the central role of consensus guidelines from the major cardiovascular societies in determining our standards of care.

Accordingly, here is some critical information about the guidelines.

- ESC Guidelines for the diagnosis and treatment of acute and chronic heart failure 2012 were published in *European Heart Journal.* 2012;33:1787-1847.
- The 2013 ACCF/AHA Guideline for the Management of Heart Failure was published in the *Journal of the American College of Cardiology.* 2013;62:e147-e239 and in *Circulation.* 2013;128:e240-e327.
- The 2016 ESC Guidelines for the diagnosis and treatment of acute and chronic heart failure became available online May 20, 2016 from *European Heart Journal.* 2016;18(8):891-975.[1]
- A 2016 ACC/AHA/HFSA Focused Update on New Pharmacological Therapy for Heart Failure: An Update of the 2013 ACCF/AHA Guideline for the Management of Heart Failure: A Report of the American College of Cardiology/American Heart Association Task Force on Clinical Practice Guidelines and the Heart Failure Society of America was released online from *J Am Coll Cardiol.* 2016;68(13):1476-1488 and from *Circulation.* 2016;134(13):e292-e293.[2]

The 2013 ACCF/AHA document and the 2016 ESC Guidelines are the most recent comprehensive practice guidelines; the 2016 ACC/AHA/HFSA publication focuses on two new pharmacologic treatments for heart failure, sacubitril/valsartan and ivabradine, now approved for use in the United States.

Much to their credit, the ESC and the ACC/AHA/HFSA have evolved toward more consistent methods for evaluation of strength of evidence and the ranking of their recommendations. This facilitates comparison between recommendations from the two organizations. The current ACC/AHA approach is shown in detail in **Table 1**.

The ACC/AHA update, as mentioned above, is limited to recommendations on the use of sacubitril/valsartan and ivabradine. With regard to the former, the update states:

- This ARNI has recently been approved for patients with symptomatic HF-rEF and is intended to be substituted for ACE inhibitors or ARBs. HF effects and potential off-target effects may be complex with inhibition of the neprilysin enzyme, which has multiple biological targets. Use of an ARNI is associated with hypotension and a low-frequency incidence of angioedema.
- ARNI should not be administered concomitantly with ACE inhibitors or within 36 hours of the last dose of an ACE inhibitor.
- ARNI therapy should not be administered in patients with a history of angioedema because of the concern that it will increase the risk of a recurrence of angioedema.

With regard to ivabradine, the update recommends that given the well-proven mortality benefits of beta-blocker therapy, it is important to initiate and up titrate these agents to target doses, as tolerated, before assessing the resting heart rate for consideration of ivabradine initiation.

Important points from the newest ESC guidelines include:

TABLE 1 — ACC/AHA Recommendation System: Applying Class of Recommendation and Level of Evidence to Clinical Strategies, Interventions, Treatments, or Diagnostic Testing in Patient Care[a] (Updated August 2015)

Class (Strength) of Recommendation

Class I (Strong) — Benefit >>> Risk

Suggested phrases for writing recommendations:
- Is recommended
- Is indicated/useful/effective/beneficial
- Should be performed/administered/other
- Comparative-Effectiveness Phrases[b]:
  - Treatment/strategy A is recommended/indicated in preference to treatment B
  - Treatment A should be chosen over treatment B

Class IIa (Moderate) — Benefit >> Risk

Suggested phrases for writing recommendations:
- Is reasonable
- Can be useful/effective/beneficial
- Comparative-Effectiveness Phrases[b]:
  - Treatment/strategy A is probably recommended/indicated in preference to treatment B
  - It is reasonable to choose treatment A over treatment B

Class IIb (Weak) — Benefit ≥ Risk

Suggested phrases for writing recommendations:
- May/might be reasonable
- May/might be considered
- Usefulness/effectiveness is unknown/unclear/uncertain or not well established

Class III: No Benefit (Moderate) — Benefit = Risk
(Generally, LOE A or B use only)

Suggested phrases for writing recommendations:
- Is not recommended
- Is not indicated/useful/effective/beneficial
- Should not be performed/administered/other

Class III: Harm (Strong) — Risk > Benefit

Suggested phrases for writing recommendations:
- Potentially harmful
- Causes harm
- Associated with excess morbidity/mortality
- Should not be performed/administered/other

Continued

TABLE 1 — Continued

Level (Quality) of Evidence[c]

Level A

High-quality evidence[c] from more than 1 RCT
- Meta-analyses of high-quality RCTs
- One or more RCTs corroborated by high-quality registry studies

Level B-R (Randomized)

- Moderate-quality evidence[c] from 1 or more RCTs
- Meta-analyses of moderate-quality RCTs

Level B-NR (Nonrandomized)

- Moderate-quality evidence[c] from 1 or more well-designed, well-executed nonrandomized studies, observational studies, or registry studies
- Meta-analyses of such studies

Level C-LD (Limited Data)

- Randomized or nonrandomized observational or registry studies with limitations of design or execution
- Meta-analyses of such studies
- Physiological or mechanistic studies in human subjects

Level C-EO (Expert Opinion)

- Consensus of expert opinion on clinical experience

Key: COR, Class of Recommendations; EO, expert opinion; LD, limited data; LOE, level of Evidence; NR, nonrandomized; R, randomized; and RCT, randomized controlled trial.

COR and LOE are determined independently (any COR may be paired with any LOE).

A recommendation with LOE C does not imply that the recommendation is weak. Many important clinical questions addressed in guidelines do not lend themselves to clinical trials. Although RCTs are unavailable, there may be a very clear clinical consensus that a particular test or therapy is useful or effective.

[a] The outcome or result of the intervention should be specified (an improved clinical outcome or increased diagnostic accuracy or incremental prognostic information).

[b] For comparative-effectiveness recommendations (COR I and IIa; LOE A and B only), studies that support the use of comparator verbs should involve direct comparisons of the treatments or strategies being evaluated.

Continued

TABLE 1 — Continued

c The method of assessing quality is evolving, including the application of standardized, widely used, and preferably validated evidence grading tools; and for systematic reviews, the incorporation of an Evidence Review Committee

Halperin JL, et al. *J Am Coll Cardiol.* 2016;67:1572-1574

- The goals of treatment in patients with HF are to improve their clinical status, functional capacity and quality of life, prevent hospital admission, and reduce mortality.
  - It is only in patients with HF-rEF that therapies have been shown to reduce both morbidity and mortality.
- Patients with an LVEF in the range of 40% to 49% represent a "grey area" which we now define as heart failure with mid-range ejection fraction (HF-mrEF).
- Neuro-hormonal antagonists (ACEIs, MRAs and beta-blockers) have been shown to improve survival in patients with HF-rEF and are recommended for the treatment of every patient with HF-rEF, unless contraindicated or not tolerated. A new compound (LCZ696) that combines the moieties of an ARB (valsartan) and a neprilysin (NEP) inhibitor (sacubitril) has recently been shown to be superior to an ACEI (enalapril) in reducing the risk of death and of hospitalization for HF in a single trial with strict inclusion/exclusion criteria. Sacubitril/valsartan is therefore recommended to replace ACEIs in ambulatory HF-rEF patients who remain symptomatic despite optimal therapy and who fit these trial criteria.
  - To minimize the risk of angioedema caused by overlapping ACE and neprilysin inhibition, the ACEI should be withheld for at least 36 hours before initiating sacubitril/valsartan. Combined treatment with an ACEI (or ARB) and sacubitril/valsartan is contraindicated.

- ARBs have not been consistently proven to reduce mortality in patients with HF-rEF and their use should be restricted to patients intolerant of an ACEI or those who take an ACEI but are unable to tolerate an MRA.
  - ARBs are indicated for the treatment of HF-rEF only in patients who cannot tolerate an ACEI because of serious side effects.
- Ivabradine reduces the elevated heart rate often seen in HF-rEF and has also been shown to improve outcomes, and should be considered when appropriate.
  - The European Medicines Agency (EMA) approved ivabradine for use in Europe in patients with HF-rEF with LVEF $\leq 35\%$ and in sinus rhythm with a resting heart rate ≥ 75 bpm, because in this group ivabradine conferred a survival benefit based on a retrospective subgroup analysis requested by the EMA.
- Depression is common and is associated with worse clinical status and a poor prognosis in HF. It may also contribute to poor adherence and social isolation. A high index of suspicion is needed to make the diagnosis, especially in the elderly. Routine screening using a validated questionnaire is good practice.
  - Psychosocial intervention and pharmacological treatment are helpful, as well as exercise training, in patients with HF-rEF and depression. Cognitive behavioral therapy delivered in patients with HF and major depression beyond standard care and a structured education program were able to reduce depression severity, anxiety, and fatigue symptoms, as well as improve social functioning and mental and HF-related quality of life.
  - Selective serotonin reuptake inhibitors are thought to be safe, although the Sertraline Antidepressant Heart Attack Randomized Trial did not confirm that sertraline provides a greater reduction in depressive symptoms

or improvement in cardiovascular status compared with placebo in HF-rEF patients, but this trial was not powered enough to prove the latter.
- Escitalopram had no effect on either depression or clinical outcomes during the 24-month follow-up compared with placebo in patients with HF-rEF and depression.
- Importantly, tricyclic antidepressants should be avoided because they may cause hypotension, worsening HF and arrhythmias.

The published guidelines represent a consensus view from experts from North America and Europe, and serve as an authoritative resource for the heart failure community. They are generally consistent in their recommendations, and the ACC/AHA update and the new ESC guidelines are similar with regard to sacubitril/valsartan and ivabradine.

In their approach to the management of depression in HF patients, the authors of the ESC guidelines clearly recognize the importance of specific guidance on management of comorbidities, an important contribution. On the other hand, the utility of creating the HF-mrEF category seems questionable; time will tell.

REFERENCES

1. Ponikowski P, Voors AA, Anker SD, et al; Authors/Task Force members; Document Reviewers. 2016 ESC Guidelines for the diagnosis and treatment of acute and chronic heart failure. The Task Force for the diagnosis and treatment of acute and chronic heart failure of the European Society of Cardiology (ESC). Developed with the special contribution of the Heart Failure Association (HFA) of the ESC. *Eur J Heart Fail.* 2016;18(8):891-975.

2. Yancy CW, Jessup M, Bozkurt B, et al. 2016 ACC/AHA/HFSA focused update on new pharmacological therapy for heart failure: an update of the 2013 ACCF/AHA guideline for the management of heart failure. *J Am Coll Cardiol.* 2016;68(13):1476-1488.

1 Clinical Diagnosis of Heart Failure

Introduction

The primary focus of this book is the clinical management of patients with heart failure (HF). However, the first critical step in that process is efficiently developing a correct and detailed diagnosis. The diagnostic process often requires acquisition of a substantial amount of data over time.

Clinicians must keep in mind Heraclitus' adage that one never steps into the same river twice. Patients differ, and even the same patient changes over time.

Presentation

Patients' presentations with HF vary in both acuity and severity, and both the diagnosis and management should be appropriate to the individual situation (**Table 1.1**).

Diagnosis

The diagnosis of HF almost always involves the investigation of salt and water retention, exercise intolerance, and dyspnea. The tools available for the investigation are shown in **Table 1.2**.

As the American College of Cardiology Foundation/American Heart Association (ACCF/AHA) guidelines emphasize, "There is no single diagnostic test for HF because it is largely a clinical diagnosis based on a careful history and physical examination."[1]

TABLE 1.1 — Heart Failure Patients May Present With Any Possible Combination of Variables From These Categories

Ejection fraction	Reduced (HF-rEF)
	Preserved (HF-pEF)
Timing	Acute
	Chronic
Symptoms	Cardiogenic shock
	Pulmonary edema
	Volume overload
	Exercise intolerance
	Dyspnea

TABLE 1.2 — The Evaluation of Salt and Water Retention, Exercise Intolerance, and Dyspnea

- History and physical examination
- Laboratory evaluation
- Imaging studies
- Functional testing

History and Physical Examination

Standard texts and HF guidelines cover the components of the history and physical examination in some detail. The points in the history listed in **Table 1.3** have particular relevance for clinicians evaluating patients with suspected HF.

Familial heart disease may not manifest itself until well into adulthood. A careful family history may reveal hereditary cardiovascular disease (CVD) or familial neuromuscular disease with cardiovascular (CV) manifestations (**Table 1.4**).

Detailing the onset of exercise intolerance by reviewing milestones in the patient's history often reveals that modest limitations have existed for months

TABLE 1.3 — Cardiovascular History

Family history	Heart failure
	Sudden death
Critical markers for individual	Participation in sports
	Service in the military
	Pregnancies and outcomes
	Insurance and employment exams
	History of an abnormal EEG (RBBB, LBBB)
	Cancer treatment: chest radiation or cardiotoxic chemotherapy
	Substance abuse: particularly alcohol or cocaine
	Involuntary weight gain or weight loss
	Onset of diabetes
	Signs or symptoms of sleep-related breathing disorders

or years and with increased survival after initial treatment for cancer, patients often fail to make the connection between thoracic radiation or prior chemotherapy and new-onset cardiac failure.

For patients presenting with suspected HF, the basic goal of the physical examination is to assess volume status, adequacy of peripheral perfusion, and to differentiate cardiac pressure vs volume overload, if possible. Careful attention to the findings listed above will help with the assessment of these key factors. In addition, the physical examination should include assessment of body mass index (BMI), respiratory rate and respiratory pattern, and a search for signs of comorbid illnesses.

Clinical Laboratory

A pre-determined strategy should structure the clinical approach to laboratory testing, despite the fact

TABLE 1.4 — Cardiovascular Physical Examination

Volume status	Neck veins
	Rales or effusion
	Gallop rhythm
	Hepatomegaly
	Peripheral edema
Pulmonary examination	Periodic respiration
	Prolonged expiratory phase (COPD?)
Peripheral perfusion	Skin temperature
	Capillary refill
	Mental status
Pressure vs volume	Heart rate, rhythm
	Pulse pressure
	Sustained vs hyperkinetic apex
	S4 vs S3 gallop
General health	Cachexia, obesity, morbid obesity
	Signs of systemic illness (psoriasis, connective tissue disease)

that clinical laboratory tests are often ordered as an undifferentiated series of blood tests. The laboratory can offer clues to the CV diagnosis, to comorbid processes exacerbating HF, and to the individual patient's prognosis. **Table 1.5** outlines the context for interpretation of the most commonly available clinical laboratory studies.

The 12-Lead Resting Electrocardiogram

The routine resting 12-lead contains a treasure trove of highly relevant information for the evaluation of patients with suspected HF. **Table 1.6** lists important points to look for on the electrocardiogram (ECG). Assessment of the ECG should include assessment of

TABLE 1.5 — Routine Laboratory Studies in the Evaluation of Suspected HF Patients

Hemoglobin/hematocrit	Anemia of any type reduces oxygen-carrying capacity and exacerbates heart failure
White blood cell count	Leukocytosis may be the first clue to occult infection exacerbating heart failure
Iron/iron-binding capacity	Iron deficiency suggests occult bleeding Iron overload suggests further evaluation for hemochromatosis
Thyroid functions/thyroid-stimulating hormone	Thyroid dysfunction, either hyper- or hypothyroidism, may be a primary cause of heart failure or an important exacerbating factor
Renal function	An estimated glomerular filtration rate or creatinine clearance provides important baseline and prognostic information. Caveat: the estimating equations are not reliable in unstable patients
Electrolytes	Heart failure itself, comorbidities such as renal disease, and, most importantly, drugs such as diuretics, ACEi/ARBs, and anti-aldosterone agents all cause serious, and sometimes fatal, electrolyte disorders
Blood glucose and glycosylated hemoglobin	Diabetes is a critical underlying comorbidity in heart failure Both the diabetic disease and its treatment may substantially impact treatment and outcomes
Biomarkers	BUN, B-type natriuretic peptide (BNP), or N-terminal pro BNP (NT-pro-BNP), troponin, and possibly ST2 provide important diagnostic and prognostic data, and serial assessment may improve clinical management strategies

TABLE 1.6 — Common Findings on the Resting 12-Lead ECG in Heart Failure Patients

Rate	Is the resting rate excessively rapid (>90 bpm) or slow (<65 bpm)?
Rhythm	Are p-waves present?
	Presence of terminal p-inversion in V1 (LA abnormality) or atrial fibrillation suggests left sided heart disease
	Atrial fibrillation occurs in about 30% of all HF patients. Inadequate rate control is often an exacerbating factor in heart failure
	Multiple PACs or multifocal atrial tachycardia suggests pulmonary disease
	Multiple PVCs may be a clue to the potential for sustained ventricular arrhythmia
QRS	Duration >120 msec indicates potential for resynchronization
	Q-waves suggest prior MI
	LVH pattern suggests chronic pressure overload
	RVH pattern suggests pulmonary or right-heart disease
	Low voltage suggests pericardial effusion or diffuse myopathic process
ST-T waves	Acute ST-T wave changes suggest pericarditis, myocarditis, ischemia
	Chronic ST-elevation suggests ventricular aneurysm
T waves, U-waves	QT_c (Fridericia) prolongation may indicate potential problems with drugs, electrolytes, etc
	T wave abnormalities are often nonspecific; peaked T-waves suggest hyperkalemia; U-waves suggest hypokalemia

both positive (what is seen) and important negative (not present) findings. For example, HF due to coronary artery disease (CAD) is a low probability diagnosis when the ECG shows no evidence of prior myocardial infarction (MI).

An orderly, systematic review of the routine ECG is as critical as the history, physical examination, and routine laboratory studies to the evaluation of the patient with suspected HF.

Chest X-Ray

The "routine" posteroanterior (PA) and lateral chest X-ray, taken during deep inspiration at 6 feet with the patient standing, continues to merit a class one recommendation in the latest guidelines. Why, in this era of sophisticated specialized imaging, do we still get a chest film? **Table 1.7** lists many of the very nonspecific but important reasons.

The lack of specificity of many of the findings on the routine chest film enhances its utility as an important screening tool in clinical medicine. When the

TABLE 1.7 — Important Findings on Routine Chest X-ray

Shortness of breath	Alternative diagnoses such as infectious, neoplastic, or infiltrative pulmonary disease
Heart	Document heart size and configuration; valvular or pericardial calcification (specialized imaging required to determine LVEF)
Lungs	Increased venous pressure; interstitial, peribronchial, or alveolar edema; parenchymal lung disease
Great vessels	Size and shape of aorta; vascular calcification
Pleura, chest wall	Pleural thickening, effusion; chest wall deformity

chest film suggests non-cardiac or combined cardiopulmonary pathology, specialized imaging and functional studies will almost certainly be required to arrive at an accurate diagnosis and prognosis.

Cardiac Imaging Studies

In the 15 years that have passed since the second edition of this book, technical advances in echocardiography have led to a consensus that the 2-dimensional comprehensive echocardiogram represents "the most useful diagnostic test in the evaluation of patients with, or at risk for, HF." Echocardiography has a class one guideline recommendation for the initial evaluation of patients with suspected HF.[1] Echocardiography is widely available, does not expose patients to ionizing radiation and, along with a Doppler flow study, provides physiologic as well as anatomic information (**Table 1.8**).

TABLE 1.8 — Important Data from 2D and Doppler Echocardiography

- LV ejection fraction
- LV size and shape, wall thickness, volumes, regional wall motion
- RV size, function
- Estimated RA and RV-systolic pressure
- R and L atrial dimensions
- Valve anatomy and flow patterns (all valves)
- Mitral inflow, pulmonary venous inflow, mitral annular velocity, tricuspid regurgitant gradient, IVC diameter, and response to respiration

Serial echocardiographic studies can document response to treatment or progression of disease, but echocardiography should not be performed without a change in clinical status or a change in treatment. **Table 1.9** lists additional specialized cardiac imaging studies that may be useful and the various clinical situations in which the data may be important.

TABLE 1.9 — Specialized Cardiac Imaging Studies

Cardiac magnetic resonance imaging	High resolution required
	Quantify extent myocardial fibrosis
	Document myocardial perfusion and viability for revascularization
	Document changes specific for amyloid, sarcoidosis, iron storage, other infiltrative diseases
Cardiac computed tomography	Implanted device; high resolution required
	Implanted device; characterize myocardium
	CT angiography may be useful for the noninvasive documentation of coronary artery disease
Radionucleotide ventriculography	Useful for serial evaluation of LVEF; detection of cardiotoxicity

The extent and severity of comorbidities may impact the choice of specialized imaging modalities for individual patients. For example, an estimated 25% of HF patients in the United States have implanted electrophysiologic devices, which may limit the use of cardiac magnetic resonance imaging (cMRI).[2] Also, HF patients have a high prevalence of renal dysfunction and require caution in the selection of studies that require intravascular contrast administration.

Functional Studies

Functional evaluation of lung volumes and airway mechanics has an important role in the assessment of HF patients (**Table 1.10**). Pulmonary function testing may demonstrate important comorbid pulmonary disease that may hamper the clinical evaluation, limit the options for HF treatment, or even more importantly, limit the degree of improvement that may be attained with HF therapy alone. In HF patients with known or

TABLE 1.10 — Functional Cardiopulmonary Testing

Pulmonary function studies	Spirometry and lung volumes, pre- and post-bronchodilators
	Diffusing capacity
Stress testing for myocardial ischemia	Exercise testing with radionuclide or echo imaging for extent, severity of ischemia
	Pharmacologic (adenosine, dobutamine) with radionuclide or echo imaging for extent, severity of ischemia
Cardiopulmonary exercise evaluation	Documents maximal functional capacity (MVO_2)
	Serial studies may be used to assess response to therapy

suspected CAD, stress testing may help with the decision to pursue invasive studies (coronary angiography) and revascularization or alternatively to intensify medical measures for CAD.

Finally, for stage C or stage D patients, maximal cardiopulmonary exercise testing is important in order to document the individual patient's functional status, objectively assess the patient's response to treatment, and assess the appropriateness of assist device implantation or cardiac transplantation.

Invasive Studies: Cardiac Catheterization and Endomyocardial Biopsy

Left heart catheterization, contrast ventriculography, and selective coronary angiography are rarely required as part of the initial diagnostic evaluation of HF patients. Generally, these studies should be employed in two situations. First, when other attempts to document or exclude obstructive CAD as the etiology of impaired LV function have been unproductive, diagnostic coronary angiography may be the only technique that can provide a definitive diagnosis. Second, when a HF patient has either symptomatic ischemia or a large volume of viable but ischemic myocardium, coronary angiography provides important information for decisions on the appropriateness and feasibility of myocardial revascularization.

In recent years, right heart catheterization has probably been under-utilized in the diagnosis and management of HF. The assessment of right heart hemodynamics, including PCWP, and cardiac output using a Swan-Ganz catheter is a relatively quick, easy, and safe procedure that provides important and reliable hemodynamic data, including bi-ventricular filling pressures and both pulmonary and systemic resistances. These data are often not well correlated with the patient's clinical findings, particularly after intensive medical treatment.

Endomyocardial biopsy (essentially limited to right ventricular EMB) is subject to major limitations due to sampling error. In addition, although quite safe in cardiac transplant recipients, the procedure carries a small but definite risk in patients with an intact pericardium. EMB is reasonable for patients with a high pre-test likelihood of having systemic amyloidosis or giant cell myocarditis. EMB should not be a part of the "routine" evaluation of HF patients.[1]

Summary

A complete evaluation of the dyspneic, exercise-intolerant patient with suspected HF, including assessment of the initial response to therapy, may take several weeks. A well-documented conclusion that the patient's symptoms, physical findings, and laboratory data are or are not consistent with HF is the primary objective of the diagnostic evaluation. If the patient does indeed have HF, then a complete and accurate diagnosis, along with *at least* the specific data listed in **Table 1.11** should be available.

TABLE 1.11 — Outcomes of the Heart Failure Evaluation

- Comprehensive and accurate etiologic diagnosis
- Left ventricular function (ejection fraction)
- Volume status ("wet" vs "dry") and renal function
- Electrophysiologic status:
  – Atrial fibrillation?
  – Rate vs rhythm control?
  – Candidate for resynchronization?
  – Candidate for defibrillator implant?
- Functional status: described by AHA stage, NYHA Class, MVO_2. See *Chapter 2*
- Prognosis: based on previous hospitalizations, biomarkers, functional status

REFERENCES

1. Yancy CW, Jessup M, Bozkurt B, et al; American College of Cardiology Foundation; American Heart Association Task Force on Practice Guidelines. 2013 ACCF/AHA guideline for the management of heart failure: a report of the American College of Cardiology Foundation/American Heart Association Task Force on Practice Guidelines. *J Am Coll Cardiol.* 2013;62(16):e147-239.

2. Mills RM, Zhu V, Cody RJ, Yuan Z. Estimated prevalence of implanted electrophysiologic devices in patients with heart failure. *Am Heart J.* 2015;169(1):188-189.

2 Clinical Syndromes and Staging of Heart Failure

Introduction

Before embarking on a fairly detailed chapter that describes the various clinical syndromes of HF and the two widely accepted HF staging systems, we want to emphasize the importance of clinical classification and severity staging.

The HF population consists of patients with widely varying clinical characteristics, who also have a wide spectrum of signs and symptoms. In the era of evidence-based medicine, appropriate management strategies differ for patients with HF and preserved left ventricular function compared to those with HF and reduced left ventricular function, and, within these two syndromes, for those at different stages of HF.

In the early 1960s, the treatment options for HF included little more than digitalis and thiazide or mercurial diuretics. Today, 50 years after the commercial introduction of furosemide, HF treatment options have expanded substantially. However, the evidence supporting efficacy and safety for these options varies substantially among the different HF syndromes and stages. It is critical, therefore, first to gather the diagnostic data described in *Chapter 1*, and second, to use that data to accurately determine where each individual patient fits in the spectrum of HF.

In addition to providing the information required for evidence-based therapy, the process of classification and staging allows physicians to give better answers to the four questions that every patient either asks or wants to ask: "What's wrong with me?" "How bad is it?" "What can you do about it?" and "What's going to happen to me?"

Classification based on the timing of HF onset is shown in **Figure 2.1**.

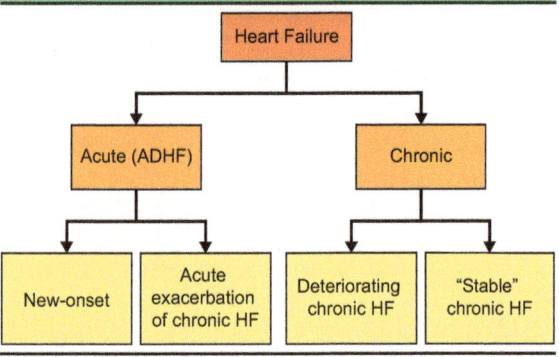

FIGURE 2.1 — Classification of Heart Failure Based on Timing of Symptoms

Acutely decompensated HF (ADHF) is an urgent medical problem, usually presenting for emergency care and often requiring subsequent hospital admission. The numbers of HF hospital discharges increased steadily from 1979 through 2006, as shown in **Figure 2.2**.

However, more recently, in a 100% sample of Medicare beneficiaries analyzed in order to identify

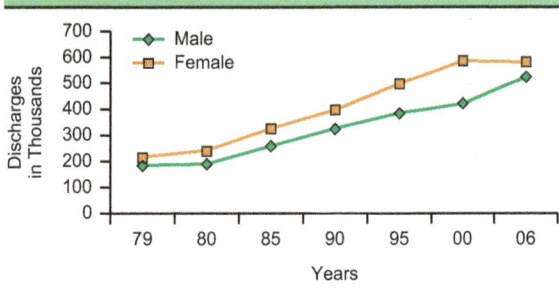

FIGURE 2.2 — Hospital Discharges for Heart Failure, 1979-2006

Lloyd-Jones D, et al. *Circulation*. 2010;121:e46-e215.

trends in HF hospitalization rates between 1998 and 2008, the overall risk-adjusted HF hospitalization rate decreased from 2845 per 100 000 person-years in 1998 to 2007 (95% CI, 1974-2041) per 100 000 in 2008, a relative decline of 29.5% ($P<0.001$ for trend).[1] These more detailed data, that differentiated ADHF from chronic stable HF, showed that hospitalization rates for acutely decompensated HF varied by race and gender. Black men had the highest incidence and recurrence rates of hospitalized ADHF; white women had the lowest rates.

The distinction between an acute exacerbation of chronic HF and the slowly progressive deterioration that many HF patients experience is not clear. Worsening of comorbid processes such the onset of atrial fibrillation, acute bronchitis in chronic obstructive pulmonary disease (COPD), deterioration of chronic kidney disease (CKD), or chronic GI blood loss with anemia often precipitates acute exacerbations of HF. On the other hand, the progression of coronary disease with increasing myocardial ischemic injury or the process of progressive remodeling of the failing heart with increasing wall stress, increasing subendocardial ischemia, and increasing functional mitral regurgitation often drive the slow deterioration of patients with chronic HF. *Chapter 8* will discuss with the management of ADHF in detail.

Table 2.1 shows recent overall demographic data for the HF population.

Figure 2.3 shows a classification of HF syndromes in which the primary distinction is based on differentiation of primary left ventricular failure from primary right ventricular failure.

The clinical picture of primary right ventricular (RV) failure most commonly occurs in one of two settings. In the first, congenital heart disease results in pressure or volume overload of the RV, for example, RV outflow obstruction or left-to-right shunts. These patients are usually recognized and managed by pediatric subspecialists with structural interventions in

TABLE 2.1 — Demographics of Heart Failure

	1999–2000	2001–2002	2003–2004	2005–2006	2007–2008
Number of HF hospitalizations	1017410	1026363	1048103	953706	820727
Age (mean, SD)	79.0 (7.7)	79.1 (7.8)	79.3 (7.8)	79.6 (7.9)	79.9 (8.0)
Female	598993 (58.9)	599416 (58.4)	601251 (57.4)	536431 (56.2)	457174 (55.7)
White	860860 (84.6)	864831 (84.3)	880764 (84.0)	798581 (83.7)	688680 (83.9)
Black	114804 (11.3)	119665 (11.7)	123185 (11.8)	113358 (11.9)	95707 (11.7)
Other race	41746 (4.1)	41867 (4.1)	44154 (4.2)	41767 (4.4)	36340 (4.4)
Comorbidities					
Cardiovascular Conditions and Risk Factors					
Coronary artery disease	564365 (55.5)	583036 (56.8)	602460 (57.5)	541162 (56.7)	454815 (55.4)
Prior heart failure	309219 (30.4)	322255 (31.4)	334472 (31.9)	306133 (32.1)	264651 (32.2)
Prior myocardial infarction	73613 (7.2)	76880 (7.5)	75265 (7.2)	63452 (6.7)	55166 (6.7)
Unstable angina	63460 (6.2)	57987 (5.6)	48696 (4.6)	35535 (3.7)	26455 (3.2)
Peripheral vascular disease	72217 (7.1)	77437 (7.5)	80431 (7.7)	72063 (7.6)	63020 (7.7)
Stroke	16627 (1.6)	16275 (1.6)	15581 (1.5)	14134 (1.5)	12354 (1.5)
Cerebrovascular disease other than stroke	50941 (5.0)	48807 (4.8)	44433 (4.2)	35473 (3.7)	29676 (3.6)
Hypertension	487460 (47.9)	532256 (51.9)	564108 (53.8)	502223 (52.7)	499978 (60.9)
Diabetes mellitus	373151 (36.7)	397640 (38.7)	408184 (38.9)	366621 (38.4)	307059 (37.4)

Geriatric Conditions					
Dementia	94031 (9.2)	102191 (10.0)	109615 (10.5)	102154 (10.7)	91619 (11.2)
Functional disability	24392 (2.4)	24045 (2.3)	22636 (2.2)	18106 (1.9)	17606 (2.1)
Malnutrition	31327 (3.1)	31241 (3.0)	35052 (3.3)	36011 (3.8)	40134 (4.9)
Other Medical Conditions					
Chronic obstructive pulmonary disease	331241 (32.6)	353538 (34.4)	376219 (35.9)	352487 (37.0)	286107 (34.9)
Pneumonia	147932 (14.5)	158486 (15.4)	168679 (16.1)	180319 (18.9)	185769 (22.6)
Respiratory failure	46759 (4.6)	49056 (4.8)	52755 (5.0)	56480 (5.9)	66693 (8.1)
Liver disease	10806 (1.1)	11397 (1.1)	12522 (1.2)	11772 (1.2)	10246 (1.2)
Renal failure	80998 (8.0)	96289 (9.4)	116556 (11.1)	146920 (15.4)	164497 (20.0)
Other Non-medical Conditions					
Majo psychiatric disorder	21094 (2.1)	21732 (2.1)	21237 (2.0)	17252 (1.8)	16861 (2.1)
Depression	59387 (5.8)	68443 (6.7)	74062 (7.1)	62283 (6.5)	51582 (6.3)
Trauma in past year	47445 (4.7)	52321 (5.1)	58493 (5.6)	54851 (5.8)	49036 (6.0)
Mean length of stay, days (SD)	6.8 (5.8)	6.8 (5.6)	6.6 (5.4)	6.5 (5.2)	6.4 (5.2)

Other race includes Asian, Hispanic, North American Native, or other not specified. Comparison across years of patient characteristics using Mantel-Haenszel chi-squared test for linear association for categorical variables and Cuzick test for continuous variables using 2-sided test. All P values <0.001.

Chen J, et al. *JAMA*. 2011;306(15):1669-1678.

FIGURE 2.3 — Classification of Adults with Heart Failure on the Basis of Anatomy and Function

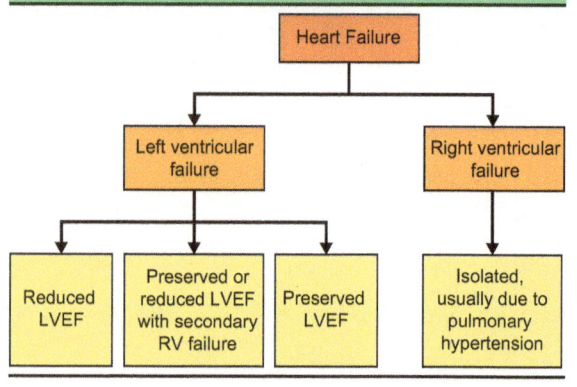

```
                        Heart Failure
                       /            \
           Left ventricular      Right ventricular
               failure                failure
          /      |      \               |
   Reduced   Preserved or  Preserved   Isolated,
   LVEF      reduced LVEF  LVEF        usually due to
             with secondary            pulmonary
             RV failure                hypertension
```

childhood. In the second, patients develop right HF as a consequence of chronic pulmonary hypertension due to a wide spectrum of disease processes including connective tissue disease, primary pulmonary hypertension, or chronic thromboembolic pulmonary hypertension (CTEPH). These patients require management focused on the pharmacologic reduction of the pulmonary vascular resistance, often combined with surgical intervention in the CTEPH patients. Fortunately, patients with isolated pulmonary hypertension and primary RV failure are rare, particularly compared to HF due to left ventricular (LV) dysfunction. Their management is beyond the scope of this volume.

In contrast, left HF is a final common pathway for a wide variety of diseases that impact LV structure and function. The population of HF patients with impaired or reduced LV systolic function (HF-rEF) is often more easily recognized. These patients often have had prior MI or cardiomyopathy with cardiac enlargement that can be appreciated on physical examination and chest X-ray. Largely because this population can be easily defined clinically, HF-rEF patients have formed the study population for most clinical trials of HF treatment, and the evidence base for their management is far more substantial.

With the introduction and widespread adoption of echocardiography, a population of patients with clinical signs and symptoms of HF who have relatively preserved LV systolic function in conjunction with impaired diastolic function was recognized (HF-rEF). These patients now comprise about half of the HF population.[2]

Table 2.2 shows the hemodynamic patterns in HF. Bedside right heart (Swan-Ganz) catheterization may occasionally be indicated in order to firmly establish the hemodynamic status of an individual with HF; however, as experience with "tailored therapy" accumulated in the 1980s, the correlation of clinical pictures and hemodynamic patterns in HF patients became clearer. Clinical assessments improved, and eventually the Evaluation Study of Congestive Heart Failure and Pulmonary Artery Catheterization Effectiveness (ESCAPE) trial[3] demonstrated that right heart catheterization did not improve clinical outcomes in comparison to noninvasive management for most patients.

TABLE 2.2 — Hemodynamic Patterns in Heart Failure

Cardiogenic shock	High filling pressure
	Low forward output
"Cool and dry" heart failure	Low filling pressure
	Low forward output
"Warm and wet" heart failure	High filling pressure
	Near-normal forward output
Acute pulmonary edema	Marked elevation of filling pressure
	Near-normal cardiac output

Today, hemodynamically guided management is usually reserved for hospitalized patients who are particularly difficult to manage or who may require mechanical support with a left ventricular assist device. However, clinicians caring for ADHF patients should make a practice of estimating each patient's hemodynamic status on the basis of the clinical findings and managing pharmacologic treatment accordingly.

The NYHA Classification and the ACC/AHA Stages of Heart Failure

The New York Heart Association (NYHA) classification system, first developed in 1928 for assessment of patients with rheumatic heart disease, requires highly subjective physician interpretation of patient-reported information in order to classify patients.[4] Remarkably, NYHA class correlates modestly well with 6-minute walk test performance[5] and with survival data based on maximal oxygen uptake[6] (**Figure 2.4** and **Table 2.3**). Despite its limitations, the NYHA classification remains in active use[7] in both clinical care and clinical trials.

In 2001, the ACC/AHA proposed a new "staging system" for HF (**Table 2.4**).[8] The new ACC/AHA classification uses stages that are much more inclusive than the older NYHA classification, and thereby extending the classification to persons considered "at risk" for HF.

FIGURE 2.4 — NYHA Classification and Peak Oxygen Uptake in Heart Failure Patients

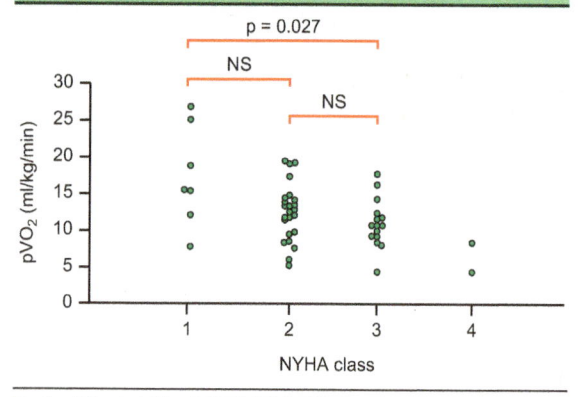

Raphael C, et al. *Heart*. 2007;93(4):476-482.

TABLE 2.3 — The NYHA Classification

NYHA Class I	Asymptomatic
	No limitation of usual activity
NYHA Class II	Symptoms with usual levels of exertion
	Slightly limited
NYHA Class III	Symptoms with less than ordinary exertion
	Marked limitation
NYHA Class IV	Symptoms at rest

TABLE 2.4 — ACC/AHA Stages of Heart Failure

ACC/AHA Stage A	At high risk for heart failure
	No symptoms or structural disease
ACC/AHA Stage B	Structural disease (including LA enlargement or LV hypertrophy)
	No signs, symptoms of heart failure
ACC/AHA Stage C	Structural disease
	Current or prior heart failure symptoms
ACC/AHA Stage D	Refractory heart failure requiring special interventions

Figure 2.5 graphically presents the relationship between the ACC/AHA stages and the NYHA classes. Both have important uses and limitations. The ACC/AHA system with very broad stages A and B emphasizes the potential for primary prevention of HF with measures such as broad-based control of risk factors including hypertension, hypercholesterolemia, and type 2 diabetes.

The appropriate ACC/AHA classification and the optimal management of patients who present with HF-rEF and subsequently have improvement of left

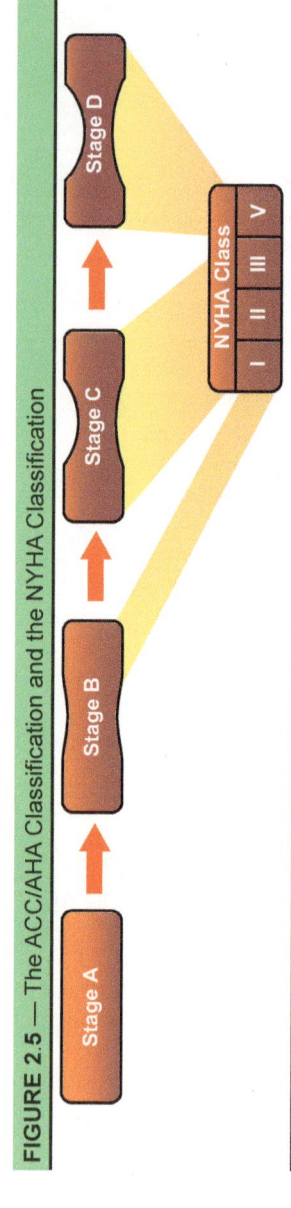

FIGURE 2.5 — The ACC/AHA Classification and the NYHA Classification

The new ACC/AHA classification includes, for the first time, persons "at risk" for heart failure (Stage A), and those with early changes in heart structure and function who have no clinical evidence of disease (Stage B). Stages C and D encompass the range of disease described by the earlier NYHA classification.

ventricular function ("recovered systolic function") on treatment remains uncertain. In a study of 174 patients with initial LV dysfunction who had LVEF ≥45% after beta-adrenergic blocker treatment, approximately one quarter of the population had recurrent LV dysfunction after an 8-year follow-up.[9] A recent review of management of patients with recovered systolic function recommends weaning of diuretics as tolerated, but continued use of neurohormonal antagonists in most situations.[10]

Summary

The various descriptors and classification systems for HF help clinicians to add context to the diagnosis of "HF" to better inform evidence-based management. **Table 2.5** gives three examples to clarify this concept. Recent observational studies support the concept that each of the patients described above is likely to have a distinctive phenotype[11,12] (**Figure 2.6**).

Patients presenting with acute pulmonary edema often have hypertension and also have a relatively high prevalence of self-admitted substance abuse.[13] The patient with HF-pEF and new-onset AF is likely to be an older obese hypertensive diabetic female. The patient with chronic biventricular failure is likely to be a late middle-aged male with CAD and prior MI, who has undergone revascularization and ICD implantation.

Despite their obvious clinical differences, these patients have many pathophysiologic processes in common. In *Chapter 3*, we will explore this further.

TABLE 2.5 — Examples of the Context Provided by Detailed Classification and Staging Systems

Heart Failure	Acute, new onset
	Left ventricular failure, reduced EF (HF-rEF)
	Acute pulmonary edema
	Stage C/NYHA IV
	Acute exacerbation of chronic heart failure due to new-onset atrial fibrillation
	Preserved LV function (HF-pEF)
	"Warm and wet"
	Stage C/NYHA IV
	Stable, chronic heart failure
	HF-rEF with secondary RV failure
	"Cool and dry"
	Stage C/NYHA III

REFERENCES

1. Chen J, Normand ST, Wang Y, Krumholz HM. National and regional trends in heart failure hospitalization and mortality rates for Medicare beneficiaries, 1998-2008. *JAMA*. 2011;306(15):1669-1678.

2. Owan TE, Hodge DO, Herges RM, et al. Trends in prevalence and outcome of heart failure with preserved ejection fraction. *N Engl J Med*. 2006;355:251-259.

3. Binanay C, Califf RM, Hasselblad V, et al; ESCAPE Investigators and ESCAPE Study Coordinators. Evaluation study of congestive heart failure and pulmonary artery catheterization effectiveness: the ESCAPE trial. *JAMA*. 2005;294(13):1625-1633.

4. Raphael C, Briscoe C, Davies J, et al. Limitations of the New York Heart Association functional classification system and self-reported walking distances in chronic heart failure. *Heart*. 2007;93(4):476-482.

5. Yap J, Lim FY, Gao F, et al. Correlation of the New York Heart Association Classification and the 6-minute walk distance: a systematic review. *Clin Cardiol*. 2015;38(10):621-628.

6. van den Broek SA, van Veldhuisen DJ, de Graeff PA, et al. Comparison between New York Heart Association classification and peak oxygen consumption in the assessment of functional status and prognosis in patients with mild to moderate chronic congestive heart failure secondary to either ischemic or idiopathic dilated cardiomyopathy. *Am J Cardiol.* 1992;70(3):359-363.

7. McMurray JJ, Adamopoulos S, Anker SD, et al. ESC guidelines for the diagnosis and treatment of acute and chronic heart failure 2012: the Task Force for the Diagnosis and Treatment of Acute and Chronic Heart Failure 2012 of the European Society of Cardiology. Developed in collaboration with the Heart Failure Association (HFA) of the ESC [published correction appears in Eur J Heart Fail. 2013;15:361-362]. *Eur J Heart Fail.* 2012;14:803-869.

8. Hunt SA, Baker DW, Chin MH, et al. ACC/AHA guidelines for the evaluation and management of chronic heart failure in the adult: executive summary. A report of the American College of Cardiology/American Heart Association Task Force on Practice Guidelines (Committee to revise the 1995 Guidelines for the Evaluation and Management of Heart Failure). *J Am Coll Cardiol.* 2001;38(7):2101-2113.

9. de Groote P, Fertin M, Pentiah AD, et al. Long-term functional and clinical follow-up of patients with heart failure with recovered left ventricular ejection fraction after β-blocker therapy. *Circ Heart Fail.* 2014;7:434-439.

10. Basuray A, Fang JC. Management of patients with recovered systolic function. *Prog Cardiovasc Dis.* 2016;58:434-443.

11. Samson R, Jaiswal A, Ennezat PV, Cassidy M, Le Jemtel TH. Clinical phenotypes in heart failure with preserved ejection fraction. *J Am Heart Assoc.* 2016;5(1). pii: e002477.

12. Ahmad T, Desai N, Wilson F, et al. Clinical implications of cluster analysis-based classification of acute decompensated heart failure and correlation with bedside hemodynamic profiles. *PLoS One.* 2016;11(2):e0145881.

13. Diercks DB, Fonarow GC, Kirk JD, et al. Illicit stimulant use in a United States heart failure population presenting to the emergency department (from the Acute Decompensated Heart Failure National Registry Emergency Module). *Am J Cardiol.* 2008;102(9):1216-1219.

FIGURE 2.6 — Phenotypes ("Clusters") in the HF-ACTION Study

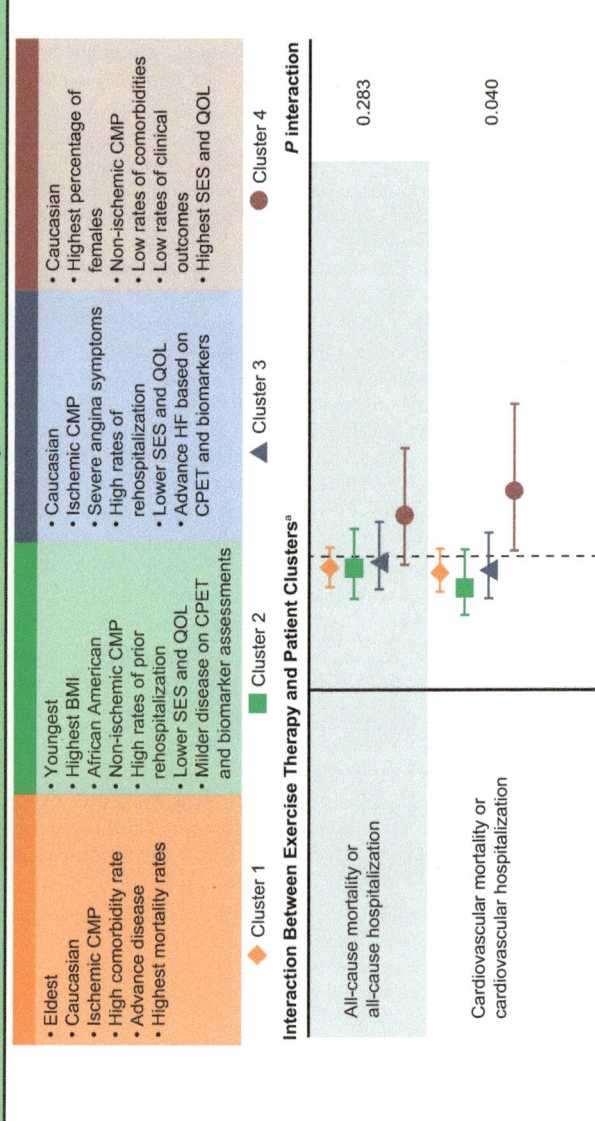

Cluster 1
- Eldest
- Caucasian
- Ischemic CMP
- High comorbidity rate
- Advance disease
- Highest mortality rates

Cluster 2
- Youngest
- Highest BMI
- African American
- Non-ischemic CMP
- High rates of prior rehospitalization
- Lower SES and QOL
- Milder disease on CPET and biomarker assessments

Cluster 3
- Caucasian
- Ischemic CMP
- Severe angina symptoms
- High rates of rehospitalization
- Lower SES and QOL
- Advance HF based on CPET and biomarkers

Cluster 4
- Caucasian
- Highest percentage of females
- Non-ischemic CMP
- Low rates of comorbidities
- Low rates of clinical outcomes
- Highest SES and QOL

◆ Cluster 1 ■ Cluster 2 ▲ Cluster 3 ● Cluster 4

Interaction Between Exercise Therapy and Patient Clusters[a]

	P interaction
All-cause mortality or all-cause hospitalization	0.283
Cardiovascular mortality or cardiovascular hospitalization	0.040

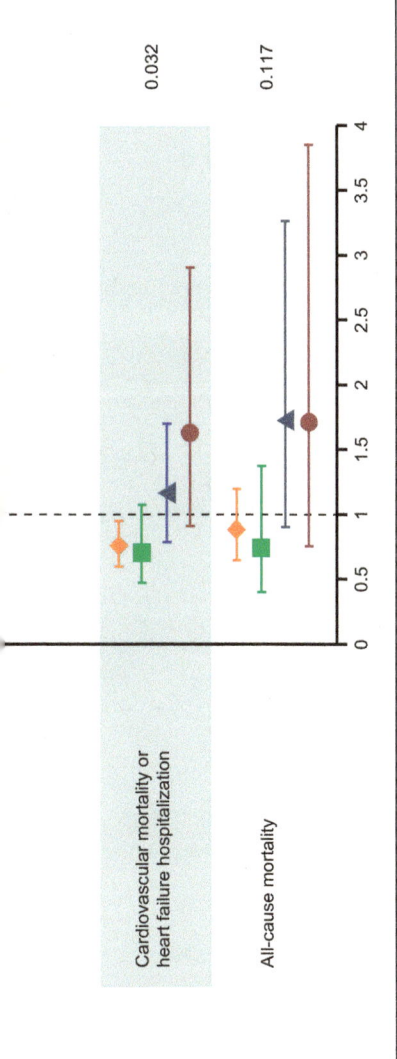

a Symbols represent hazard ratios (HR), with HR <1.00 denoting benefit from exercise, and HR >1.00 denoting harm.

Ahmad T, et al. *PLoS One.* 2016;11(2):e0145881.

3 Pathophysiology of Heart Failure

Introduction

As the 2013 ACCF/AHA Guideline for the Management of Heart Failure publication clearly stated, "Randomized controlled trials in patients with HF have mainly enrolled patients with HF-rEF...and it is only in these patients that efficacious therapies have been demonstrated to date."[1] The profound difference in response to pharmacologic interventions in patients with HF-rEF compared to those with HF-pEF dictates that we consider pathophysiology of the two conditions separately.

Although both syndromes fall under the topic of "heart failure," this chapter introduces the concept that myocardial injury initiates the HF-rEF syndrome and that the negative feedback properties of the renin-angiotensin-aldosterone system and the sympathetic nervous system perpetuate it and are responsible for progressive deterioration.

In contrast, the tightly linked processes of reduction in left ventricular compliance and alterations in ventricular-vascular coupling that characterize HF-pEF appear to be causally related to the multiple comorbid processes that accompany the phenotype, in particular, hypertension, diabetes, impairment of vascular function, and obesity. The mechanisms of the causal relationship remain unclear at this point.

Feedback Cycles in HF-rEF

Extensive laboratory and clinical data support the role of negative feedback cycles in the pathophysiology of HF-rEF. **Figure 3.1** illustrates the critical cycle in which systemic arterial underfilling results in activation

FIGURE 3.1 — Primary Negative Feedback Cycle in HF-rEF

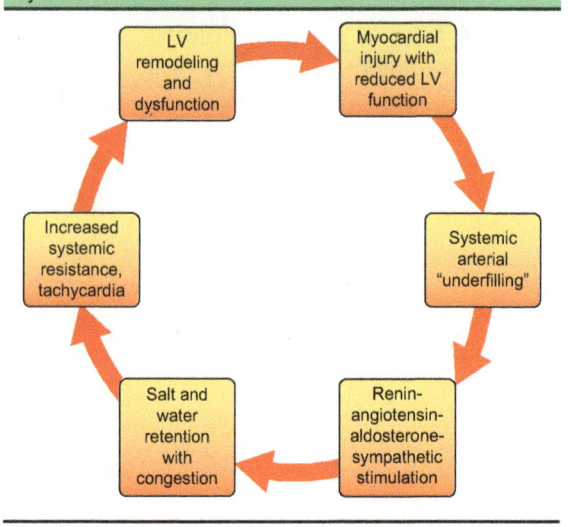

of the renin-angiotensin-aldosterone system (RAAS) and the sympathetic nervous system. This activation results in two adverse outcomes. First, salt and water retention leads to expansion of extracellular volume and increased cardiac filling pressures with systemic and pulmonary congestion. Second, increased levels of renin and angiotensin lead to increased systemic vascular resistance, imposing additional afterload on the failing left ventricle, while sympathetic activation raises heart rate with increased myocardial oxygen demand.

The process of salt and water retention can be considered as a continuum that begins with hemodynamic changes and progresses to overt clinical congestion.[2] Hemodynamic congestion refers to the state of increased intra-cardiac filling pressures due to cardiopulmonary volume overload that may occur without clinically evident signs/symptoms. In contrast, clinical congestion occurs when there are signs and/or symptoms that reflect the elevated intracardiac filling pressures. Data from ambulatory pressure monitoring demonstrate that filling pressures may begin to rise days to weeks before the onset of symptoms.[3]

RAAS activation also stimulates many other physiologic processes, including the important "counter-regulatory" secretion of the cardiac natriuretic peptide hormones, A-type natriuretic peptide (ANP), and B-type natriuretic peptide (BNP) (**Figure 3.2**).

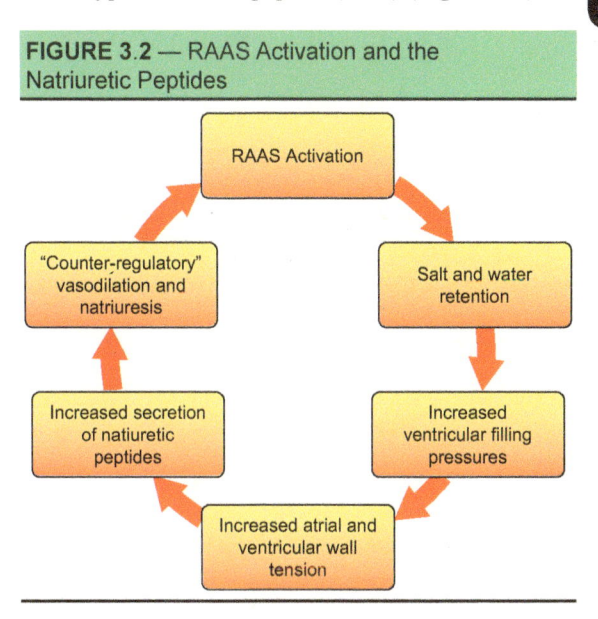

FIGURE 3.2 — RAAS Activation and the Natriuretic Peptides

RAAS Activation → Salt and water retention → Increased ventricular filling pressures → Increased atrial and ventricular wall tension → Increased secretion of natiuretic peptides → "Counter-regulatory" vasodilation and natriuresis → RAAS Activation

■ **Cardiovascular Responses to HF-rEF**

Although HF is a syndrome rather than a specific disease, once the HF-rEF syndrome is established, the process tends to become self-perpetuating through HF-driven continuing myocardial remodeling with atrial and ventricular enlargement, subendocardial ischemia, and the development of functional AV-valve regurgitation. At the cellular level, myocardial fibrosis and apoptosis occur, and at the subcellular metabolic level, impairment of energy production and sarcomere calcium handling become critical (**Figure 3.3**).

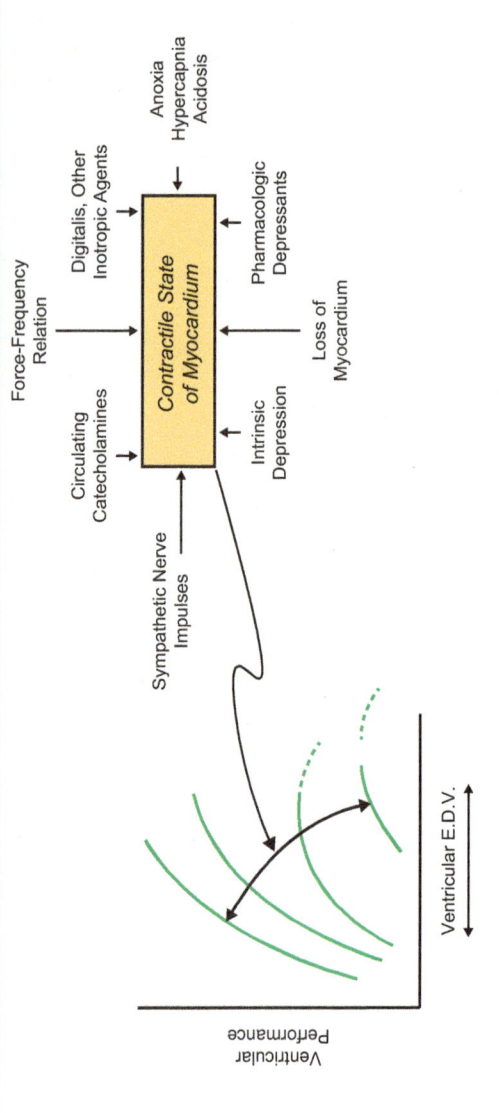

FIGURE 3.3 — Relationship of Cardiac Performance and End Diastolic Volume

The relationship of cardiac performance and end-diastolic volume is characterized by a family of curves reflecting the contractile state of the heart.

Right. Diagram showing the major influences that elevate or depress the contractile state of the myocardium.

Left. The way in which alterations in the contractile state of the myocardium affect the level of ventricular performance at any given level of ventricular end-diastolic volume.

Braunwald E, et al. *Mechanisms of Contraction of the Normal and Failing Heart.* 2nd ed. Boston, IL: Little Brown & Co: 1976.

In many ways, the myocardial "stretch–squeeze" relationship exemplified in the family of Sarnoff curves shown in the figure reproduced above is the most fundamental physiologic concept in HF. Ventricular EDV, on the horizontal axis, is analogous to the degree of "stretch" to which the cardiomyocytes are subjected. Ventricular performance, on the vertical axis, is analogous to the force of the "squeeze" that the cardiomyocytes develop when they contract.

Under the impact of the underlying heart disease, the neurohumoral response to HF, associated comorbidities, and hemodynamic stress, the HF-rEF heart undergoes progressive structural remodeling, with dilation, increased sphericity, and the development of functional mitral regurgitation due to annular dilation and adverse re-orientation of the papillary muscles. The severity of functional mitral regurgitation may vary substantially under different loading conditions. Exercise may increase the severity of functional MR, and the degree of MR at the anaerobic threshold or peak exercise is a strong determinant of exercise capacity, independent of resting EF.[4]

Less well understood, electrical remodeling also occurs. The dilated left atrium is prone to paroxysmal and ultimately persistent atrial fibrillation, and the failing left ventricle becomes susceptible to ventricular arrhythmia, particularly with underlying coronary heart disease. In addition, chronotropic incompetence is common in both HF-rEF and HF-pEF.[4]

■ Pulmonary Abnormalities in HF-rEF

Patients with HF have significant ventilatory abnormalities that can contribute to exercise intolerance.[4,5] In 1988, Sullivan and colleagues studied 64 subjects with HF-rEF, mean EF $20 \pm 6\%$ and demonstrated intact ventilator control. The correlation between decreased cardiac output and increased ventilation in the patient group suggested that attenuated pulmonary perfusion may play a role in causing exercise hyperpnea in the presence of chronic HF by producing ventilation perfusion abnormalities and thereby increasing physiologic pulmonary dead space.[5]

■ Renal Responses to HF-rEF

Large scale observational data from the ADHERE-HF registry made it clear that a complex interaction existed between HF and impaired renal function. In an attempt to clarify the possible interactions, Ronco and coworkers proposed five categories of cardio-renal syndromes (CRS), as shown in **Table 3.1**.

TABLE 3.1 — Categories of Cardio-Renal Syndrome	
CRS Type 1	Rapid worsening of cardiac function, leading to acute kidney injury (AKI)
CRS Type 2	Chronic abnormalities in cardiac function (eg, chronic congestive HF) causing progressive CKD
CRS Type 3	Abrupt and primary worsening of kidney function (eg, AKI, ischemia, or glomerulonephritis), leading to acute cardiac dysfunction
CRS Type 4	Primary CKD (eg, chronic glomerular disease) contributing to decreased cardiac function, ventricular hypertrophy, diastolic dysfunction, and/or increased risk of adverse cardiovascular events
CRS Type 5	Combined cardiac and renal dysfunction due to acute or chronic systemic disorders

The type 1 and type 2 syndromes are most important to understanding HF pathophysiology. **Table 3.2** lists some of the multiple mechanisms involved in the development of renal function impairment in patients with HF. An analysis of hemodynamics and renal function data from 575 HF-rEF patients who participated in the ESCAPE (Evaluation Study of Congestive Heart Failure and Pulmonary Artery Catheterization Effectiveness) trial demonstrated that "reduction in cardiac index is not the primary mechanism responsible for renal dysfunction in patients hospitalized for HF."[6]

TABLE 3.2 — Suggested Mechanisms of Renal Impairment in Heart Failure

- Hemodynamic and clinical congestion:
  - Reduced mesenteric and renal perfusion
  - Elevation of intra-abdominal pressure (>8 mm Hg)
- Elevated right atrial and central venous pressure
- Reduced forward cardiac output
- Activation of inflammatory pathways
- Comorbid pre-existing chronic kidney disease
- Drug effects: NSAIDs, diuretics, antibiotics, etc.

Elevated central venous or right atrial pressure results in elevated pressures in the renal veins and increased renal interstitial pressure, with ensuing renal dysfunction (**Figure 3.4**).[7] This may lead to both impaired GFR and hypoxic damage similar to congestive liver dysfunction in HF.[8]

In summary, these recent findings suggest that clinicians managing decompensated HF-rEF should give top priority to treatment strategies that reduce venous pressures and lead to decongestion, thereby increasing renal perfusion pressure, rather than strategies focused on increasing forward cardiac index.

Musculoskeletal Responses to HF-rEF

Patients with chronic HF, like those with COPD and CKD, experience shortness of breath and fatigue related to peripheral muscle abnormalities.[9] **Table 3.3** lists a number of proposed mechanisms that may play a role in the development of peripheral muscle abnormalities in HF.[9,10]

Pathophysiology of HF-pEF

The general diagnosis of HF is based on symptoms and signs typical for HF, accompanied by objective evidence of resting structural or functional heart abnormalities including increased BNP levels and an abnormal echocardiogram.[11] The specific definition of HF-pEF also requires an LVEF >50%, LV end-diastolic volume index <97 ml/m^2, and evidence of diastolic dysfunction[12] (**Figure 3.5**).

In contrast to the depression of systolic myocardial function seen in HF-rEF, a general consensus favors the concept that reduced LV compliance (dV/dP) with resulting abnormality in the LV diastolic pressure volume relationship represents the primary pathophysiologic alteration in HF-rEF.

The conceptual basis of HF-pEF is neither firmly established or nor widely agreed upon. **Figure 3.6** is an attempt to summarize current thinking. Although the RAAS system is activated in patients with HF-pEF, RAAS activity does not drive a negative feedback cycle of ventricular remodeling and progressive myocardial dysfunction as it does in HF-rEF. Instead, the presence of HF-pEF seems to substantially increase the patient's vulnerability to comorbidities.

As expressed by S. Mohamed, "In HF with preserved ejection fraction, potentially modifiable factors (obesity, anemia, and chronotropic incompetence) are strongly associated with exercise capacity, whereas resting measures of ventricular and vascular structure and function are not."

Figure 3.7 shows that patients with HF-pEF experience marked increases in filling pressure in response to increases in volume. Thus they are uniquely susceptible to stress in the form of increased cardiac output occurring in response to hypoxemia, increased work of breathing, fever, anemia, etc.

■ Pulmonary Responses to HF-pEF

In contrast to HF-rEF, marked exercise intolerance dominates the clinical picture of HF-pEF even when patients appear well compensated at rest. This can be documented by decreased peak oxygen uptake at maximal exercise (peak VO$_2$), and is a strong determinant of prognosis and reduced quality of life[13] (**Figure 3.8, Table 3.4**).

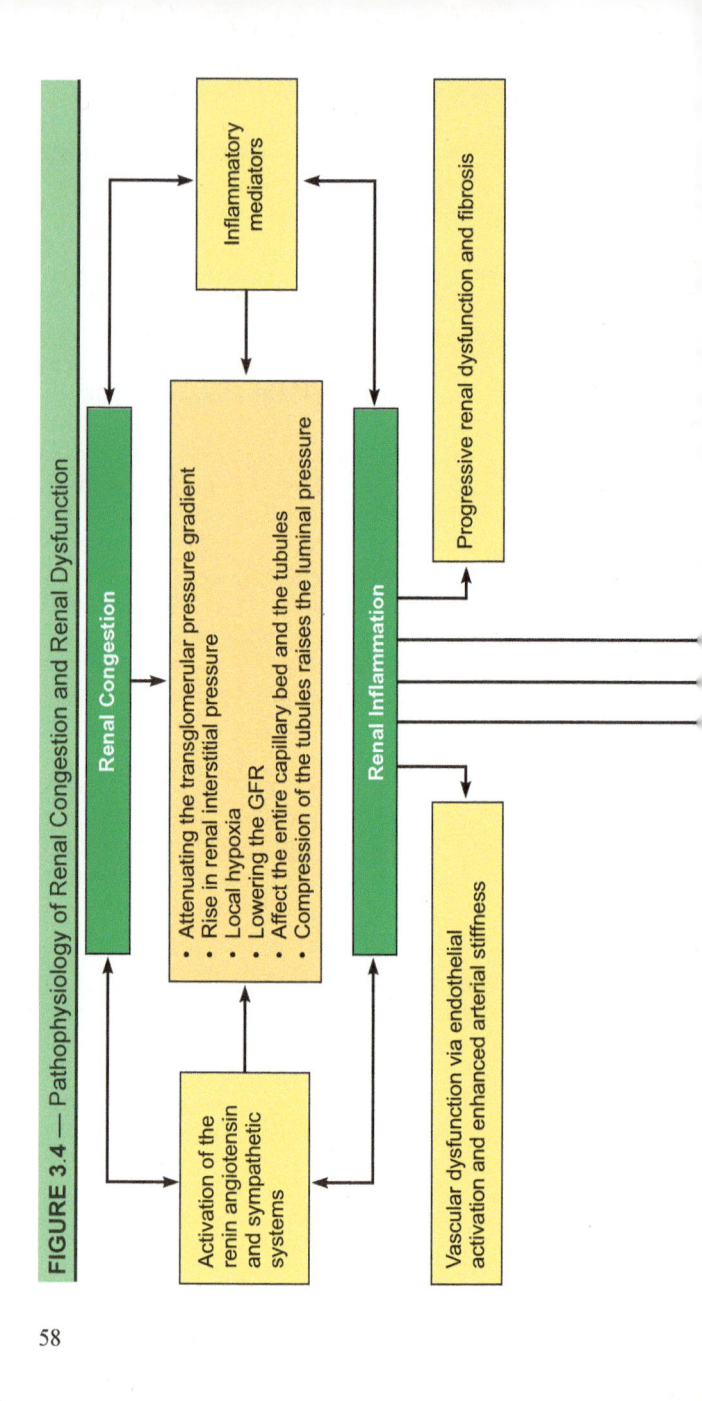

FIGURE 3.4 — Pathophysiology of Renal Congestion and Renal Dysfunction

- Attenuating the transglomerular pressure gradient
- Rise in renal interstitial pressure
- Local hypoxia
- Lowering the GFR
- Affect the entire capillary bed and the tubules
- Compression of the tubules raises the luminal pressure

Renal Congestion

Renal Inflammation

Inflammatory mediators

Activation of the renin angiotensin and sympathetic systems

Progressive renal dysfunction and fibrosis

Vascular dysfunction via endothelial activation and enhanced arterial stiffness

Increase the permeability of the endothelium allowing extravasation of fluids into the alveolar space of the lungs

Absorption of pro-inflammatory endotoxin from the bowel

Reduce myocardial contractility by functional suppression of the contractile apparatus and by increased myocardial cell death

Afsar B, et al. *Clin Kidney J.* 2016;9:39-47.

TABLE 3.3 — Possible Mechanisms of Peripheral Muscle Abnormality in Heart Failure

Loss of Muscle Mass	
Metabolic abnormalities	Phosphocreatine depletion
	Reduced oxidative capacity
Impaired Calcium Handling	
Coordinated down regulation	Increased sympathetic nerve activity

From Mentz 2014: "An alternative explanation for the close association between COPD and HF-pEF involves coupling between impaired LV filling and pulmonary venous changes due to lung parenchymal abnormalities. Moreover, HF may result in pulmonary function changes and patient symptoms that mimic COPD. Because patients with preserved EF do not have the alternative diagnosis of low EF, they may be more likely to receive a COPD diagnosis as an explanation for dyspnea. Despite the potential for bias related to increased COPD diagnosis in HF-pEF patients, the consistent observation of increased COPD prevalence in HF-pEF patients suggests that concomitant pulmonary and cardiac dysfunction may be particularly important in the preserved EF group."[14]

Development of chronic pulmonary hypertension in HF-pEF is associated with poor prognosis.

■ Renal Responses to HF-pEF

Because the HF-pEF phenotype includes advanced age and multiple comorbidities, the relationship between HF-pEF physiology and renal dysfunction is complex. With a prevalence of 30% to 60%, renal dysfunction is one of the most common comorbidities in HF-pEF.[15] Gori and associates recently reported on associations between albuminuria and/or low eGFR and comprehensive echocardiographic findings in subjects in the PARAMOUNT trial, a prospective study comparing the efficacy of therapy with an angiotensin receptor blocker (ARB) vs an angiotensin receptor neprilysin inhibitor (ARNI) in patients with HF-pEF. They found that compared with subjects with preserved renal function, patients with either reduced eGFR or elevated urinary albumin/creatinine ratio had greater LV wall thickness and LV mass, a higher prevalence of abnormal LV geometry and higher NT-proBNP.

Similarly, observational data from an 11-year cohort study in the Netherlands demonstrated that higher age, urinary albumin and cystatin C levels were strong risk factors for new onset HF-pEF.[16]

In summary, when both albuminuria and eGFR are considered, impairment of renal function is strongly associated with, and may often precede, clinical evidence of HF-pEF.

■ Musculoskeletal Responses to HF-pEF

At this time, the majority of evidence suggests more similarities than differences when comparing the impact of HF-rEF and HF-pEF on peripheral muscle function. **Table 3.5** lists some of the skeletal muscle abnormalities which may be more characteristic of HF-pEF. In addition, we will explore this topic in more detail in the chapter on nonpharmacologic therapies.

FIGURE 3.5 — Physiology of HF-pEF

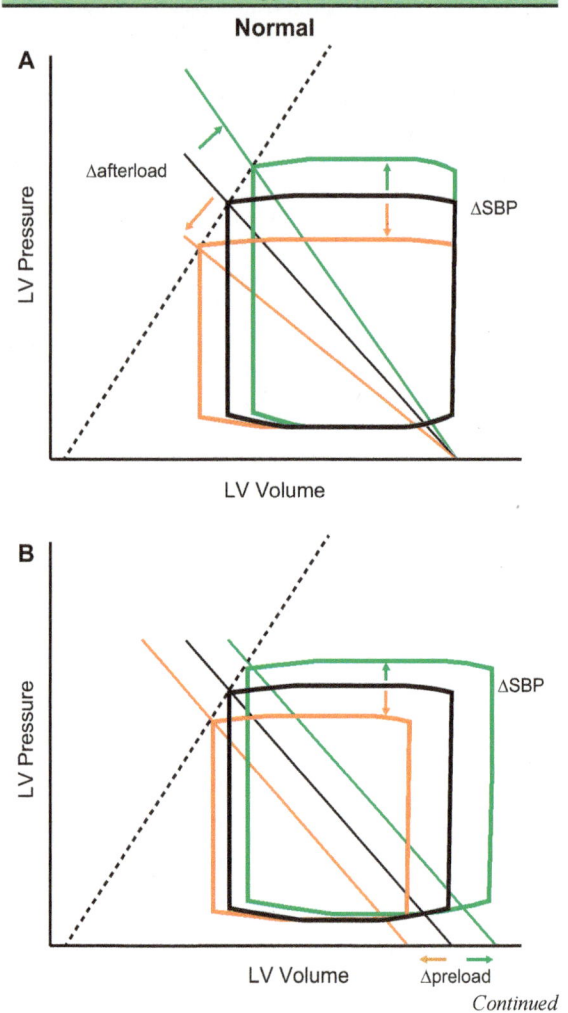

Normal

A

Δafterload

ΔSBP

LV Pressure

LV Volume

B

ΔSBP

LV Pressure

LV Volume Δpreload

Continued

62

FIGURE 3.5 — Continued

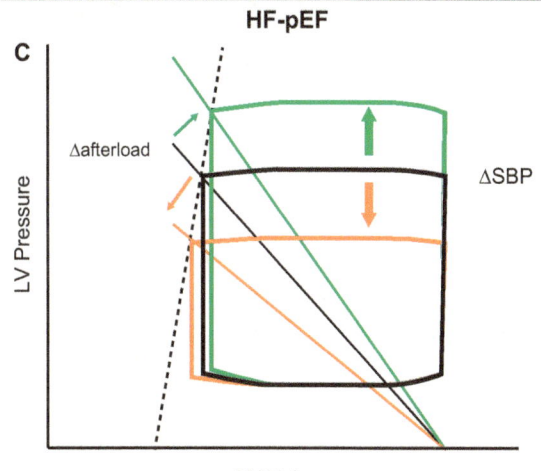

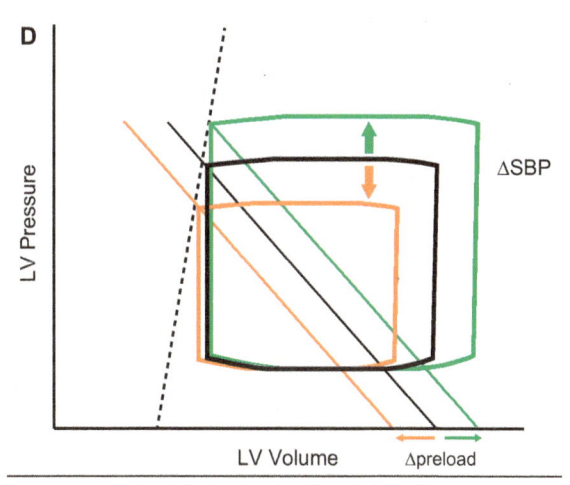

HF-pEF

C

Δafterload

ΔSBP

LV Pressure

LV Volume

D

ΔSBP

LV Pressure

LV Volume   Δpreload

Borlaug BA, Paulus WF. *Eur Heart J.* 2011;32:670-679.

FIGURE 3.6 — Pathophysiology of HF-pEF

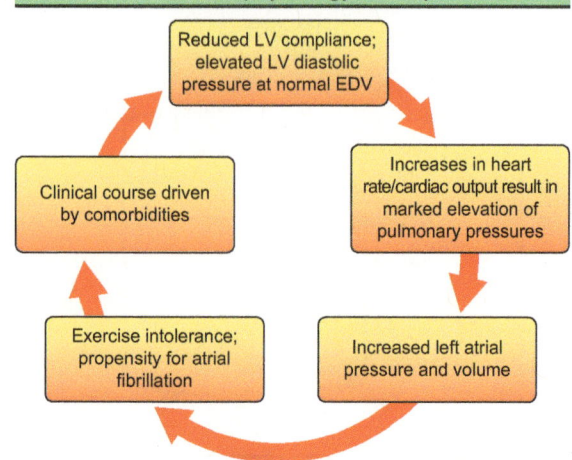

Reduced LV compliance; elevated LV diastolic pressure at normal EDV → Increases in heart rate/cardiac output result in marked elevation of pulmonary pressures → Increased left atrial pressure and volume → Exercise intolerance; propensity for atrial fibrillation → Clinical course driven by comorbidities → (cycle continues)

FIGURE 3.7 — PV Loops and Pressure vs Time Relationship in HF-pEF

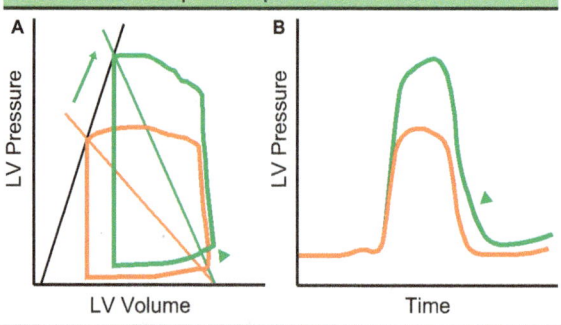

A. LV Pressure vs LV Volume

B. LV Pressure vs Time

Borlaug BA, Paulus WF. *Eur Heart J.* 2011;32:670-679.

REFERENCES

1. Yancy CW, Jessup M, Bozkurt B, et al; American College of Cardiology Foundation; American Heart Association Task Force on Practice Guidelines. 2013 ACCF/AHA guideline for the management of heart failure: a report of the American College of Cardiology Foundation/American Heart Association Task Force on Practice Guidelines. *J Am Coll Cardiol.* 2013;62(16):e147-239.

2. Gheorghiade M, Filippatos G, De Luca L, et al. Congestion in acute heart failure syndromes: an essential target of evaluation and treatment. *Am J Med.* 2006;119:S3-S10.

3. Adamson PB, Magalski A, Braunschweig F, et al. Ongoing right ventricular hemodynamics in heart failure: clinical value of measurements derived from an implantable monitoring system. *J Am Coll Cardiol.* 2003;41:565-571.

4. Shimiaie J, Sherez J, Aviram G, et al. Determinants of effort intolerance in patients with heart failure: combined echocardiography and cardiopulmonary stress protocol. *JACC Heart Fail.* 2015;3(10):803-814.

5. Sullivan MJ, Higginbotham MB, Cobb FR. Increased exercise ventilation in patients with chronic heart failure: intact ventilatory control despite hemodynamic and pulmonary abnormalities. *Circulation.* 1988;77(3):552-559.

6. Hanberg J, Sury K, Wilson F, et al. Reduced cardiac index is not the dominant driver of renal dysfunction in heart failure. *J Am Coll Cardiol.* 2016;67:2199-2208.

7. Afsar B, Ortiz A, Covic A, et al. Focus on renal congestion in heart failure. *Clin Kidney J.* 2016;9:39-47.

8. Damman K, Navis G, Smilde TD, et al. Decreased cardiac output, venous congestion and the association with renal impairment in patients with cardiac dysfunction. *Eur J Heart Fail.* 2007;9:872-878.

9. Middlekauf HR. Making the case for skeletal myopathy as the major limitation of exercise capacity in heart failure. *Circ Heart Fail.* 2010;3(4):537-546.

10. Hirai DM, Musch TI, Poole DC. Exercise training in chronic heart failure: improving skeletal muscle O2 transport and utilization. *Am J Physiol Heart Circ Physiol.* 2015;309(9):H1419-1439.

11. Penicka M, Bartunek J, Trakalova H, et al. Heart failure with preserved ejection fraction in outpatients with unexplained dyspnea: a pressure-volume loop analysis. *J Am Coll Cardiol.* 2010;55(16):1701-1710.

FIGURE 3.8 — Interplay Between HF-pEF and Comorbidities

Comorbidity	Bidirectional Impact on Disease Progression	Heart Failure Specifics
Chronic obstructive pulmonary disease	Inflammation; hypoxia; parenchymal changes; airflow limitation, leading to pulmonary congestion; abnormal LV diastolic filling; inhaled beta-agonist cardiovascular effects Elevated LV end-diastolic pressure and beta-blocker use may compromise lung function	More prevalent in preserved ejection fraction (HF-pEF), compared to reduced (HF-rEF) Higher mortality risk in HF-pEF
Anemia	Adverse LV remodeling; adverse cardiorenal effects; increased neurohormonal and inflammatory cytokines Inflammation; hemodilution; renal dysfunction; metabolic abnormalities exacerbate	More prevalent in HF-pEF Similar increased risk for mortality in both groups
Diabetes	Diabetic cardiomyopathy; mitochondrial dysfunction; abnormal calcium homeostasis; oxidative stress; RAAS activation; atherosclerosis; coronary artery disease Incident and worsening diabetes mellitus via sympathetic and RAAS activation	More prevalent in HF-pEF Similar increased risk for mortality in both groups

Renal dysfunction	Sodium and fluid retention; anemia; inflammation; RAAS and sympathetic activation	Similar prevalence in both groups
	Cardiorenal syndrome through low cardiac output; accelerated atherosclerosis; inflammation; increased venous pressure	Similar increased risk for mortality in both goups
Sleep-disordered breathing	Hypoxia; systemic inflammation; sympathetic activation; arrhythmias; hypertension (pulmonary and systemic); RV dysfunction; worsening congestion	Similar prevalence in both groups
	Rostral fluid movement may worsen pharyngeal obstruction; instability of ventilatory control system	Unknown mortality differential associated with HF-pEF vs HF-rEF
Obesity	Inflammation; reduced physical activity and deconditioning; hypertension; metabolic syndrome; diabetes mellitus	More prevalent in HF-pEF
	Fatigue and dyspnea may limit activity; spectrum of metabolic disorders including nutritional deficiencies	Obesity paradox; potential for a U-shaped association with mortality

Mentz RJ, et al. *J Am Caroll Cardiol.* 2014; 64(21):2281-2293.

TABLE 3.4 — Cardiac Changes in HF-pEF

Molecular changes	Collagen
	Titin
	Slowing of active relaxation
Altered ventricular-arterial coupling, vascular dysfunction	Acute afterload elevation in the setting of ventricular–arterial stiffening causes greater increase in blood pressure, which may then feedback to further impair diastolic relaxation—leading to dramatic increases in filling pressures during stress
Chronotropic incompetence and cardiovascular reserve dysfunction	Chronotropic reserve is depressed in HF-pEF
	Blunted increases in preload volume with exertion, despite marked elevations in filling pressure
Functional mitral regurgitation	May occur with stress, not related to degree of MR at baseline
Left atrial dysfunction	LA dilation, increased susceptibility to AF

TABLE 3.5 — Skeletal Muscle Impairment in HF-pEF

Abnormalities of muscle structure[a]	Reduced type I-to-type II fiber ratio
	Reduced capillary-to-fiber ratio
Vascular dysfunction[b]	Reduced oxygen delivery
Diaphragmatic muscle weakness[c]	Reduced ventilatory capacity

[a] Kitzman DW, et al. *Am J Physiol Heart Circ Physiol.* 2014;306:H1364-H1370.
[b] Zamani P, et al. *Circulation.* 2015;131:371-380.
[c] Yamada K, et al. *J Cardiol Fail.* 2016;22:38-47.

12. Paulus WJ, Tschöpe C, Sanderson JE, et al. How to diagnose diastolic heart failure: a consensus statement on the diagnosis of heart failure with normal left ventricular ejection fraction by the Heart Failure and Echocardiography Associations of the European Society of Cardiology. *Eur Heart J.* 2007;28(20):2539-2550.

13. Upadhya B, Haykowsky MJ, Eggebeen J, Kitzman DW. Exercise intolerance in heart failure with preserved ejection fraction: more than a heart problem. *J Geriatr Cardiol.* 2015;12:294-304.

14. Mentz RJ, Kelly JP, von Lueder TG, et al. Noncardiac comorbidities in heart failure with reduced versus preserved ejection fraction. *J Am Coll Cardiol.* 2014;64(21):2281-2293.

15. Gori M, Senni M, Gupta DK, et al; PARAMOUNT Investigators. Association between renal function and cardiovascular structure and function in heart failure with preserved ejection fraction. *Eur Heart J.* 2014;35(48):3442-3451.

16. Brouwers FP, de Boer RA, van der Harst P, et al. Incidence and epidemiology of new onset heart failure with preserved vs. reduced ejection fraction in a community-based cohort: 11-year follow-up of PREVEND. *Eur Heart J.* 2013;34(19):1424-1431.

4. Nonpharmacologic Management of Chronic Heart Failure: Diet, Activity, and Environment

Patients with clinically overt HF (ACC/AHA Stage C) may benefit substantially from nonpharmacologic management (NPM), although NPM alone is not sufficient to significantly improve long-term outcomes.[1]

Dietary Interventions

Sodium Limitation

Although almost all practitioners advise HF patients to limit salt intake, the evidence for recommending dietary sodium limitation is largely based on observational studies in white patients with HF-rEF. These evidence shortcomings make it difficult to give precise recommendations about daily sodium intake and whether or how it should vary with respect to the type of HF (eg, HF-rEF vs HF-pEF), disease severity (eg, NYHA class), HF-related comorbidities (eg, renal dysfunction), or other characteristics (eg, age or race). A recently published review[2] reached similar conclusions.

Although the ACC/AHA guidelines cite three randomized studies of dietary sodium restriction, all three publications[3-5] are from the same institution with various combinations of authors. The data from the studies are consistent in showing that in patients receiving high doses of furosemide (250-500 mg/day), additional restriction of sodium intake is associated with RAAS activation.

The authors support the statement in the ACC/AHA guidelines, "Because sodium intake is typically high (>4 g/d) in the general population, clinicians should consider some degree (eg, <3 g/d) of sodium restriction in patients with stage C and D HF for symptom improvement." **Table 4.1** lists some useful conversion factors.

TABLE 4.1 — Useful Conversion Factors for Prescribing Sodium Limitations

- To convert milligrams of sodium to milligrams of salt, multiply mg of sodium × 2.5
- To convert millimols of sodium to milligrams of sodium, multiply mmol × 23
- To convert millimols of sodium to mg of sodium chloride, multiply mmol of sodium by 58.5

Fluid Restriction

Increased thirst frequently accompanies Stage C HF, and is seldom recognized or discussed.[6,7] Two recently published reviews that included randomized trials of fluid restriction vs liberal fluid intake for HF patients found no differences in re-hospitalization or mortality rates between the two strategies; however, BNP levels were higher in the group with free fluid intake.[8,9]

In contrast, a small randomized trial in hyponatremic HF patients (serum sodium ≤137 meq/dL) showed subjective improvement in functional status and "A strong trend for reduced HF ED visits and all-cause death and a weaker trend for reduced HF hospitalizations" in the group randomized to a 1000 mL/d fluid restriction. A recent randomized trial in patients with acute HF showed no differences in weight loss or clinical improvement but a marked increase in thirst with more severe (800 mL/day) fluid restriction.[10]

Based on the available evidence, there is little support for fluid restriction as an across-the-board recommendation for all HF patients; however, moderate fluid restriction may be beneficial in hyponatremic patients.

Caloric Restriction

Weight loss should clearly be recommended and supported for ACC/AHA Stage A obese individuals without cardiac pathology to prevent the development of future cardiomyopathy. Obesity is common in HF-pEF, which has become the most common form of HF among older persons. However, a recently published trial[11] showed no improvements in quality of life among 100 participants randomized to diet and/or exercise interventions.

Obesity is a risk factor for the development of HF but has been associated with improved survival in patients with established HF. Overweight and mildly obese HF patients with BMI between 25-35 kg/m^2 may be somewhat protected from cardiac cachexia. Weight loss is not expected to enhance their survival but may offer symptomatic benefit.

A recent meta-analysis that included almost 23,000 patients[12] largely confirmed the now widely-recognized obesity paradox seen in patients with established HF: "In conclusion, risk for total mortality and CV mortality and hospitalization was highest in patients with chronic HF who were underweight as defined by low BMI, whereas risk for CV mortality and hospitalization was lowest in overweight subjects." Another recent meta-analysis reached similar conclusions[13] although, importantly, the data demonstrated a worse prognosis for patients with extreme obesity defined as BMI >40 kg/m^2.

For extremely obese patients, clinical recommendations are also relatively clear. For morbidly obese individuals, defined as those with BMI $\geq$40 kg/m^2, who are younger than 50 years with severely depressed systolic function and NYHA class III-IV symptoms, expert opinion favors consideration for bariatric surgery at an experienced center. The goal of this approach is to achieve either improvement in systolic function and symptoms or sufficient weight loss for heart transplant eligibility.

Further, individual HF patients and their family members who are involved in meal preparation should have the opportunity to consult with a knowledgeable dietitian about an appropriate diet. **Table 4.2** shows a summary of dietary recommendations for HF patients.

TABLE 4.2 — Summary of Dietary Recommendations for Heart Failure Patients

Sodium restriction	Suggested intake ≤3 g/day
	Avoid combination of extreme restriction and high dose diuretic
Fluid restriction	Not recommended for all patients
	Consider 1000 mL/day fluid restriction for hyponatremic patients
Caloric restriction	Yes, for stage A; not required for stage C patients with BMI 25 to 35
	Consider bariatric surgery for younger patients with morbid obesity and severe HF-rEF

■ Alcohol Intake

Confusion about the clinical importance of limiting alcohol intake in patients with HF continues despite large numbers of publications and frequent discussion. There is a firm consensus that individuals who have a clinical diagnosis of alcoholic cardiomyopathy should be counseled to abstain from alcohol. However, there are almost no data on the impact of alcohol consumption on hard outcomes in HF due to other etiologies.

Our Canadian neighbors[14] give very clear recommendations for alcohol intake by healthy individuals to avoid hypertension. "Healthy adults should limit alcohol consumption to two drinks or less per day, and consumption should not exceed 14 standard drinks per week for men and nine standard drinks per week for women (grade B) (**Figure 4.1**). (Note: one standard drink is considered to be 13.6 g or 17.2 mL of ethanol, or approximately 44 mL of 80 proof [40%] spirits, 355 mL of 5% beer or 148 mL of 12% wine.)" The

FIGURE 4.1 — Canadian Hypertension Alcohol Intake Recommended Limits for Healthy Adults

Intake per week

- **Men**
  - Spirits → 21 fluid oz; 1.3 pints
  - Beer → 168 fluid oz; 14 standard 12-oz cans
  - Wine → 70 fluid oz; 2.75 standard 750-mL bottles
- **Women**
  - Spirits → 16 fluid oz; 1.0 pint
  - Beer → 108 fluid oz; 9 standard 12-oz cans
  - Wine → 45 fluid oz; 1.75 standard 750-mL bottles

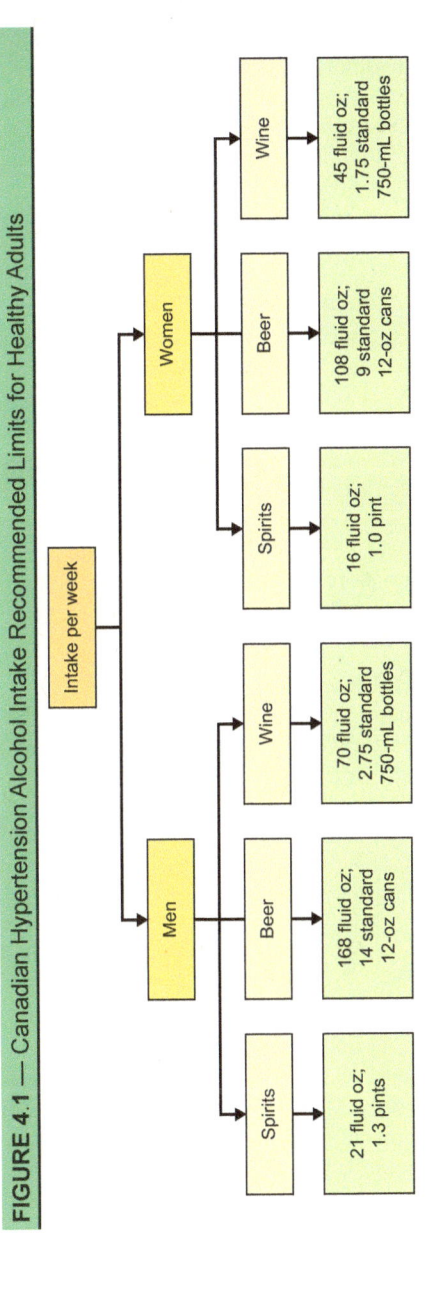

following table converts these recommendations into frequently used volume measures in the United States.

Since hypertension is one of the most common risk factors for HF, these recommendations are probably appropriate for individuals who could be classified as having ACC/AHA Stage A and Stage B HF as well.

The evidence base for recommendations about alcohol intake for individuals with non-alcohol–related HF is strikingly limited; however, an analysis of 6973 patients in the GISSI-HF study (older Italian patients who, if drinkers, consumed almost exclusively wine) showed no relationship between wine intake (none, occasional, 1-2 glasses/day, ≥3 glasses/day) and hard outcomes including death, sudden death, and readmission for HF. In addition, in a subgroup of 1235 patients circulating biomarkers of inflammation were decreased with higher regular wine consumption even after adjustment for age, sex, and severity of HF.[15]

In summary, there appears to be no reason to recommend severe curtailment of moderate wine intake in Class C HF patients.

■ Dietary Supplements

The search for credible evidence supporting the use of any specific dietary supplements in patients with HF is both time-consuming and unrewarding. Experienced clinicians will likely agree that questions about dietary supplementation most frequently involve coenzyme Q10. The CORONA investigators carefully addressed this topic.[16] They concluded, "Coenzyme Q10 is not an independent prognostic variable in HF. Rosuvastatin reduced coenzyme Q10, but even in patients with a low baseline coenzyme Q10, rosuvastatin treatment was not associated with a significantly worse outcome."

A small trial of acute dietary nitrate supplementation has recently demonstrated improvement in peripheral muscle function in HF-rEF patients.[17] Testing the hypothesis that skeletal muscle dysfunction may be in part related to decreased nitric oxide (NO) bioavailability, the investigators tested beetroot juice as a source of inorganic nitrate (NO_3^-) that would increase NO production and improve muscle. They showed enhanced NO bioavailability and muscle power with the active supplement compared to an inactive control.

In an era where drug costs, even for generic prescriptions, have become a topic of heated debate, it is difficult to explain why patients continue to purchase commercial dietary supplements and physicians fail to dissuade them.

Physical Activity

HF-rEF

Based largely on the risk-adjusted findings of the HF-ACTION trial, a randomized controlled trial of exercise training vs usual care in 2331 patients with LVEF ≤35% and NYHA class II to IV symptoms despite optimal HF therapy for at least 6 weeks, current guidelines recommend exercise training, regular physical activity, or cardiac rehabilitation for clinically stable patients. (ACC/AHA guidelines). Importantly, 45% of the HF-ACTION patients had received an ICD or biventricular pacemaker prior to randomization.[18]

HF-pEF

A smaller trial with a 2×2 factorial design tested 20 weeks of diet, exercise, or both in 100 subjects with HF-pEF. Those randomized to caloric restriction or aerobic exercise training showed increased peak $\dot{V}O_2$; however, neizther intervention had a significant effect on quality of life as measured by the MLHF Questionnaire.

In summary, limited exercise appears safe for HF patients. Those with HF-rEF who are compliant with an exercise program may expect modest benefits over time. Patients with HF-pEF have shown increases in functional capacity with exercise training, but the clinical benefits remain uncertain.

Environmental Conditions

■ Altitude

Altitude exposure is a frequent concern for patients with chronic HF. Commercial aircraft cabins are pressurized to the equivalent of 1800-2400 m (6000-8000 feet) above sea level, and some patients may wish to travel to destinations at altitude.

A recent study provided limited data[19] demonstrating that NYHA class I and II HF-rEF patients with an exercise capacity of at least 50% of predicted $\dot{V}O_2$ tolerated a 4- to 5-hour exposure to an altitude of 3454 m (11,000 ft) after a 3.5-hour ascent by public transport from 540 m. The altitude exposure included two exercise tests; the subjects mean peak $\dot{V}O_2$ decreased by 22.2% at altitude and two of the 29 subjects had mild mountain sickness. The subjects in this study probably had more severe baseline exercise impairment than those previously studied in a simulated altitude study[20]; nonetheless, the findings of the two studies are consistent in suggesting that patients with more severe baseline impairment of functional capacity experience greater reductions in performance at altitude.

These limited data suggest that stable ACC/AHA Stage C patients with HF-rEF can tolerate altitudes of 3000 m or 10,000 feet safely; however, patients should be advised to limit activity at altitude and to descend promptly if symptoms worsen at altitude.

■ Temperature

Extremes of environmental temperature, both heat and cold, are associated with increased CV mortality. In a review of 36 studies published between 2001 and 2008, elevated environmental temperature was associated with increased risk of death from CV, respiratory, cerebrovascular disease, including ischemic heart disease, CHF, and MI.[21]

In a recent European study, increases in the 2-day average temperature from the 90th (20.0°C) to the 99th percentiles (24.8°C) was associated with a 10% increase of cardiovascular mortality (95% CI: 5% to

15%) and decreases from the 10th (-1.0°C) to the 1st percentiles (-7.5°C) in the 15-day average temperature were associated with an 8% increase in CV mortality (95% CI: 2% to 14%). Importantly, the strongest risk estimates were associated with high 2-day average temperatures and mortality due to heart diseases including arrhythmias and HF.[22] Data from New England also show adverse impacts from both heat and cold[23] with increased mortality associated with warmer summers and cooler winters.

In an era when greater extremes of environmental temperatures are expected, HF patients should be advised of these findings and advised to limit their exposure to extremes of heat or cold as much as possible.

Particulate Pollution

Much of the literature related to adverse cardiovascular effects of particulate air pollution has focused on the triggering of acute MI.[24] However, recent data from studies in Detroit and Beijing show that a brief exposure to coarse particulate matter also raises arterial BP.[25,26]

Based on a growing body of evidence, HF patients as well as the elderly, diabetics and those with pulmonary disease should limit outdoor activities when air pollution is high.[27]

Summary

Patients with Stage C HF will encounter many situations that engender questions about nonpharmacologic management of their condition. Physicians and other health care professionals should attempt to provide answers based on up-to-date data whenever possible, particularly since those answers may differ substantially for HF-rEF vs HF-pEF patients.

REFERENCES

1. Yancy CW, Jessup M, Bozkurt B, et al; American College of Cardiology Foundation; American Heart Association Task Force on Practice Guidelines. 2013 ACCF/AHA guideline for the management of heart failure: a report of the American College of Cardiology Foundation/American Heart Association Task Force on Practice Guidelines. *J Am Coll Cardiol.* 2013;62(16):e147-239.

2. Colin-Ramirez E, Ezekowitz JA. Salt in the diet in patients with heart failure: what to recommend. *Curr Opin Cardiol.* 2016;31(2):196-203.

3. Paterna S, Gaspare P, Fasullo S, et al. Normal-sodium diet compared with low-sodium diet in compensated congestive heart failure: is sodium an old enemy or a new friend? *Clin Sci (Lond).* 2008;114:221-230.

4. Paterna S, Parrinello G, Cannizzaro S, et al. Medium term effects of different dosage of diuretic, sodium, and fluid administration on neurohormonal and clinical outcome in patients with recently compensated heart failure. *Am J Cardiol.* 2009;103:93-102.

5. Parrinello G, Di Pasquale P, Licata G, et al. Long-term effects of dietary sodium intake on cytokines and neurohormonal activation in patients with recently compensated congestive heart failure. *J Card Fail.* 2009;15:864-873.

6. Waldreus N, Hahn RG, Jaarsma T. Thirst in heart failure: a systematic literature review. *Eur J Heart Fail.* 2013;15(2):141-149.

7. Waldreus N, van der Wal MH, Hahn RG, van Veldhuisen DJ, Jaarsma T. Thirst trajectory and factors associated with persistent thirst in patients with heart failure. *J Card Fail.* 2014;20(9):689-695.

8. De Vecchis R, Baldi C, Cioppa C, Giasi A, Fusco A. Effects of limiting fluid intake on clinical and laboratory outcomes in patients with heart failure: results of a meta-analysis of randomized controlled trials. *Herz.* 2016;41:63-75.

9. Li Y, Fu B, Qian X. Liberal versus restricted fluid administration in heart failure patients. A systematic review and meta-analysis of randomized trials. *Int Heart J.* 2015;56(2):192-195.

10. Aliti GB1, Rabelo ER, Clausell N, Rohde LE, Biolo A, Beck-da-Silva L. Aggressive fluid and sodium restriction in acute decompensated heart failure: a randomized clinical trial. *JAMA Intern Med.* 2013;173(12):1058-1064.

11. Kitzman DW, Brubaker P, Morgan T, et al. Effect of caloric restriction or aerobic exercise training on peak oxygen consumption and quality of life in obese older patients with heart failure with preserved ejection fraction: a randomized clinical trial. *JAMA*. 2016;315(1):36-46.

12. Sharma A, Lavie CJ, Borer JS, et al. Meta-analysis of the relation of body mass index to all-cause and cardiovascular mortality and hospitalization in patients with chronic heart failure. *Am J Cardiol*. 2015;115:1428-1434.

13. Oga EA, Eseyin OR. The obesity paradox and heart failure: a systematic review of a decade of evidence. *J Obes*. 2016;2016:9040248.

14. Khan NA, Hemmelgarn B, Herman RJ, et al. The 2008 Canadian Hypertension Education Program recommendations for the management of hypertension: Part 2 – therapy. *Can J Cardiol*. 2008;24(6):465-475.

15. Cosmi F, Di Giulio P, MSc; Masson S, et al. Regular wine consumption in chronic heart failure. Impact on outcomes, quality of life, and circulating biomarkers. *Circ Heart Fail*. 2015;8:428-437.

16. McMurray JV, Dunselman P, Wedel H, et al. Coenzyme Q10, rosuvastatin, and clinical outcomes in heart failure: a pre-specified substudy of CORONA (Controlled Rosuvastatin Multinational Study in Heart Failure. *J Am Coll Cardiol*. 2010;56:1196-1204.

17. Coggan AR, Leibowitz JL, Spearie CA, et al. Acute dietary nitrate intake improves muscle contractile function in patients with heart failure: a double-blind, placebo-controlled, randomized trial. *Circ Heart Fail*. 2015;8:914-920.

18. O'Connor CM, Whelan DL, Lee KL, et al. Efficacy and safety of exercise training in patients with chronic heart failure: HF-ACTION Randomized Controlled Trial. *JAMA*. 2009;301:1439-1450.

19. Schmid JP, Nobel D, Brugger N, et al. Short-term high altitude exposure at 3454 m is well tolerated in patients with stable heart failure. *Eur J Heart Fail*. 2015;17:182-186.

20. Agostoni P, Cattadori G, Guazzi M, et al. Effects of simulated altitude-induced hypoxia on exercise capacity in patients with chronic heart failure. *Am J Med*. 2000;109:450-455.

21. Basu R. High ambient temperature and mortality: a review of epidemiologic studies from 2001 to 2008. *Environ Health*. 2009;8:40.

22. Breitner S, Wolf K, Peters A, Schneider A. Short-term effects of air temperature on cause-specific cardiovascular mortality in Bavaria, Germany. *Heart*. 2014;100:1272-1280.
23. Shi L, Kloog I, Zanobetti A, et al. Impacts of temperature and its variability on mortality in New England. *Nat Clim Chang*. 2015;5:988-991.
24. Pope CA, Muhlestein JB, Anderson JL, et al. Short-term exposure to fine particulate matter air pollution is preferentially associated with the risk of ST-segment elevation acute coronary events. *J Am Heart Assoc*. 2015;4:e002506.
25. Byrd JB, Morishita M, Bard RL, et al. Acute increase in blood pressure during inhalation of coarse particulate matter air pollution from an urban location. *J Am Soc Hypertens*. 2016;10(2):133-139.
26. Wu S1, Deng F, Huang J, et al. Does ambient temperature interact with air pollution to alter blood pressure? A repeated-measure study in healthy adults. *J Hypertens*. 2015;33(12):2414-2421.
27. Franklin BA, Brook R, Arden Pope C 3rd. Air pollution and cardiovascular disease. *Curr Probl Cardiol*. 2015;40(5):207-238.

5. Pharmacologic Management of Chronic Heart Failure

Skillful use of approved medications is the single most important tool for the management of chronic HF in the physician's toolbox. Our discussion will, with a few exceptions, focus on classes of drugs rather than on specific agents. Because HF patients will inevitably receive multiple drugs, this chapter will first review the key issues involved in the use of each class, then discuss issues involved in polypharmacy. In *Chapter 7*, we will address specific issues in the management of HF patients with important comorbidities.

The evidence supporting pharmacologic recommendations for HF-rEF is substantially stronger than that supporting recommendations for HF-pEF. In fact, the 2016 ESC guidelines state that treatment has only been demonstrated to reduce morbidity and mortality in HF-rEF. This dichotomy reflects the central role of the RAAS in HF-rEF, as discussed in *Chapter 3*. Therefore, recommendations for pharmacologic management of chronic HF-rEF are addressed first for each class of agent. The classes of pharmacologic agents available for HF treatment are shown in **Table 5.1**.

Angiotensin-Converting Enzyme Inhibitors (ACEi-s), Angiotensin-Receptor Blockers (ARBs), and Valsartan-Sacubitril (Val-Sac)

The critical role of neurohormonal negative feedback cycles in HF-rEF was first recognized in the 1970s and became widely accepted in the 1980s.[1,2] ACE inhibitors interfere with the upstream conversion of Ang I to Ang II. In contrast, ARBs competitively inhibit the downstream binding of Ang II to AT1

TABLE 5.1 — Classes of Pharmacologic Agents Available for Heart Failure Treatment

- ACEi/ARB and sacubitril/valsartan
- β-Blockers and ivabradine
- Mineralocorticoid receptor antagonists
- Hydralazine-nitrates
- Loop-blocking diuretics
- Digitalis glycosides
- Anti-thrombotic agents: antiplatelet agents, warfarin, novel anticoagulants
- Agents specifically targeting pulmonary hypertension

receptors in heart, kidney, and vascular tissue. Because of these differences in mechanism of action, *the two classes of drugs are not equivalent and should be considered separately.*[3]

In HF patients, the safety and efficacy of ACEi-s and the safety and efficacy of ARBs are considered as class effects, since clinical trials with several agents from each drug class have demonstrated similar benefit.[4]

■ ACEi-s

Evidence and experience with ACEi agents in severe HF now spans almost 3 decades, dating from the CONSENSUS trial[5] and the SOLVD trial.[6] ACEi-s act more proximally in the RAAS than ARBs (**Figure 5.1**) and have distinctly different pharmacology. In addition to suppression of Ang II formation, some of the effects of ACE inhibitors may be related to the accumulation of kinins, particularly bradykinin, due to ACE inhibition.[7]

Clinical trial data in HF-rEF patients show that ACEi treatment is associated with reduction in both mortality and hospitalizations across the spectrum of severity and in both ischemic and non-ischemic patients. As a consequence, ACE-inhibition remains the recommended first step in constructing a pharmacologic approach to HF-rEF in both the ACC/AHA[8] and ESC 2016 guidelines[9] updates. On the other hand,

FIGURE 5.1 — The Renin-Angiotensin Cascade

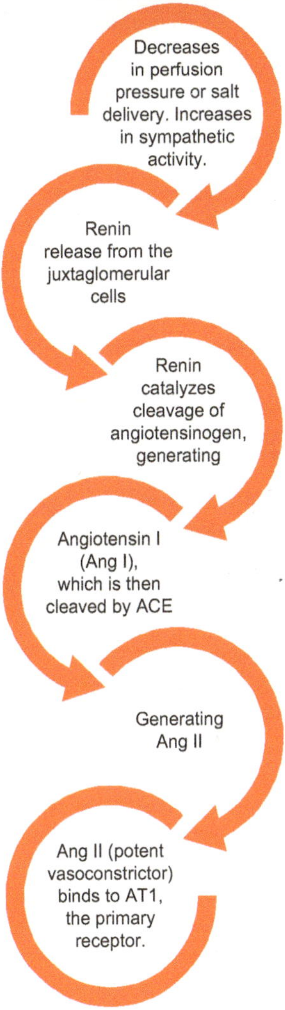

Decreases in perfusion pressure or salt delivery. Increases in sympathetic activity.

Renin release from the juxtaglomerular cells

Renin catalyzes cleavage of angiotensinogen, generating

Angiotensin I (Ang I), which is then cleaved by ACE

Generating Ang II

Ang II (potent vasoconstrictor) binds to AT1, the primary receptor.

ACE inhibition is associated with a more significant burden of adverse effects. **Table 5.2** lists the common adverse effects of ACEi-s and ARBs and **Table 5.3** lists contraindications and cautions in prescribing these agents.[4,10]

TABLE 5.2 — Adverse Effects of ACE Inhibitors and ARBs

	ACE Inhibitors	ARBs
Hypotension	✔	✔
Azotemia	✔	✔
Hyperkalemia	✔	✔
Angioedema	✔	
Cough	✔	
Taste disorder	✔	

TABLE 5.3 — ACE Inhibitors and ARB Contraindications and Cautions

- Prior angioedema (contraindication)
- Pregnancy or planned pregnancy (contraindication)
- Systolic BP ≤80 mm Hg (caution)
- Serum creatinine ≥3.0 mg/dL
- Hyperkalemia ≥5 meq/L
- Bilateral renal artery stenosis

■ ARBs

As a class of therapeutic agents, the ARBs are remarkably well-tolerated. In clinical practice, ACEi-related annoying cough and taste disturbance are probably the most common reasons for substitution of an ARB for an ACEi. Before considering switching because of cough, physicians should confirm that the cough is drug-related and not due to worsening pulmonary congestion or comorbid pulmonary disease. When switching from an ACEi to an ARB, as a reasonable clinical practice, physicians should first stop the ACEi for a period approximately equal to three to four times the half-life of the drug, then initiate ARB dosing.

Importantly, abrupt withdrawal from ACEi therapy without introduction of an ARB may result in rapid worsening of HF symptoms.[8]

There are limited data directly comparing the safety and efficacy of an ACEi vs an ARB. The ONTARGET Trial[11] involved more than 25,000 subjects in a three-way comparison of ramipril, telmisartan, or the combination in patients with vascular disease or high-risk diabetes. The primary composite outcome was death from CV causes, MI, stroke, or hospitalization for HF. The median follow-up was 56 months. The primary outcome occurred in 1412 patients in the ramipril group (16.5%) compared with 1423 patients in the telmisartan group (16.7%; RR, 1.01; 95% confidence interval [CI], 0.94 to 1.09).

Compared with subjects in the ramipril group, those receiving telmisartan had less cough (1.1% vs 4.2%, $P<0.001$) and angioedema (0.1% vs 0.3%, $P=0.01$) and more hypotensive symptoms (2.6% vs 1.7%, $P<0.001$); the occurrence of syncope was 0.2% in both groups (0.2%). Combination therapy with both active agents had no additional benefit and was associated with more adverse events and a greater number of total study discontinuations, including discontinuations due to hypotension and syncope.

Because the ONTARGET subjects did not have established HF-rEF, these data should not be interpreted as demonstrating that ACEi-s and ARBs have similar efficacy profiles in the management of HF-rEF.

The CHARM-Alternative trial compared candesartan to placebo in 2028 ACE-intolerant (primarily cough) HF-rEF patients. The median follow-up was 33.7 months, during which 33% of 1013 patients in the candesartan group and 40% of 1015 in the placebo group had either CV death or hospital admission for CHF (unadjusted HR 0.77 [95% CI 0.67-0.89], $P=0.0004$; covariate adjusted 0.70 [0.60-0.81], $P<0.0001$).[12] The findings from ONTARGET and CHARM-Alternative offer support for the practice of switching to an ARB when side effects of ACE inhibition warrant discontinuing that strategy.

With regard to HF-pEF, in the CHARM-Preserved Trial, the primary outcome was CV death or hospitalization for heart failure. Three thousand twenty-three HF-pEF patients were randomized to candesartan or placebo with a median follow-up of 36.6 months. CV death rate was the same in both groups, but fewer patients in the candesartan group than in the placebo group were admitted to hospital for CHF once (230 vs 279, $P=0.017$) or multiple times.[13]

In a meta-analysis of 30 studies that included 53,878 HF-pEF patients, treatment with standard agents for HF-pEF including ACEi-s and ARBs improved exercise tolerance but did not have the dramatic impact on mortality that is seen in HF-rEF.[14] Since hypertension often plays a major role in the development of HF-pEF, current thinking favors careful control of blood pressure in HF-pEF with the use of ACEi or ARB agents as primary antihypertensives.

■ Sacubitril/Valsartan

The combination of sacubitril, a neprilysin inhibitor, and valsartan, an ARB, is a unique chemical entity, since the combination actually crystalizes in a fixed ratio. This agent represents a first of a new drug class, the combined angiotensin receptor blocker/neprilysin inhibitor or ARNI.

The two major human natriuretic peptides (NPs), ANP and BNP, play an important counter-regulatory role to the RAAS. Small proof-of-concept studies using 12 weeks of twice-daily subcutaneous rh-BNP have shown improvement in patients with both diastolic and systolic dysfunction, confirming the utility of chronic natriuretic peptide augmentation in HF.[15,16] However, because twice-daily subcutaneous injection is a challenging mode of drug delivery, this approach to HF treatment has not generated great enthusiasm.

ANP and BNP are cleared from the circulation by different mechanisms. BNP is largely cleared by cell surface clearance receptors. However, ANP is predominantly cleared by a circulating enzyme called neprilysin.

Sacubitril, an orally effective neprilysin inhibitor (NEPi), was described in 1995.[17] Neprilysin inhibition with sacubitril is associated with increases in circulating ANP and the typical effects of ANP on CV physiology. However, sacubitril also inhibits the degradation of angiotensin II and when administered as a single agent, it showed limited efficacy in the treatment of HF or high blood pressure.

An important breakthrough came when sacubitril was combined with valsartan, an angiotensin receptor blocker. The combination was designated LCZ626 in 2003.[18] Because six molecules of valsartan and six molecules of sacubitril combine in a unique crystal structure, LCZ696 was recognized as a new drug rather than a fixed-dose combination of existing agents[19] (**Figure 5.2**).

Based on the encouraging results from small early trials, LCZ696 was tested in the PARADIGM-HF trial.[20] PARADIGM-HF included 8442 HF patients (NYHA Class II, III, or IV and ejection fraction ≤40%) randomly assigned to receive either LCZ696 (200 mg twice daily) or enalapril (10 mg twice daily) in addition to recommended therapy. The primary efficacy endpoint was a composite of death from CV causes or hospitalization for HF. With a mean follow-up of 27 months, the trial was stopped because the statistical boundary for an overwhelming benefit with LCZ696 had been crossed. The efficacy composite had occurred in 914 patients (21.8%) in the LCZ696 group and 1117 patients (26.5%) in the enalapril group (HR for the LCZ696 group = 0.80; 95% CI, 0.73 to 0.87; $P<0.001$) (**Figure 5.3**).

The FDA approved LCZ696, trade named Entresto, on July 7, 2015 to reduce the risk of cardiovascular death and hospitalization for HF in patients with chronic HF (NYHA Class II-IV) and reduced ejection fraction. Importantly, Entresto is contraindicated in patients with a history of ACE inhibitor or ARB-induced angioedema.[21] The FDA-approved prescribing information includes detailed instructions

FIGURE 5.2 — Molecular Structure of Entresto (Sacubitril and Valsartan)

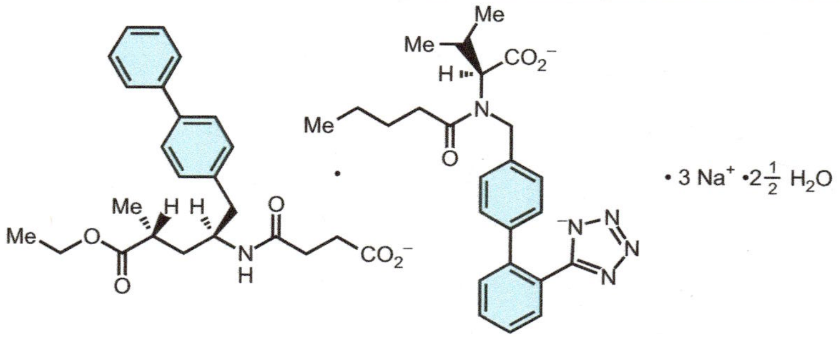

Entresto [package insert]. East Hanover, NJ: Novartis Pharmaceuticals Corporation. 2015.

on initiating therapy with this agent in patients taking ACEi or ARBs, and in those who are treatment-naive to these agents. The information is shown in **Figure 5.4**. Based on the evidence from PARADIGM-HF, 2016 ACC/AHA updated guidelines include recommendations use of ACEI, or ARB, or ARNI as a class I recommendation among patients with HF-rEF. The guidelines additionally give a class I recommendation for patients on ACEI or ARB with reasonable BP to be switched to sacubitril/valsartan for mortality and morbidity benefit.

Medical economic issues are beyond the scope of this book and beyond the expertise of the authors. However, the value of reduction of HF hospitalization appears to extend beyond financial savings and may include improvement of prognosis. These issues should be considered and communicated to the patient when considering alternatives, including patient-assistance programs. Establishing an evidence-based role for this new agent in the management of HF-rEF will require more than a single trial. However, the initial clinical experience with it seems quite promising.

Sacubitril/valsartan has also been tested in patients with HF-pEF. The Prospective comparison of ARNi (angiotensin receptor neprilysin inhibitor) with ARB on Management of Heart Failure With Preserved Ejection Fraction (PARAMOUNT) trial included 301 patients randomly assigned to LCZ696 or valsartan.[22] Independent of reduction of blood pressure, LCZ696 was more effective than valsartan in reducing levels of NT-proBNP, reducing left atrial size, and improving NYHA class and eGFR at 36 weeks.

A subgroup analysis of the PARAMOUNT trial examined the effect of sacubitril/valsartan in 164 patients who had elevated high-sensitivity troponin T (hs-TnT) >0.014 mg/L.REF Those with an elevated hs-TnT were older, more likely to have diabetes, and were less likely to be receiving β-blockers. The hs-TnT levels declined in both the valsartan and sacubitril/valsartan-treated groups, however, the effect was greater in the latter, as shown in **Figure 5.5**.

FIGURE 5.3 — Hazard Ratios for the Composite Endpoint and Components for LCZ vs Enalapril Displayed by Ejection Fraction (≤28%, >28%-33%, and ≥33%)

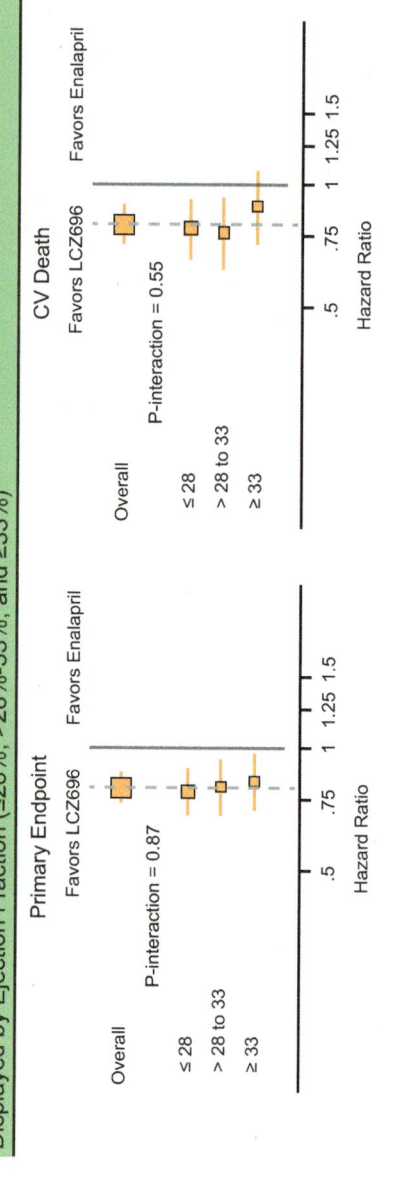

HF Hospitalization

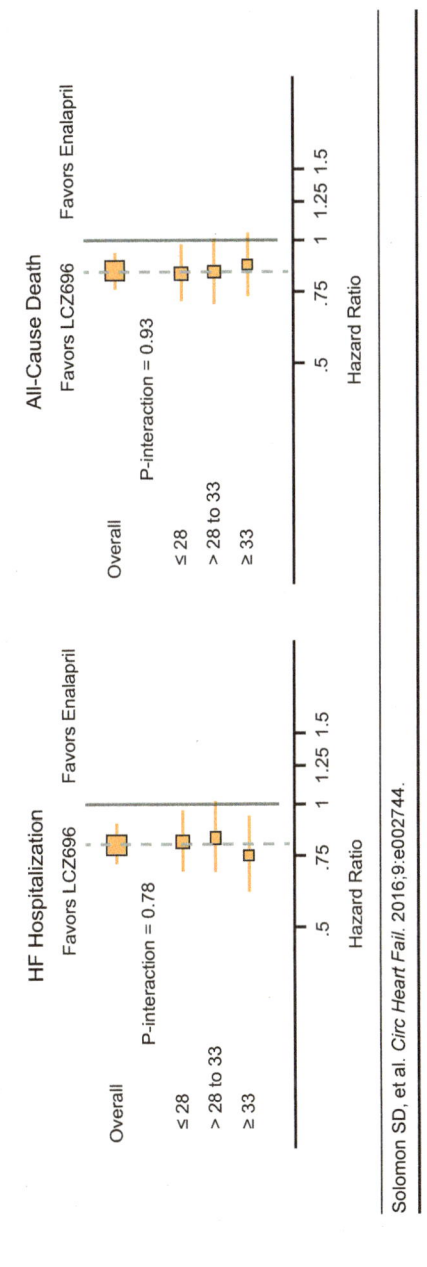

	Favors LCZ696	Favors Enalapril

Overall

P-interaction = 0.78

≤ 28

> 28 to 33

≥ 33

.5   .75   1   1.25 1.5
Hazard Ratio

All-Cause Death

	Favors LCZ696	Favors Enalapril

Overall

P-interaction = 0.93

≤ 28

> 28 to 33

≥ 33

.5   .75   1   1.25 1.5
Hazard Ratio

Solomon SD, et al. *Circ Heart Fail.* 2016;9:e002744.

FIGURE 5.4 — Algorithm for Choosing Dosing for Sacubitril/Valsartan Based on Current Treatment

Angiotensin-converting enzyme inhibitor (ACEI)

- Patients receiving a total daily dose of >10 mg of enalapril or therapeutically equivalent doses of another ACEi, for example:
  - Lisinopril >10 mg
  - Ramipril >5 mg

  → Stop ACEi 36 hours before starting sacubitril/valsartan → Start sacubitril/valsartan at the recommended dose of 49/51 mg twice daily

- Patients receiving a total daily dose of ≤10 mg of enalapril or therapeutically equivalent doses of another ACEi, for example:
  - Lisinopril ≤10 mg
  - Ramipril ≤5 mg

  → Stop ACEi 36 hours before starting sacubitril/valsartan → Start sacubitril/valsartan at the recommended dose of 24/26 mg twice daily → Double the dose after 2-4 weeks to 49/51 mg twice daily, as tolerated by the patient

Angiotensin II receptor blockers (ARB)

- Patients receiving a total daily dose of >160 mg of valsartan or therapeutically equivalent doses of another ARB, for example:
  - Losartan >50 mg
  - Olemsartan >10 mg

  → Start sacubitril/valsartan at the recommended dose of 49/51 mg twice daily

- Patients receiving a total daily dose of ≤160 mg of valsartan or therapeutically equivalent doses of another ARB, for example:
  - Losartan ≤50 mg
  - Olemsartan ≤10 mg

  → Start sacubitril/valsartan at the recommended dose of 24/26 mg twice daily → Double the dose after 2-4 weeks to 49/51 mg twice daily, as tolerated by the patient

Not on ACEI or ARB

→ Not currently taking ACEIs or ARBs → Start sacubitril/valsartan at the recommended dose of 24/26 mg twice daily → Double the dose after 2-4 weeks to 49/51 mg twice daily, as tolerated by the patient

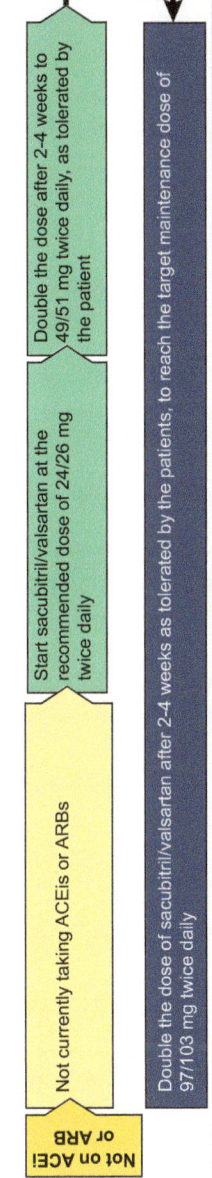

Double the dose of sacubitril/valsartan after 2-4 weeks as tolerated by the patients, to reach the target maintenance dose of 97/103 mg twice daily

Adapted and modified from Entresto (sacubitril/valsartan) Dosing and Titration Guide. Entresto Web site. https://www.entrestohcp.com/sfc/servlet.shepherd/version/download/06812000001NqWHAA0. Accessed August 25, 2016.

FIGURE 5.5 — Decline in High-Sensitivity Troponin T Over 36 Weeks With LCZ696 and With Valsartan in the PARAMOUNT Trial

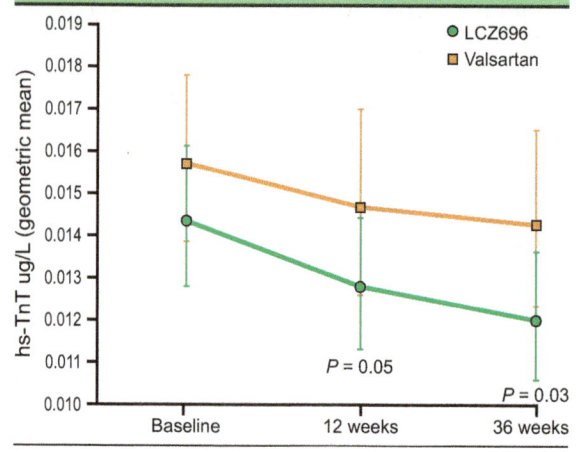

Pardeep S, et al. *Circ Heart Fail.* 2014;7:953-959.

The investigators suggested that LCZ696 may have been more effective in hs-TnT reduction by potentiating the known effects of natriuretic peptides. Further studies in HF-pEF patients are required to determine whether these interesting phase 2 findings will have an impact on long-term hard clinical outcomes. Nonetheless, these results are encouraging for a subset of patients who are difficult to manage.

β-Blockers and Ivabradine

In the decade since the previous edition of this book, β-adrenergic blocking agents have become widely accepted as first-line therapy for HF-rEF. In the 2013 ACC/AHA guidelines, the recommendation for "use of one of the three β-blockers proven to reduce mortality (eg, bisoprolol, carvedilol, and sustained-release metoprolol succinate) is recommended for all patients with current or prior symptoms of HF-rEF, unless contraindicated, to reduce morbidity and mortality" has Class 1 status with an A-level of evidence.

Nonetheless, carvedilol, metoprolol succinate, and bisoprolol, the available β-blockers differ in their selectivity for adrenergic receptors and their effects on the peripheral circulation. These differences have raised questions about whether the agents differ in efficacy, safety, or tolerability, particularly in HF-rEF patients with comorbid airway disease.

A recent randomized trial in such patients demonstrated that N-terminal pro-hormone brain natriuretic peptide was significantly lower with carvedilol than with metoprolol or bisoprolol (mean: carvedilol 1001 [95% CI: 633-1367] ng/l; metoprolol 1371 [95% CI: 778 to 1964] ng/l; bisoprolol 1349 [95% CI: 782-1916] ng/l; $P<0.01$), but in subjects with COPD, forced expiratory volume in 1 s was lowest with carvedilol and highest with bisoprolol (carvedilol 1.85 [95% CI: 1.67-2.03] l/s; metoprolol 1.94 [95% CI: 1.73-2.14] l/s; bisoprolol 2.0 [95% CI: 1.79-2.22] l/s; $P<0.001$).[23] There were no long-term data to indicate whether the observed differences were clinically significant.

In the absence of robust head-to-head trials, several groups have attempted to explore potential differences in β-blockers for HF-rEF using meta-analysis approaches. Chatterjee and colleagues used network meta-analysis, a special type of meta-analysis allowing them to make indirect comparisons of two β-blockers via a common comparator.[24] Their analysis included 23,122 patients and showed, "no obvious differences when comparing the different β-blockers head to head for the risk of death, sudden cardiac death, death due to pump failure, or drug discontinuation." In addition, "improvements in left ventricular ejection fraction were also similar irrespective of the individual study drug." However, carvedilol showed the greatest absolute risk reduction for mortality, 6.6%, with a number needed to treat of 15 to prevent one death.

In a traditional meta-analysis comparing carvedilol to the β-1 selective β-blockers to evaluate effects on mortality, CV events, and hospital readmissions in the setting of AMI or systolic HF, the results favored carvedilol. Compared to β(1)-selective β-blockers used in HF (eight trials, $n=4563$), carvedilol significantly reduced all-cause mortality (risk ratio 0.85, 95% CI 0.78 to 0.93, $P=0.0006$).[25]

The most recent study was a comparison of carvedilol vs metoprolol on all-cause mortality and hospitalizations in patients with HF that included four prospective controlled and six cohort studies with 30,943 patients who received carvedilol and 69,925 patients who received metoprolol (tartrate and succinate).[26] The findings included a reduction in all-cause mortality in prospective studies with carvedilol vs metoprolol tartrate. However, neither all-cause mortality nor hospitalizations differed between carvedilol and metoprolol succinate in the cohort studies. A summary of β-blocker comparisons is shown in **Table 5.4**.

TABLE 5.4 — Summary of β-Blocker Comparisons

	Carvedilol	Metoprolol Succinate	Bisoprolol
Mortality reduction	++	+	+
Improved ejection fraction	+	+	++
NT-proBNP reduction	++	+	+
FEV_1	--	-	-

In summary, based on the patterns observed in these studies, carvedilol may offer some modest advantages over the other agents for patients who do not have COPD; however, all three agents, carvedilol, metoprolol succinate, and bisoprolol, have been tested extensively and found to be superior to placebo in patients with chronic HF.

A recent meta-analysis of the impact of β-blockers on mortality and morbidity in HF-pEF patients included 15 observational studies and two randomized control trials involving a total of 27,099 patients. In the observational studies, β-blockers were associated with lower all-cause mortality (RR 0.81 [0.72-0.90], $P<0.001$) but not with reductions in HF hospitalization (RR 0.79 [0.57-1.10], $P<0.001$). Most importantly, in the RCTs, β-blockers were not associated with improvement in all-cause mortality (RR 0.94 [0.67-1.32], $P=0.72$) or rates of HF hospitalization (0.90 [0.54-1.49], $P=0.68$).[27] Given the demonstrated role of chronotropic incompetence in the pathophysiology of HF-pEF,[28] perhaps this is not surprising.

The recent introduction of ivabradine (Corlanor, Amgen) for management of chronic HF represents a novel pharmacologic approach. An elevated HR, probably reflecting activation of the sympathetic nervous system, has been associated with worse CV outcomes.[29-31] Although β-blockers reduce HR in HF treatment, uptitration of β-blockers can be associated with an increased risk of adverse reactions.[32] Ivabradine lowers HR by inhibiting the specific sinus node pacemaker I_f current[33] and does not adversely affect echocardiographic indices of LV function in patients with LV dysfunction.[34]

The SHIFT (Systolic HF Treatment with I_f Inhibitor Ivabradine) trial was an RCT with 6558 patients with HF-rEF (LVEF ≤35%) in sinus rhythm with HR ≥70 bpm.[35] In SHIFT, ivabradine significantly reduced the primary efficacy endpoint, the composite of CV death or hospital admission for worsening HF and deaths due to HF (**Figure 5.6**).

One criticism of the SHIFT trial is that many patients did not receive so-called "target doses" of β-blockers. If, as the data suggest, these patients had not tolerated higher doses of β-blockers, then these results are relevant to clinical management. Given its promising therapeutic value, ivabradine should be considered for HF-rEF patients with an elevated HR and intolerance to β-blockers.

Ivabradine received FDA approval in April 2015 for reduction of worsening HF. Establishing an evidence-based role for this new agent in the management of HF-rEF will require more clinical experience with it;

FIGURE 5.6 — SHIFT: Kaplan-Meir Plots for the Composite Endpoint, Cardiovascular Death, and Hospitalization, and Each Component Separately

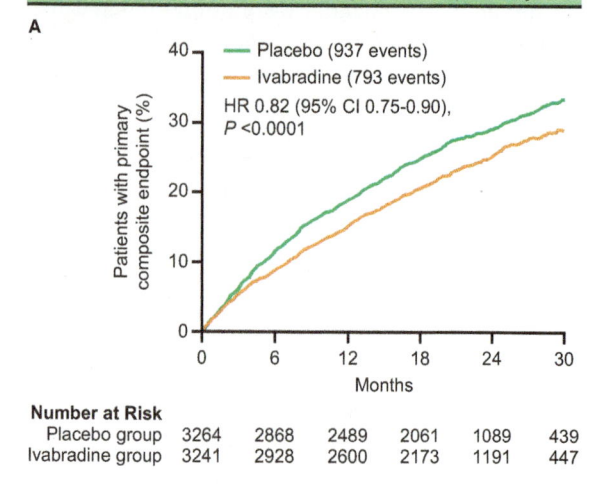

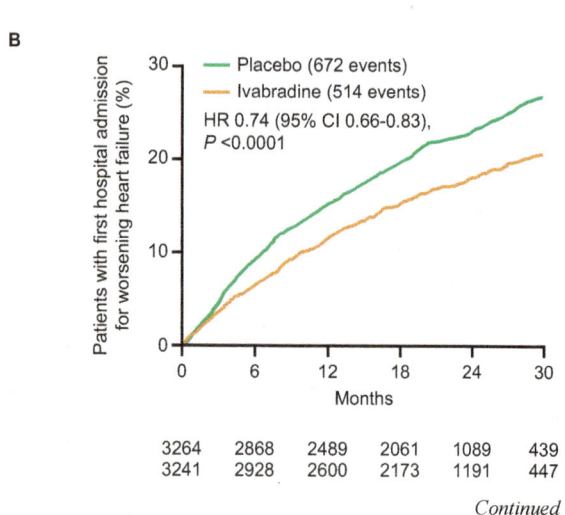

A

- Placebo (937 events)
- Ivabradine (793 events)

HR 0.82 (95% CI 0.75-0.90), $P < 0.0001$

Number at Risk

Placebo group	3264	2868	2489	2061	1089	439
Ivabradine group	3241	2928	2600	2173	1191	447

B

- Placebo (672 events)
- Ivabradine (514 events)

HR 0.74 (95% CI 0.66-0.83), $P < 0.0001$

3264	2868	2489	2061	1089	439
3241	2928	2600	2173	1191	447

Continued

FIGURE 5.6 — *Continued*

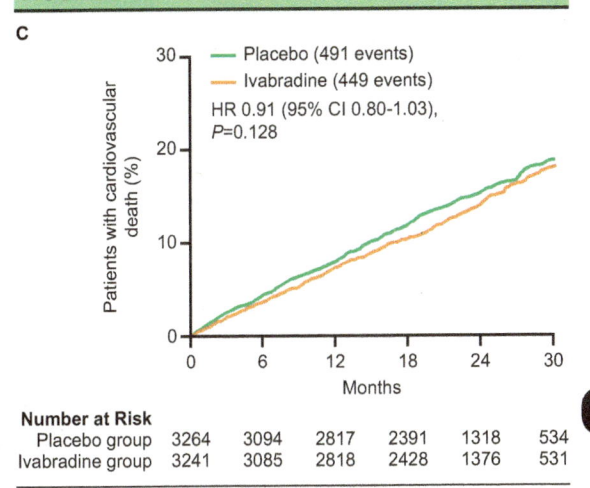

C

[Graph showing Patients with cardiovascular death (%) vs Months]
- Placebo (491 events)
- Ivabradine (449 events)
- HR 0.91 (95% CI 0.80-1.03), $P=0.128$

Number at Risk

	0	6	12	18	24	30
Placebo group	3264	3094	2817	2391	1318	534
Ivabradine group	3241	3085	2818	2428	1376	531

Swedberg K, et al. *Lancet.* 2010;376:875-885.

however, it also seems quite promising. In a therapeutic area where cost issues are critical, the comments above with regard to cost and sacubitril/valsartan also apply to ivabradine. Ivabradine may be particularly useful in patients with coexisting HF-rEF and COPD, as discussed in more detail in *Chapter 7*. Both the ACC/AHA 2016 update and the ESC 2016 guidelines discuss its use. The ACC/AHA document emphasizes that because β-blockers have proven mortality benefit, it is important to initiate and uptitrate β-blockers to target doses if possible before considering ivabradine. The ESC guidelines also recommend considering ivabradine for patients on ACEi or ARB treatment who are unable to tolerate or have contraindications for a β-blocker.

In contrast, a recent randomized, crossover study comparing selective heart rate reduction with ivabradine (7.5 mg twice daily) vs placebo for 2 weeks each in 22 symptomatic patients with HF-pEF showed that ivabradine significantly reduced peak heart rate compared with placebo, but significantly worsened the change in O_2 peak in the HF-pEF cohort (-2.1 vs 0.9 mL/kg(-1)/min(-1); $P=0.003$) and significantly reduced submaximal exercise capacity, as determined by the oxygen uptake efficiency slope.[36] Again, given the demonstrated role of chronotropic incompetence in the pathophysiology of HF-pEF,[37] perhaps this is not surprising.

Mineralocorticoid Receptor Antagonists (MRAs)

In addition to Ang II (**Figure 5.1**), aldosterone is the other potent effector hormone of the RAAS. Aldosterone is a steroid hormone released primarily from the adrenal cortex in response to increased Ang II and increased plasma [K+]. Aldosterone binds to a mineralocorticoid receptor (MR), and activation of the receptor is associated with increased salt and water reabsorption, increased blood volume, and alterations in ion-channel expression. The currently approved receptor antagonists, spironolactone and eplerenone, competitively inhibit aldosterone binding to mineralocorticoid receptors in the heart, kidney, and peripheral vasculature.

■ MRAs in HF-rEF

The current ACC/AHA guidelines give MRAs a class 1 recommendation, level of evidence A, for, "NYHA class II–IV HF and who have LVEF of 35% or less, unless contraindicated, to reduce morbidity and mortality. Patients with NYHA class II HF should have a history of prior CV hospitalization or elevated plasma natriuretic peptide levels to be considered for aldosterone receptor antagonists."

However, perhaps more than for any other pharmacologic approach to HF, the decision to employ an MRA for management of chronic HF-rEF is complicated by comorbidities and polypharmacy, since treatment-related hyperkalemia is a significant concern. **Table 5.5** gives recommendations for MRA dosing.

All HF patients should have regular, frequent monitoring of electrolytes and renal function; however, this is particularly important in those receiving MRAs. In addition, patients should discontinue MRA therapy if they experience diarrhea or dehydration, or while loop diuretic therapy is interrupted.

The major clinical differentiation between eplerenone and spironolactone is in their selectivity of aldosterone receptor antagonism, not their receptor blocking activity. The Randomized Aldactone Evaluation Study (RALES) trial randomized 822 HF-rEF patients to receive 25 mg of spironolactone daily, and 841 to receive placebo (27% of both groups were female). There was a 32% reduction in the risk of the composite end point of death from cardiac causes or hospitalization for cardiac causes in the spironolactone group compared with the placebo group (RR, 0.68; 95% CI, 0.59 to 0.78; $P<0.001$). Serious hyperkalemia occurred in 14 spironolactone patients vs 10 patients in the placebo group. However, gynecomastia or breast pain was reported by 10% of the men in the spironolactone group vs 1% of the men in the placebo group ($P<0.001$), with the result that more men in the spironolactone group discontinued treatment (10 vs 1, $P=0.006$).[38]

In the Eplerenone Post–Acute Myocardial Infarction Heart Failure Efficacy and Survival Study (EPHESUS), 6642 patients were randomized to eplerenone (25 mg per day) or matching placebo for 4 weeks, then the eplerenone dose was increased to a maximum of 50 mg per day. 885 patients in the eplerenone group (26.7%) and 993 patients in the placebo group (30.0%) had an end point event, death from CV causes or hospitalization for CV events (RR, 0.87; $P=0.002$). The incidence of gynecomastia in males was 0.5% and 0.6% for eplerenone and control patients, respectively.[39]

A systematic review and meta-analysis of eight trials involving 3929 patients concluded that MRAs were superior to the control for reduction of all-cause

TABLE 5.5 — Dosing Recommendations for MRAs

	Eplerenone		Spironolactone		Time Points for Potassium and Serum Creatinine Monitoring	
	eGFR ≥50 mL/min/1.73 m²	eGFR 30-49 mL/min/1.73 m²	eGFR ≥50 mL/min/1.73 m²	eGFR 30-49 mL/min/1.73 m²	Interim	Routine
Initial dose	25 mg once daily	25 mg once every other day	12.5-25 mg once daily	12.5 mg once daily or every other day	Within 72 hours to 1 week of the initial dose, with any dose titrations, or with any alterations in other concomitant drugs, diseases, or acute illnesses that may influence potassium levels	Monthly for first 3 months, then regularly at 3- to 4-month intervals
Maintenance dose after 4 weeks (if K ≤5 mmol/L)	50 mg once daily	25 mg once daily	25 mg once or twice daily	12.5-25 mg once daily		
For K 5.5-5.9 mmol/L[a]	25 mg once daily	25 mg once every other day	12.5-25 mg once daily or every other day	12.5-25 mg once every other day		
For K >6.0 mmol/L	Hold until K <5.0 mmol/L	Hold until K <5.0 mmol/L	Hold until K <5.0 mmol/L	Hold until K <5.0 mmol/L		

| Reassess after 72 hours, and for K that returns to <5.0 mmol/L | Restart at 25 mg once daily | Restart at 25 mg once every other day | Restart at 12.5-25 mg once daily | Restart at 12.5 mg once daily or every other day |

[a] These dosing guidelines were used in the EMPHASIS-HF trial under the close supervision and monitoring typical of a randomized controlled, clinical trial. In clinical practice, a more conservative approach may be warranted, such as holding the aldosterone antagonist until serum potassium is ≤5.5 mmol/L.

Adapted from Butler J, et al. *J Card Fail.* 2012;18:265-281.

mortality (RR 0.79, 95% CI 0.66, 0.95) and in reduction of re-hospitalization for cardiac causes (RR 0.62, 95% CI 0.52, 0.74, $P=0.52$).[40] In a detailed review of the literature aimed at integrating evidence into clinical practice, a group of expert trialists concluded that "The morbidity and mortality benefits of MRAs may be mediated by several proposed actions, including antifibrotic mechanisms that slow HF progression, prevent or reverse cardiac remodeling, or reduce arrhythmogenesis. Both eplerenone and spironolactone have demonstrated survival benefits in individual clinical trials. Pharmacologic differences exist between the drugs, which may be relevant for therapeutic decision making in individual patients. Although serious hyperkalemia events were reported in the major MRA clinical trials, these risks can be mitigated through appropriate patient selection, dose selection, patient education, monitoring, and follow-up. When used appropriately, MRAs significantly improve outcomes across the spectrum of patients with HF-rEF."[41]

■ MRAs in HF-pEF

MRAs, such as spironolactone and eplerenone, reduce myocardial fibrosis in animal models. A recent meta-analysis that included 11 randomized controlled trials with 942 participants (weighted mean follow-up of 9.1 ± 3.0 months) assessed the impact of MRA therapy on echocardiographic parameters, surrogate measures for myocardial fibrosis (markers of collagen turnover such as carboxy-terminal peptide of procollagen type I [PICP] and amino-terminal peptide of pro-collagen type II [PIIINP]), and surrogate clinical outcomes (exercise capacity and serum potassium levels) in patients with HF-pEF or asymptomatic LVDD. Six trials included patients with symptomatic HF-pEF and five included patients with asymptomatic LVDD and/or LVH. Eight of the trials used spironolactone; two used eplerenone and one used canrenone. The principal findings were that MRA therapy was associated with improved diastolic function, blood pressure, and markers of myocardial fibrosis without significant changes in indexed LV mass or LV cavity size.[42]

These positive findings with surrogate endpoints in HF-pEF provided the rationale for the Treatment of Preserved Cardiac Function Heart Failure With an Aldosterone Antagonist (TOPCAT) trial. TOPCAT randomized 3445 patients to spironolactone or placebo: 1767 in North and South America (United States, Canada, Brazil, and Argentina) and 1678 in Russia and the Republic of Georgia. The primary efficacy outcome was the composite of CV death, aborted cardiac arrest, or hospitalization for HF. In the patients randomized from North and South America, this endpoint occurred in 11.5 of 100 patients per year, while in patients from Russia and Georgia, it was only 2.4 of 100 patients per year[43] (**Figure 5.7**).

A retrospective analysis showed that the baseline characteristics of patients enrolled in the two regions were "distinctly different for almost every variable," and the outcomes data showed that in the Americas, 522 patients (29.5%) had at least one confirmed primary outcome event (CV death, aborted cardiac arrest, or hospitalization for the management of HF) compared to 149 patients (8.9%) in Russia/Georgia, for incidence rates of 11.5 and 2.4 per 100 patient-years ($P<0.001$). "In the Americas, the HR for treatment with spironolactone was 0.82 (95% CI, 0.69-0.98), whereas in Russia/Georgia, it was 1.10 (95% CI, 0.79-1.51)" These findings suggested "possible clinical benefits with spironolactone in patients with HF and preserved ejection fraction from the Americas."[44]

In a recent review of these data, Pfeffer and Braunwald concluded, "From a strictly statistical point of view, the results of TOPCAT must be regarded as neutral. However, HF-pEF is often a disabling and life-shortening condition. Other than the administration of diuretics for fluid accumulation and the management of hypertension (if present), there is little to offer these patients. Based on the findings in TOPCAT in North and South America and in the absence of other

FIGURE 5.7 — TOPCAT Results by Region

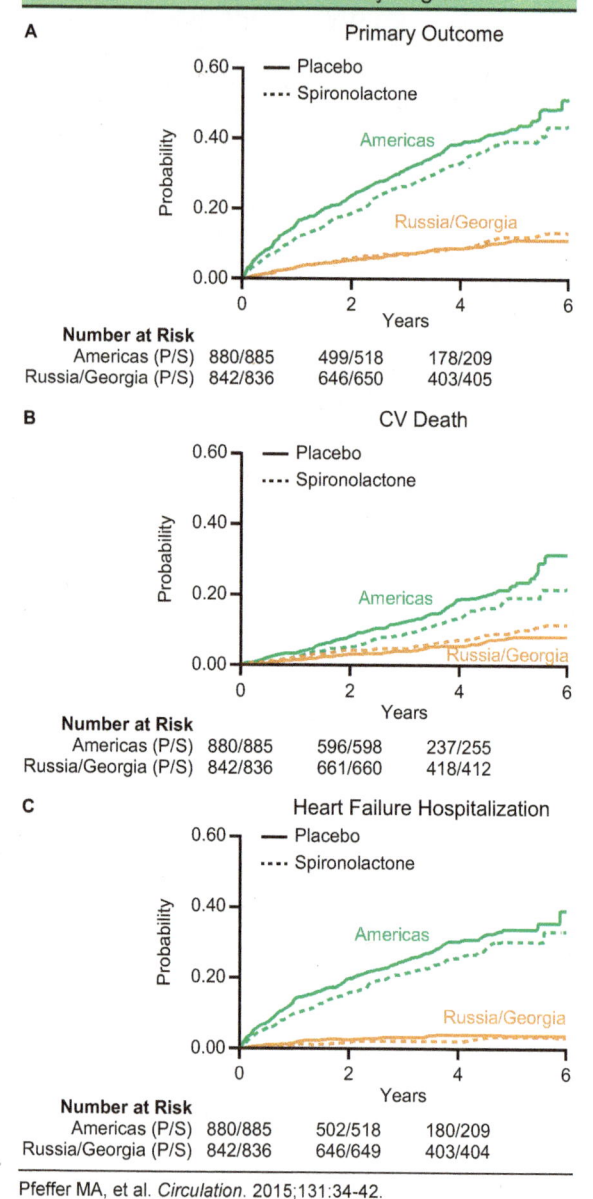

A Primary Outcome

Number at Risk
Americas (P/S)	880/885	499/518	178/209
Russia/Georgia (P/S)	842/836	646/650	403/405

B CV Death

Number at Risk
Americas (P/S)	880/885	596/598	237/255
Russia/Georgia (P/S)	842/836	661/660	418/412

C Heart Failure Hospitalization

Number at Risk
Americas (P/S)	880/885	502/518	180/209
Russia/Georgia (P/S)	842/836	646/649	403/404

Pfeffer MA, et al. *Circulation*. 2015;131:34-42.

more definitive data, it now appears reasonable to treat patients with HF-pEF resembling those enrolled in North and South America with spironolactone to improve outcomes. This drug is generic, inexpensive, and generally well tolerated, although periodic monitoring of electrolytes and creatinine must be conducted to detect the occasional development of hyperkalemia and renal dysfunction."[45]

Monitoring for Patients Receiving MRAs

Patients with either HF-rEF or HR-pEF who are candidates for MRA therapy are, by definition, receiving multiple drugs that significantly impact renal function and electrolyte balance. A recent claims data study included 10,443 Medicare beneficiaries who had started MRA therapy for HF. Appropriate laboratory monitoring was defined as a claim for a specific test or laboratory panel including creatinine and potassium within 120 days before initiation, two or more measurements during the early post-initiation period (days 1 through 10), and three or more measurements during the extended post-initiation period (days 11 through 90), consistent with current ACC/AHA guideline recommendations. After the onset of MRA therapy, 1384 patients (13.3%) received appropriate testing in early follow up and 3122 patients (29.9%) received appropriate testing in extended follow-up. Five thousand seven hundred eight-two patients (55.4%) and 2328 (22.3%) received no testing in early or extended follow-up, respectively[46] (**Table 5.6**).

These data suggest that laboratory monitoring of patients receiving MRAs in the community setting may not be adequate to avoid significant fluid and electrolyte disturbances. Physicians who initiate MRA therapy should emphasize the importance of regular laboratory monitoring with their patients.

Hydralazine/Nitrates

The rationale for the use of hydralazine and nitrates in combination rests on a hemodynamic

TABLE 5.6 — Observed Laboratory Testing of Potassium and Creatinine Levels Among Patients Initiating Mineralocorticoid Receptor Antagonist Therapy for Heart Failure

	No. (%) of Patients (N = 10,443)
Preinitiation Testing (120 days before drug initiation)	
Appropriate[a]	9564 (91.6)
None	879 (8.4)
Early Post-initiation Testing (1-10 days after drug initiation)	
Appropriate[b]	1384 (13.3)
Any	4661 (44.6)
None	5782 (55.4)
Extended Post-initiation Testing (11-90 days after drug initiation)	
Appropriate[c]	3122 (29.9)
Any	8115 (77.7)
None	2328 (22.3)
Received all appropriate testing	756 (7.2)
No preinitiation or post-initiation testing	280 (2.7)

[a] Defined by the presence of at least one laboratory claim (or hospitalization) within 120 days before drug initiation.
[b] Defined by the presence of two laboratory claims (or hospitalizations or one laboratory claim plus hospital discharge within 3 days before initial outpatient prescription fill) within 10 days after drug initiation.
[c] Defined by the presence of three laboratory claims (or hospitalizations) within 11 to 90 days after drug initiation

Cooper LB, et al. *JAMA*. 2015;314(18):1973-1975.

approach to HF. As stated in the 1986 publication reporting the outcome of a Veterans Administration Cooperative Study of vasodilators in HF, "The rationale for vasodilator therapy for HF is evidence that vasoconstriction in the systemic arterial and venous beds raises impedance to left ventricular ejection and shifts blood centrally from the venous capacitance vessels. The result of these circulatory effects is increased preload and afterload that adversely affect left ventricular performance and contribute to the low cardiac output and venous congestion that characterize HF. Studies of the hemodynamic effects of sodium nitroprusside have revealed that the relaxing effect of the drug on the arteries and veins could produce a profoundly favorable effect on left ventricular performance. Subsequent studies indicated that orally administered prazosin or hydralazine, given in combination with isosorbide dinitrate (ISDN), could produce a similar hemodynamic effect."[47]

In fact, in patients receiving digitalis and diuretics the combination of hydralazine and nitrates reduced all-cause mortality over 3 years compared to either prazosin or placebo. However, the complexity of taking both drugs three times daily, a relatively high incidence of adverse effects, and the superior efficacy of ACEi/ARB and β-blocker management pushed hydralazine/ISDN into a second-line position.

A retrospective subgroup analysis of the data from the two Veterans Administration HF trials, V-HeFT-I and V-HeFT-II, suggested that black vs white racial differences in HF etiology, and neurohormonal and pharmacologic responses existed, and that hydralazine/ISDN was as effective as ACEi in black patients.[48] These findings prompted the African-American Heart Failure Trial (A-HeFT), a randomized, placebo-controlled, double-blind trial to evaluate the efficacy of a fixed dose of hydralazine/ISDN in 1050 self-identified black patients who had New York Heart Association (NYHA) class III or IV HF-rEF and who were receiving background therapy that included neurohormonal blockers. The primary efficacy endpoint was a composite of death from any cause, first hospitalization for HF, and a change in the quality of life.

The trial was stopped early because of significantly higher mortality in the placebo arm than in the group given isosorbide dinitrate plus hydralazine, as shown

111

in **Figure 5.8**. When the trial was discontinued with a mean duration of follow-up of 10 months, 54 patients had died in the placebo arm (10.2%) compared to 32 patients in the combination-therapy group (6.2%), a 43% improvement in survival (HR, 0.57; $P=0.01$ by the log-rank test). The Kaplan-Meier survival analysis showed that the survival difference appeared at approximately 180 days, then widened progressively ($P=0.01$ by log-rank test).[49]

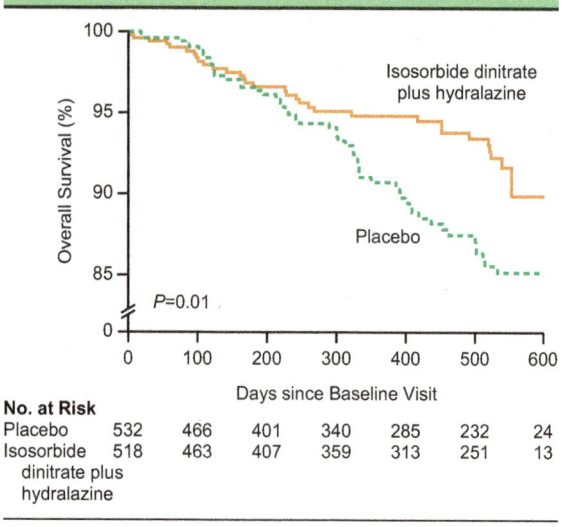

FIGURE 5.8 — Kaplan-Meier Survival Curves from A-HeFT

	0	100	200	300	400	500	600
No. at Risk							
Placebo	532	466	401	340	285	232	24
Isosorbide dinitrate plus hydralazine	518	463	407	359	313	251	13

Taylor AL, et al. *N Engl J Med.* 2004;351(20):2049-2057.

Based primarily on the A-HeFT data, hydralazine/ISDN is recommended for patients self-described as African-American who are receiving optimal ACEi and β-blocker treatment, and also for patients of any race who are ACEi/ARB intolerant.

In addition to the specific data related to hydralazine/ISDN, A-HeFT had an important contribution to the field of clinical research by targeting a specific patient population based on phenotype in which there was a high likelihood of successfully establishing efficacy. This trial was an initial step toward a much more personalized approach to medical care.

How hydralazine/ISDN will fit in clinical practice for HF-rEF with the advent of sacubitril/valsartan and with ivabradine is uncertain. With regard to HF-pEF, there are pathophysiologic arguments to support the use of hydralazine/ISDN.[50] However, the authors are not aware of any large scale randomized trials of hydralazine/ISDN specifically in HF-pEF.

Diuretics

Thiazide diuretics are a cornerstone of antihypertensive treatment, and thus in the management of Stage A and B HF, both HF-rEF and HF-pEF. Both of the commonly used thiazide diuretics, hydrochlorothiazide and chlorthalidone, have received increased attention recently because of newer evidence suggesting that chlorthalidone may be a more effective agent. **Table 5.7** compares PK and PD information for the two agents.

In the Antihypertensive and Lipid-Lowering Treatment to Prevent Heart Attack Trial (ALLHAT),[51] a randomized, double-blind, active-controlled clinical trial, a total of 33,357 participants aged 55 years or older with hypertension and at least one other CHD risk factor were randomized to treatment with chlorthalidone, 12.5 to 25 mg/day ($n=15,255$); amlodipine, 2.5 to 10 mg/day ($n=9048$); or lisinopril, 10 to 40 mg/day ($n=9054$) for planned follow-up of approximately 4 to 8 years. The primary outcome was combined fatal CHD or nonfatal MI, analyzed by intent-to-treat. Systolic blood pressure was lower with chlorthalidone, and the primary outcome occurred in 2956 participants, with no difference between treatments.

In a randomized, single-blinded, active treatment, crossover study comparing chlorthalidone 12.5 mg/day (force-titrated to 25 mg/day) and hydrochlorothiazide 25 mg/day (force-titrated to 50 mg/day) in 30

TABLE 5.7 — Comparison of PK and PD for Hydrochlorothiazide and Chlorthalidone

	Hydrochlorothiazide	Chlorthalidone
Onset	2 hours	2.6 hours
Peak effect	4-6 hours	1.5-6 hours
Absorption	Well absorbed[a]	65%
Duration	6-12 hours	48-72 hours
Protein binding	40%-68%	75%
Metabolism	Not metabolized	Hepatic
Elimination half-life	10-12 hours[b]	40-89 hours
Excretion pathway	Urine (as unchanged drug)	Urine[c]

[a] When taken with food, time to maximum concentration increases from 1.6 hours to 2.9 hours. Absorption is reduced in patients with chronic heart failure.
[b] Large variation due to biphasic elimination; may be much longer with renal impairment.
[c] Data not available on the percentage of dose as unchanged drug and metabolites, concentration of the drug in body fluids, degree of uptake by a particular organ or in the fetus, or passage across the blood-brain barrier.

Cooney D, et al. *CCJM*. 2015;82(8):527-533.

untreated hypertensive patients, chlorthalidone 25 mg/day produced a greater reduction in week 8 ambulatory systolic BP than did hydrochlorothiazide 50 mg/day (24-hour mean = -12.4 ± 1.8 mm Hg vs -7.4 ± 1.7 mm Hg; $P = 0.054$; nighttime mean = -13.5 ± 1.9 mm Hg vs -6.4 ± 1.8 mm Hg; $P = 0.009$).[52]

In a network analysis of nine randomized, controlled comparisons ($n = 78,350$) in which either hydrochlorothiazide or chlorthalidone was used as the base diuretic, chlorthalidone was associated with a 21% highly significant ($P < 0.0001$) reduction in CV events.[53]

In a propensity-matched observational cohort of 29,873 Canadian patients aged 66 years or older who were newly treated with chlorthalidone or hydrochlorothiazide and who had not been hospitalized for HF, stroke, or MI in the prior year, chlorthalidone recipients ($n=10,384$) experienced the primary outcome, a composite of death or hospitalization for HF, stroke, or MI, at a rate of 3.2 events per 100 person-years of follow-up, and hydrochlorothiazide recipients experienced 3.4 events per 100 person-years of follow-up (adjusted HR, 0.93 [95% CI, 0.81 to 1.06]). The patients receiving chlorthalidone had more frequent hospitalizations for hypokalemia or hyponatremia; however, <1% of the patient population was receiving a potassium-sparing diuretic.[54]

In summary, a moderate evidence base supports the concept that chlorthalidone may be a more effective intervention for hypertensive Stage A and B patients than hydrochlorothiazide. Clinicians should consider the theoretical and practical advantages to combining chlorthalidone with an MRA for these patients.

Although the use of loop diuretics is considered standard management for patients with Stage C HF, there are limited data to guide physician choice among the widely available loop diuretics, furosemide, and bumetanide. A comprehensive review of publications from 1966 to 2009, examined loop diuretic pharmacokinetics, comparative safety and efficacy, or comparative costs.[55] In summary, when the data in patients with HF were reviewed, torsemide was associated with decreased mortality compared with furosemide in one study (2.2% vs 4.5% in the furosemide group; $P<0.05$), decreased hospitalizations in one study (23 in the torsemide group vs 61 in the furosemide group; $P<0.01$), and improved NYHA functional classifications in two studies.

A recent authoritative reappraisal of loop diuretics[56] specifically focused on the management of HF noted that, "The majority of studies that directly compared torsemide to furosemide have been small, underpowered, and with limited end-points. Nonetheless, most have suggested benefits with torsemide use, including improved NYHA functional class, improved LV function, decreased myocardial fibrosis, decreased rates of hospitalizations, and potentially a reduction in mortality." The authors concluded that torsemide should be considered as the first-line loop diuretic over furosemide (**Figure 5.9**, **Figure 5.10**, **Table 5.8**, and **Table 5.9**).

Digoxin

Even though the landmark Digitalis Investigation Group (DIG) trial[57] showed that digoxin (added to ACE inhibitors and diuretics) had a neutral effect on mortality and was associated with fewer deaths or hospitalizations attributed to worsening HF, digoxin use has decreased since 2000.[58,59]

Much of this decline may reflect continued concerns about the possibility of increased mortality associated with digoxin use. A recent systematic review and meta-analysis, which was conducted with the hypothesis that study design would have an important impact on the observed mortality associated with digoxin, found 42 studies suitable for systematic review, including 621,845 patients allocated to digoxin treatment or control. These data represented 2,248,775 patient years of follow-up. In total, there were 144,593 patients taking digoxin (23.3%) compared with 476,984 patients in the control arms (76.7%). Twenty-six studies were retrospective or prospective cohorts, nine were post-hoc analyses of randomized trials, and seven were randomized digoxin trials. The weighted average duration follow-up was 3.7 years (SD 2.4), with a range of 0.25-8.2 years.

The pooled risk ratio for death with digoxin compared to controls was 1.76 in unadjusted analyses (1.57 to 1.97), 1.61 in adjusted analyses (1.31 to 1.97), 1.18 in propensity matched studies (1.09 to 1.26), and 0.99 in randomized controlled trials (0.93 to 1.05). The studies that employed better methods with lower risk of bias were those that were more likely to report a neutral association of digoxin with mortality ($P<0.001$). Overall, the authors concluded that, "Digoxin is associated with a neutral effect on mortality in randomized trials and a lower rate of admissions to hospital across all study types. Regardless of statistical analysis, prescription biases limit the value of observational data."

A retrospective analysis of the DIG Trial that was restricted to male subjects in sinus rhythm with clinical heart failure and LVEF of 45% or less, included 3782 patients; 2611 were randomly assigned to placebo and 1171 randomly assigned to digoxin. The outcomes associated with digoxin as compared with placebo varied based on serum digoxin concentration (SDC). Those with an SDC of 0.5 to 0.8 ng/mL had a 6.3% (95% CI, 2.1%-10.5%) lower all-cause mortality rate, a 3.7% (95% CI, 0.4%-7.7%) lower rate of CV mortality, and a 4.7% (95% CI, 2.1%-7.3%) lower rate of death due to worsening HF. With SDCs of 0.9 to 1.1 ng/mL, digoxin patients had similar rates of all-cause mortality, CV mortality, and mortality due to worsening HF as the placebo patients (**Figure 5.11**). In contrast, the digoxin patients with SDCs of 1.2 ng/mL and higher had an 11.8% (95% CI, 5.7%-18.0%) higher all-cause mortality rate and an 11.5% (95% CI, 5.4%-17.5%) higher CV mortality rate than placebo patients. The authors noted similar, but not statistically significant, findings for the smaller number of women (330) who had data available. They concluded, "Our findings suggest that an SDC of 0.5 to 0.8 ng/mL likely constitutes the optimal therapeutic range for digoxin therapy among men with stable heart failure and left ventricular dysfunction."[60]

In summary, the primary accepted indication for digoxin in HF-rEF today is for the reduction of hospitalization due to HF. With the growing emphasis on reduction of readmissions, and little evidence for increased mortality from randomized controlled trials, digoxin use may yet find a place in the therapeutic armamentarium, albeit with careful monitoring of serum digoxin levels.

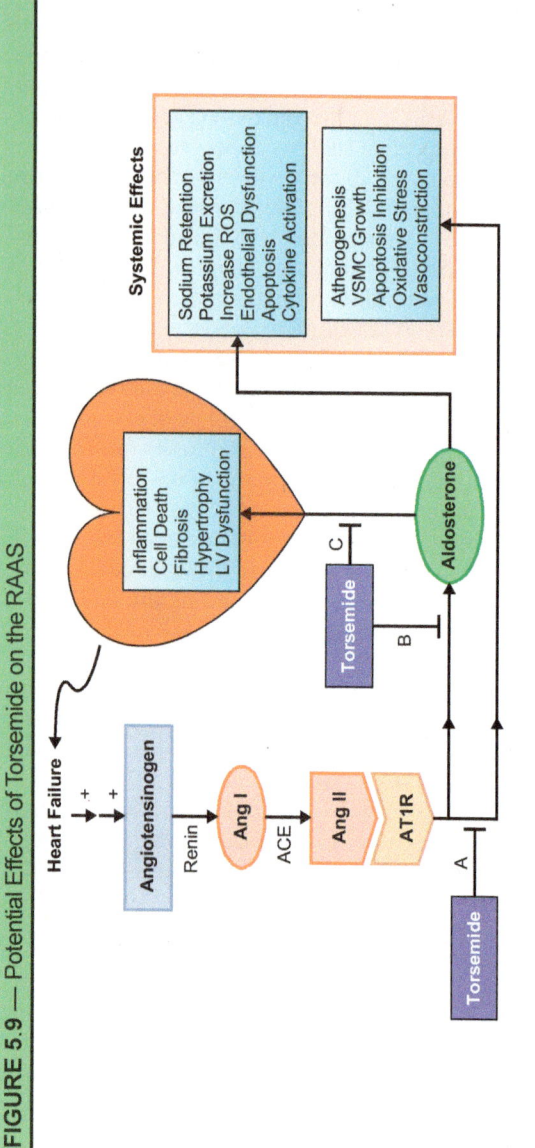

FIGURE 5.9 — Potential Effects of Torsemide on the RAAS

Heart failure leads to an up regulation of the RAAS. Renin converts angiotensinogen to Ang I, which is converted to Ang II by ACE. Ang II acts on AT1R leading to downstream effects including increasing aldosterone production and secretion, stimulating atherogenesis, VSMC growth, inhibition of apoptosis, increased oxidative stress, and promoting vasoconstriction. Circulating aldosterone acts on local myocardium receptors leading to myocardial inflammation, cell death, fibrosis, hypertrophy, and LV dysfunction leading to heart failure. Aldosterone stimulates sodium retention, potassium excretion, an increase in ROS, endothelial dysfunction, apoptosis, and increased cytokine activation. Torsemide may inhibit the downstream effects of Ang II *(A)*, the secretion of aldosterone from adrenal cells *(B)*, and aldosterone receptor binding *(C)*.

Key: ACE, Angiotensin converting enzyme; Ang I, Angiotensin; Ang II, Angiotensin II; AT1R, Angiotensin II type 1 receptor; LV, left ventricular; RAAS, renin-angiotensin-aldosterone system; ROS, reactive oxygen species; VSMC, vascular smooth muscle cell.

Buggey J, et al. *Am Heart J*. 2015;169(3):323-333.

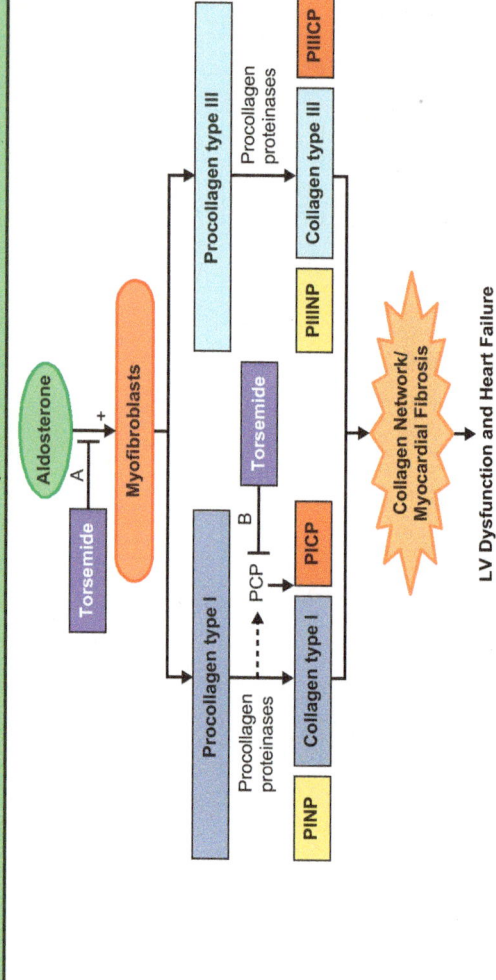

FIGURE 5.10 — Potential Effects of Torsemide on Myocardial Fibrosis

Aldosterone, as well as other cytokines, growth factors, and hormones, stimulate myofibroblasts to synthesize and secrete two main collagen precursors within the heart, procollagen type I and procollagen type III. Procollagen proteinases are enzymes that process the procollagen into collagen molecules by cleaving the terminal propeptides. The cleaved propeptides of procollagen type I (PINP and PICP) and procollagen type III (PIIINP and PIIICP) are released into circulation and can be quantified as an indirect measurement of collagen production. The mature collagen molecules are further processed and eventually form the collagen network responsible for myocardial fibrosis, subsequently leading to pathologic remodeling, LV dysfunction, and heart failure. Torsemide is thought to mainly inhibit downstream collagen synthesis through its inhibition at the level of the aldosterone receptor (A) but torsemide may also decrease the activity of the PCP enzyme, the procollagen proteinase responsible for cleavage of PICP (B).

Key: LV, left ventricular; PCP, procollagen type I carboxy-terminal proteinase; PICP, procollagen type I carboxy-terminal propeptide; PINP, procollagen type I amino-terminal propeptide; PIIICP, procollagen type III carboxy-terminal propeptide; PIIINP, procollagen type III amino-terminal propeptide.

Buggey J, et al. *Am Heart J.* 2015;169(3):323-333.

TABLE 5.8 — Torsemide vs Furosemide Studies: Hospitalizations and Mortality

Study (Year)	N	Patients	Design	Average Follow-Up	Comparison	Outcomes (Torsemide vs Furosemide)	Limitations
TORIC (2002)	1377	• Spanish-based • Average age ~68 years • NYHA class II-IV • 50% female	Open-label, non-randomized, post-marketing surveillance	9.2 months (~276 days)	Torsemide average dose 8.2 mg/day vs Furosemide average dose 35 mg/day + other diuretics	• 51.5% RR reduction in total mortality (17 vs 27 deaths) • 59.7% RR reduction in cardiac mortality (11 vs 27 deaths) • Greater improvement in ≥ 1 NYHA class	• Non-randomized • Greater concurrent use of other diuretics in furosemide group • Low use of standard HF therapies • Rural non-hospital based population • No report of hospitalization rates

| Müller et al (2003) | 237 | • Switzerland-based
• Average age ~74 years
• NYHA class II-IV
• Required ACE inhibitor use
• ~57% female | Open-label, randomized, prospective | 239 days in torsemide arm 250 days in furosemide arm | Torsemide average dose 11.36 mg/day vs furosemide average dose 40.04 mg/day | • No difference in mortality (8 vs 6 deaths)
• No difference in number of HF and CV-disease hospitalizations (10 vs 11)
• Fewer combined HF and CV-related hospital days (95 vs 146)
• Greater improvement in ≥1 NYHA class | • Small sample size
• Sample sizes in each group were not adequately powered
• Furosemide group had more renal insufficiency
• Concurrent ACE inhibitor therapy was required
• Hospitalization data skewed by a single furosemide-treated patient with prolonged hospital stay
• Lack of blinding and subjective data |

Continued

TABLE 5.8 — Continued

Study (Year)	N	Patients	Design	Average Follow-Up	Comparison	Outcomes (Torsemide vs Furosemide)	Limitations
Murray et al (2001)	234	• Indianapolis, USA-based • Average age ~64 years • NYHA class II-III • Excluded LV diastolic dysfunction only • ~53% female	Open-label, randomized, prospective	324 days in torsemide arm 318 days in furosemide arm	Torsemide average dose 72 mg/day vs furosemide average dose 136 mg/day	• No difference in mortality • 52% decrease in HF readmission rate • 34% decrease in all CV-related readmission risk • Less HF-related hospital days (106 vs 296)	• Small sample size • Torsemide group had more pre-trial HF hospitalizations in prior 1 year • High reported daily doses of loop diuretics

Buggey J, et al. *Am Heart J.* 2015;169(3):323-333.

TABLE 5.9 — Potential Benefits of Torsemide Compared With Furosemide

Preclinical Data

- Improved diuresis
- Decreased kaliuresis
- Decreased aldosterone secretion
- Inhibition of aldosterone receptor[a]
- Inhibition of Ang II effects
- Improved LV function
- Decreased myocardial collagen
- Increased survival rate

Clinical Data

- Improved diuresis and weight reduction
- Decreased transcardiac aldosterone extraction
- Less RAAS activation
- Decreased myocardial collagen
- Decreased levels of PICP[b] and PIIINP (collagen surrogates)
- Decreased PCP activity
- Decreased levels of plasma BNP
- Improved LV function
- Improved NYHA class[b]
- Improved subjective quality of life
- Decreased all-cause[c] and cardiac-associated mortality
- Decreased rates of hospitalization[c]
- Decreased length of hospital stay related to HF[a]

[a] Gravez et al found no receptor inhibition.
[b] TORAFIC study found no difference between variables.
[c] Müller et al found no difference between variables.

Buggey J, et al. *Am Heart J*. 2015;169(3):323-333.

Antithrombotic Agents

Antiplatelet Agents

Antiplatelet agents should be used as indicated for confirmed CAD. However, our primary concern in listing antiplatelet agents in this section is to warn against use of these drugs in HF patients who do *not* have coronary heart disease (CHD).

As practicing clinicians, we are aware of the adverse impact that either chronic or acute blood loss

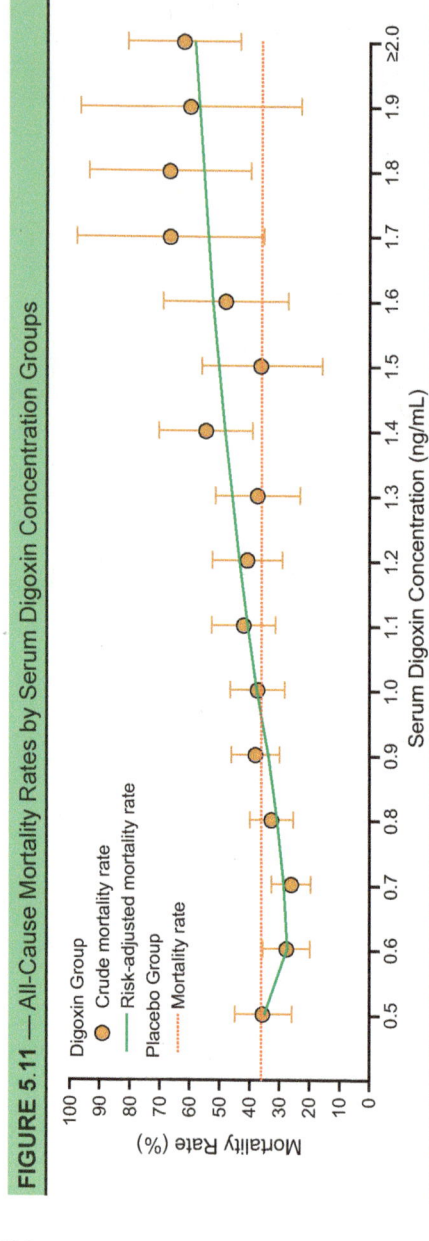

FIGURE 5.11 — All-Cause Mortality Rates by Serum Digoxin Concentration Groups

This figure presents the crude all-cause mortality rate with 95% confidence intervals and the risk-adjusted rate for patients assigned to digoxin according to their serum digoxin concentration. The mortality rate in patients assigned to placebo is presented for comparison. The risk-adjusted mortality rate was estimated using fractional polynomial modeling.

Rathore SS, et al. *JAMA*. 2003;289(7):871-878.

can have on the clinical course of HF. We are also aware that many patients view daily aspirin use as both benign and "good for your heart."

Clinicians must repeatedly inquire about use of over-the-counter pharmaceuticals, and HF patients who do not have an indication for aspirin use should be cautioned to avoid it.

■ Anticoagulants

HF and AF

The prevalence of AF in the HF population is high and increases with age. A recent British study included 6286 volunteer subjects from the general population and 782 HF patients. The majority of patients who were found to have AF in this study also had echocardiographic and clinical risk factors for stroke and thromboembolism. These data confirmed that lone AF is rare in the community, and that the majority of AF patients is found in the elderly. At age 55-64 years, about 7% of men with HF and 16% of women with HF had developed AF. In the 85 years-and over age group, the respective figures were 31% and 25%.[61] As shown in **Figure 5.12**, the prevalence of AF in the general population rises dramatically with increasing age.

HF patients with AF are likely to be classed as having high stroke risk with either the CHADS2 or CHA2DS2-VASc score, since they have HF and are in the older age groups. Their management should be appropriate to their risk scores.

A recent evaluation of warfarin management for stroke prevention in 5210 patients in a real world setting demonstrated that their overall mean and median time in therapeutic range (TTR) was 65% ± 20% and 68% (interquartile range [IQR] 53%-79%). Importantly, HF patients had significantly lower TTR than the overall population.[62]

The use of anti-Xa specific anticoagulants for these patients is clinically attractive, since these agents are generally well-tolerated, have well-defined dosing according to renal function, few drug-drug interactions,

FIGURE 5.12 — Prevalence of Atrial Fibrillation in 6286 Patients Age 45 and Older in the General Population by Age and Sex

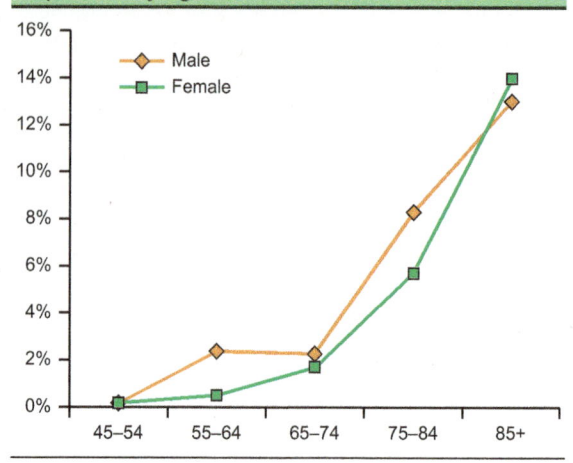

Davis RC, et al. *Europace*. 2012;14:1553-1559.

and no requirement for coagulation laboratory monitoring. In addition, although gastrointestinal bleeding is somewhat more common with these agents than with warfarin, the incidence of intracranial hemorrhage is lower with anti-Xa agents than with warfarin.

HF With AF and CAD

Co-existing comorbidities occur frequently in the HF patient population. Patients with AF who have experienced a recent acute coronary syndrome (ACS) pose a particularly difficult management problem for two reasons. First, clinical trials of antiplatelet agents for ACS have largely excluded AF patients, and second, the elderly patients with these concomitant problems are at increased risk of bleeding.

An observational description of practice patterns using multivariable logistic regressions attempted to determine predictors of AC or AP use. The investigators evaluated 5294 ACS patients in the Intermountain Heart Collaborative Study from 2004 to 2009. 923

(17%) had atrial fibrillation and 337 (6%) had a history of venous thromboembolism; 29% and 40% of these patients, respectively, received anticoagulation at discharge, and when anticoagulation was used, dual antiplatelet therapy was used significantly less often.[63]

In another descriptive study of 1159 patients with incident ACS at the Mayo Clinic, 252 (21.7%) had concomitant AF (ACS + AF). Over a median follow-up of 4.3 years, 312 bleeds, 67 ischemic strokes, and 268 deaths occurred. The overall risks of bleeding, stroke, and death were similar between those who received with double/triple vs no/single therapy antithrombotic treatment strategies. There was a suggestion of a lower risk of ischemic stroke for patients with ACS + AF on double/triple therapy. Overall, the choice of antithrombotic strategy was not associated with the risk of ischemic stroke, bleeding, or death in patients with ACS overall; however, patients with ACS + AF on double/triple therapy may have experienced reduced risks of stroke.[64]

In an observational follow-up study designed to examine the 2-year clinical outcomes of 619 patients with ACS who had an indication for anticoagulation, either due to venous thromboembolism (VTE) during hospitalization for the ACS event or a prior or new diagnosis of AF with a CHADS2 (Congestive heart failure; Hypertension; Age; Diabetes; previous ischemic Stroke) score ≥ 2, a total of 261 (42.2%) patients had a major adverse cardiac event (death, MI or stroke). However, antithrombotic treatment strategy was not a significant factor for MACE (all $P > 0.09$).[65]

A Danish registry study that included 12,165 AF patients hospitalized with MI and/or undergoing PCI focused on the safety of multiple antithrombotic treatment regimens. Within 1 year, MI or coronary death, ischemic stroke, and bleeding events occurred in 2255 patients (18.5%), 680 (5.6%), and 769 (6.3%), respectively. Relative to triple therapy (oral anticoagulation plus aspirin and clopidogrel), there was no increased risk of recurrent coronary events for the combination of OAC plus clopidogrel alone (HR: 0.69, 95% CI: 0.48 to 1.00), and when compared to triple therapy, bleeding risk was nonsignificantly lower for OAC plus clopidogrel (HR: 0.78, 95% CI: 0.55 to 1.12). The authors concluded that in AF patients with an indication for both anticoagulation and antiplatelet therapy, oral anticoagulation plus clopidogrel was equal or better for both benefit and safety outcomes compared to triple therapy.[66]

In summary, in the absence of randomized controlled trials but based on the observational data, HF patients with both AF and CHD are at high-risk for adverse events, with approximately 20% 1-year risk of death, MI, or stroke. Observational evidence suggests that the choice of antithrombotic strategy is not a major determinant of short-term outcomes for these patients, while stroke prevention remains a longer-term concern. Accordingly, until further data are available, we believe the available evidence favors the use of the combination of oral anticoagulation (warfarin or NOACs) and clopidogrel for stroke prevention and the secondary prevention of acute coronary events in these patients.

HF Without AF

The current AHA/ACC guidelines do not recommend systemic anticoagulation for HF patients without AF or other accepted indications (eg, recurrent DVT). However, the steadily accumulating evidence linking thrombosis with both inflammation and endothelial dysfunction provided the hypothesis for the COMMANDER-HF trial, an ongoing prospective, multicenter, randomized, double-blind, placebo-controlled, event-driven study of approximately 5000 patients randomized 1:1 to 2.5 mg rivaroxaban twice daily or placebo (with standard of care) after an index HF event (overnight hospitalization, emergency department or observation unit admission, or unscheduled outpatient parenteral treatment for worsening HF).[67]

The dose of rivaroxaban used in COMMANDER-HF will not result in systemic anticoagulation; however, the dose was chosen based on an unpublished subgroup analysis of ATLAS-2[68] showing that in patients diagnosed clinically with HF at the time of an ACS event, the primary outcome event of CV death, MI, or stroke after a mean follow-up of 13 months was reduced from 18.6% with placebo to 11.6% with rivaroxaban.

The results of this trial will add important information about the efficacy and safety of management of HF-rEF patients with antithrombotic measures.

Agents Specifically Targeting Pulmonary Hypertension

The development of precapillary pulmonary hypertension in HF-rEF patients, or "mixed" pulmonary hypertension with elevation of both wedge pressure and pulmonary vascular resistance, is associated with high risk. A retrospective analysis of clinical features, hemodynamics, and outcomes of pulmonary hypertension due to chronic HF with reduced ejection fraction, compared patients with no PH to those with passive PH and mixed PH. The findings demonstrated a spectrum of progressively more severe hemodynamic derangement, diastolic dysfunction, and mitral regurgitation. Over a median follow-up of 2.1 years, compared to those with no pulmonary hypertension, patients with pulmonary hypertension had a greater risk of death (HR: 2.24; confidence limits [95% CL]: 1.39, 3.98; $P<0.001$) and those with mixed PH had greater risk than those with passive PH (HR: 1.55; 95% CL: 1.11, 2.20; $P<0.001$). Those at highest risk had pulmonary vascular resistance >4 Wood units, systolic pulmonary artery pressure >35 mm Hg, pulmonary wedge pressure >25 mm Hg, and PAC <2.0 mL/mm Hg.[69]

HF-pEF may also have a component of precapillary pulmonary hypertension.[70] In a community-based echocardiographic study of 244 HF-pEF patients (age 76 ± 13 years; 45% male), 83% had pulmonary hypertension, with a median PASP of 48 (25th, 75th percentile = 37, 56) mm Hg. Pulmonary pressures were highly predictive of mortality.

In either HF-rEF or HF-pEF, demonstrated precapillary pulmonary hypertension should raise consideration for referral to a HF center. Treatment of pulmonary hypertension due to left heart disease is challenging, and requires a different approach from traditional WHO Class I PAH. Trials employing traditional PAH therapy have frequently had poor clinical responses and, in some cases, increased morbidity and mortality. The pathophysiology of pulmonary hypertension due to left heart disease differs from that of idiopathic PAH, and pharmacologic approaches that have been effective in PAH patients may increase flow through the pulmonary vasculature to the point that the left heart fails further.[71]

Table 5.10 lists the agents used in management of idiopathic pulmonary hypertension follows for reference purposes.

TABLE 5.10 — Currently Available Agents for Pulmonary Hypertension

Endothelin Receptor Antagonists
- Ambrisentan, bosentan, macitentan

Oral PDE-5Is
- Sildenafil, tadalafil

Prostanoids
- Oral, IV, subcutaneous, or inhaled; epoprostenol (intravenous), iloprost (inhaled), and treprostinil (subcutaneous or intravenous)

Selective Non-prostanoid Prostacyclin Receptor (IP receptor) Agonists (sPRAs)
- Selexipag: first-in-class orally available selective non-prostanoid IP receptor agonist

Soluble Guanylate Cyclase Stimulators (sGCSs)
- Riociguat

Adapted from Liu QQ, et al. *Ther Clin Risk Manag.* 2015;11:1731-1741.

The role of fixed or variable functional mitral regurgitation, its role in the development of pulmonary hypertension, and the potential role of catheter-based interventions for its correction, are active subjects of investigation. A post-hoc analysis of 107 patients treated in the EVEREST phase I feasibility trial and in the roll-in phase of the EVEREST II pivotal trial with mitral regurgitation and hemodynamic decompensation demonstrated that percutaneous reduction of mitral regurgitation with the MitraClip device resulted in immediate hemodynamic improvement by increasing forward CI and unloading the left ventricle.[72] The availability of percutaneous interventions for patients with multiple comorbidities is a strong argument in favor of referral to a specialized center.

REFERENCES

1. Francis GS, Goldsmith SR, Levine TB, Olivari MT, Cohn JN. The neurohumoral axis in congestive heart failure. *Ann Intern Med.* 1984;101:370-377.

2. Swedberg K. From CONSENSUS to SAVE: the early development of inhibition of the renin-angiotensin system in the treatment of chronic heart failure. *J Card Fail.* 2016;22(5):395-398.

3. Ferrari R, Rosano GM. Not just numbers, but years of science: putting the ACE inhibitor-ARB meta-analyses into context. *Int J Cardiol.* 2013;166(2):286-288.

4. Reed BN, Street SE, Jensen BC. The pathophysiologic basis of neurohormonal modulation in heart failure. *Heart Fail Clin.* 2014;10:543-557.

5. The CONSENSUS Trial Study Group. Effects of enalapril on mortality in severe congestive heart failure. Results of the Cooperative North Scandinavian Enalapril Survival Study. *N Engl J Med.* 1987;316:1429-1435.

6. The SOLVD Investigators. Effect of enalapril on survival in patients with reduced left ventricular ejection fractions and congestive heart failure. *N Engl J Med.* 1991;325:293-302.

7. Dezsi CA. Differences in the clinical effects of angiotensin-converting enzyme inhibitors and angiotensin receptor blockers: a critical review of the evidence. *Am J Cardiovasc Drugs.* 2014;14:167-173.

8. Ponikowski P, Voors AA, Anker SD, et al; Authors/Task Force members; Document Reviewers. 2016 ESC Guidelines for the diagnosis and treatment of acute and chronic heart failure. The Task Force for the diagnosis and treatment of acute and chronic heart failure of the European Society of Cardiology (ESC). Developed with the special contribution of the Heart Failure Association (HFA) of the ESC. *Eur J Heart Fail.* 2016;18(8):891-975.

9. Yancy CW, Jessup M, Bozkurt B, et al. 2016 ACC/AHA/HFSA focused update on new pharmacological therapy for heart failure: an update of the 2013 ACCF/AHA guideline for the management of heart failure. *J Am Coll Cardiol.* 2016;68(13):1476-1488.

10. ACC/AHA guidelines Yancy CW, Jessup M, Bozkurt B, et al. 2013 ACCF/AHA Guideline for the Management of Heart Failure. A report from the American College of Cardiology Foundation/American Heart Association Task Force on Practice Guidelines. *Circulation.* 2013;128:3240-e327.

11. Yusuf S, Teo KK, Pogue J, et al. Telmisartan, ramipril, or both in patients at high risk for vascular events. *N Engl J Med.* 2008;358(15):1547-1559.

12. Granger CB, McMurray JJ, Yusuf S, et al. Effects of candesartan in patients with chronic heart failure and reduced left-ventricular systolic function intolerant to angiotensin-converting-enzyme inhibitors: the CHARM-Alternative trial. *Lancet.* 2003;362:772-776.

13. Yusuf S, Pfeffer MA, Swedberg K, et al. Effects of candesartan in patients with chronic heart failure and preserved left-ventricular ejection fraction: the CHARM-Preserved Trial. *Lancet.* 2003;362:777-781).

14. Holland DJ, Kumbhani DJ, Ahmed SH, Marwick TH. Effects of treatment on exercise tolerance, cardiac function, and mortality in heart failure with preserved ejection fraction. *J Am Coll Cardiol.* 2011;57:1676-1686.

15. McKie PM, Schirger JA, Benike SL, et al. Chronic subcutaneous brain natriuretic peptide therapy in asymptomatic systolic heart failure. *Eur J Heart Fail.* 2016;18(4):433-441.

16. Wan SH, McKie PM, Schirger JA, et al. Chronic peptide therapy with B-type natriuretic peptide in patients with preclinical diastolic dysfunction (stage B heart failure). *JACC Heart Fail.* 2016;4(7):539-547.

17. Ksander GM, Ghai RD, deJesus R, et al. Dicarboxylic acid dipeptide neutral endopeptidase inhibitors. *J Med Chem.* 1995;38:1689-1700.

18. Webb RL, Ksander GM. Pharmaceutical. 2003. Pharmaceutical compositions comprising valsartan and NEP inhibitors. International Patent Application PCT/EP03/004.

19. Braunwald, EB. The path to an angiotensin receptor–neprilysn inhibitor in the treatment of heart failure. *J Am Coll Cardiol.* 2015;65:1025-1041.

20. McMurray JJ, Packer M, Desai AS, et al, PARADIGM-HF Investigators and Committees. Angiotensin-neprilysin inhibition versus enalapril in heart failure. *N Engl J Med.* 2014;371:993-1004.

21. Entresto [package insert]. East Hanover, NJ: Novartis Pharmaceuticals Corporation. 2015.

22. Jhund PS, Claggett B, Packer M, et al. Independence of the blood pressure lowering effect and efficacy of the angiotensin receptor neprilysin inhibitor, LCZ696, in patients with heart failure with preserved ejection fraction: an analysis of the PARAMOUNT trial. *Eur J Heart Fail.* 2014;16:671-677.

23. Jabbour A, Macdonald PS, Keogh AM, et al. Differences between beta-blockers in patients with chronic heart failure and chronic obstructive pulmonary disease: a randomized crossover trial. *J Am Coll Cardiol.* 2010;55:1780-1787.

24. Chatterjee S, Biondi-Zoccai G, Abbate A, et al. Benefits of β blockers in patients with heart failure and reduced ejection fraction: network meta-analysis. *BMJ.* 2013;346:f55.

25. DiNicolantonio JJ, Lavie CJ, Fares H, Menezes AR, O'Keefe JH. Meta-analysis of carvedilol versus beta 1 selective beta-blockers (atenolol, bisoprolol, metoprolol, and nebivolol). *Am J Cardiol.* 2013;111(5):765-769.

26. Briasoulis A, Palla M, Afonso L. Meta-analysis of the effects of carvedilol versus metoprolol on all-cause mortality and hospitalizations in patients with heart failure. *Am J Cardiol.* 2015;115(8):1111-1115.

27. Bavishi C, Chatterjee S, Ather S, Patel D, Messerli FH. Beta-blockers in heart failure with preserved ejection fraction: a meta-analysis. *Heart Fail Rev.* 2015;20(2):193-201.

28. Kosmala W, Rojeck A, Prewlocka-Kosmala M, et al. Contributions of nondiastolic factors to exercise intolerance in heart failure with preserved ejection fraction. *J Am Coll Cardiol.* 2016;67:659-670.

29. Butler J, Kalogeropoulos A, Georgiopoulou V, et al. Incident heart failure prediction in the elderly: the Health ABC Heart Failure Score. *Circ Heart Fail.* 2008;1:125-133.

30. Khan H, Kunutsor S, Kalogeropoulos AP, et al. Resting heart rate and risk of incident heart failure: three prospective cohort studies and a systematic meta-analysis. *J Am Heart Assoc.* 2015;4:e001364

31. Böhm M, Swedberg K, Komajda M, et al. Heart rate as a risk factor in chronic heart failure (SHIFT): the association between heart rate and outcomes in a randomised placebo-controlled trial. *Lancet.* 2010;376(9744):886-894.

32. Butler J, Arbogast PG, BeLue R, et al. Outpatient adherence to beta-blocker therapy after acute myocardial infarction. *J Am Coll Cardiol.* 2002;40(9):1589-1595.

33. Borer JS, Fox K, Jaillon P, et al. Antianginal and antiischemic effects of ivabradine, an I f inhibitor, in stable angina: a randomized, double-blind, multicentered, placebo-controlled trial. *Circulation.* 2003;107(6):817-823.

34. Manz M, Reuter M, Lauck G, et al. A single intravenous dose of ivabradine, a novel I f inhibitor, lowers heart rate but does not depress left ventricular function in patients with left ventricular dysfunction. *Cardiology.* 2003;100(3):149-155.

35. Swedberg K, Komajda M, Böhm M, et al. Ivabradine and outcomes in chronic heart failure (SHIFT): a randomised placebo-controlled study. *Lancet*. 2010;376(9744):875-885.

36. Pal N, Sivaswamy N, Mahmod M, et al. Effect of selective heart rate slowing in heart failure with preserved ejection fraction. *Circulation*. 2015;132(18):1719-1725.

37. Kosmala W, Rojeck A, Prewlocka-Kosmala M, et al. Contributions of nondiastolic factors to exercise intolerance in heart failure with preserved ejection fraction. *J Am Coll Cardiol*. 2016;67:659-670.

38. Pitt B, Zannad F, Remme WJ, et al; Randomized Aldactone Evaluation Study Investigators. The effect of spironolactone on morbidity and mortality in patients with severe heart failure. *N Engl J Med*. 1999;341:709-717.

39. Pitt B, Remme W, Zannad F, et al; Eplerenone Post-Acute Myocardial Infarction Heart Failure Efficacy and Survival Study Investigators. Eplerenone, a selective aldosterone blocker, in patients with left ventricular dysfunction after myocardial infarction. *N Engl J Med*. 2003;348(14):1309-1321.

40. Hu L, Chen Y, Deng S, et al. Additional use of an aldosterone antagonist in patients with mild to moderate chronic heart failure: a systematic review and meta-analysis. *Br J Clin Pharmacol*. 2012;75:1202-1212.

41. Zannad F, Gattis Stough W, Rossignol P, et al. Mineralocorticoid receptor antagonists for heart failure with reduced ejection fraction: integrating evidence into clinical practice. *Eur Heart J*. 2012;33:2782-2795.

42. Pandey A, Garg S, Matulevicius SA, et al. Effect of mineralocorticoid receptor antagonists on cardiac structure and function in patients with diastolic dysfunction and heart failure with preserved ejection fraction: a meta-Analysis and systematic review. *J Am Heart Assoc*. 2015;4:e002137.

43. Pitt B, Pfeffer MA, Assmann SF, et al; TOPCAT Investigators. Spironolactone for heart failure with preserved ejection fraction. *N Engl J Med*. 2014;370(15):1383-1392.

44. Pfeffer MA, Claggett B, Assmann SF, et al. Regional variation in patients and outcomes in the Treatment of Preserved Cardiac Function Heart Failure with an Aldosterone Antagonist (TOPCAT) Trial. *Circulation*. 2015;131(1):34-42.

45. Pfeffer MA, Braunwald E. Treatment of heart failure with preserved ejection fraction: reflections on its treatment with an aldosterone antagonist. *JAMA Cardiol*. 2016;1(1):7-8.

46. Cooper LB, Hammill BG, Peterson ED, et al. Consistency of laboratory monitoring during initiation of mineralocorticoid receptor antagonist therapy in patients with heart failure. *JAMA*. 2015;314:1973-1975.

47. Cohn JN, Archibald DG, Ziesche S, et al. Effect of vasodilator therapy on mortality in chronic congestive heart failure: results of a Veterans Administration Cooperative Study. *N Engl J Med*. 1986;314:1547-1552.

48. Carson P, Ziesche S, Johnson G, et al; Vasodilator-Heart Failure Trial Study Group. Racial differences in response to therapy for heart failure: analysis of the vasodilator-heart failure trials. *J Card Fail*. 1999;5:178-187.

49. Taylor AL, Ziesche S, Yancy C, et al. Combination of isosorbide dinitrate and hydralazine in blacks with heart failure. *N Engl J Med*. 2004;351:2049-2057.

50. Münzel T, Gori T, Keaney JF Jr, Maack C, Daiber A. Pathophysiological role of oxidative stress in systolic and diastolic heart failure and its therapeutic implications. *Eur Heart J*. 2015;36(38):2555-2564.

51. ALLHAT Officers and Coordinators for the ALLHAT Collaborative Research Group. The Antihypertensive and Lipid-Lowering Treatment to Prevent Heart Attack Trial. Major outcomes in high-risk hypertensive patients randomized to angiotensin-converting enzyme inhibitor or calcium channel blocker vs diuretic: The Antihypertensive and Lipid-Lowering Treatment to Prevent Heart Attack Trial (ALLHAT). *JAMA*. 2002;288(23):2981-2997.

52. Ernst ME, Carter BL, Goerdt CJ, et al. Comparative antihypertensive effects of hydrochlorothiazide and chlorthalidone on ambulatory and office blood pressure. *Hypertension*. 2006;47:352-358.

53. Roush GC, Holford TR, Guddati AK. Chlorthalidone compared with hydrochlorothiazide in reducing cardiovascular events: systematic review and network meta-analyses. *Hypertension*. 2012;59:1110-1117.

54. Dhalla IA, Gomes T, Yao Z, et al. Chlorthalidone versus hydrochlorothiazide for the treatment of hypertension in older adults: a population-based cohort study. *Ann Intern Med*. 2013;158:447-455.

55. Wargo KA, Banta WM. A comprehensive review of the loop diuretics: should furosemide be first line? *Ann Pharmacother*. 2009;43(11):1836-1847.

56. Buggey J, Mentz RJ, Pitt B, et al. A reappraisal of loop diuretic choice in heart failure patients. *Am Heart J*. 2015;169(3):323-333.

57. The Digitalis Investigation Group. The effect of digoxin on mortality and morbidity in patients with heart failure. *N Engl J Med*. 1997;336:525-533.

58. Hussain Z, Swindle J, Hauptman PJ. Digoxin use and digoxin toxicity in the post-DIG trial era. *J Card Fail*. 2006;12:343-346.

59. Patel N, Ju C, Thadani U, et al. Temporal trends of digoxin use in patients hospitalized with heart failure: analysis from the American Heart Association Get With The Guidelines-Heart Failure Registry. *JACC Heart Fail*. 2016;4(5):348-356.

60. Rathore SS, Curtis JP, Wang Y, et al. Association of serum digoxin concentration and outcomes in patients with heart failure. *JAMA*. 2003;289:871-878.

61. Davis RC, Hobbs FD, Kenkre JE, et al. Prevalence of atrial fibrillation in the general population and in high-risk groups: the ECHOES study. *Europace*. 2012;14:1553-1559.

62. Pokorney SD, Simon DN, Thomas L, et al; Outcomes Registry for Better Informed Treatment of Atrial Fibrillation (ORBIT-AF) Investigators. Patients' time in therapeutic range on warfarin among US patients with atrial fibrillation: Results from ORBIT-AF registry. *Am Heart J*. 2015;170:141-148.

63. Knight S, Klaskala W, Woller SC, et al. Antithrombotic therapy in patients with acute coronary syndrome in the intermountain heart collaborative study. *Cardiol Res Pract*. 2015;2015:270508.

64. Chamberlain AM, Gersh BJ, Mills RM, et al. Antithrombotic strategies and outcomes in acute coronary syndrome with atrial fibrillation. *Am J Cardiol*. 2015;115(8):1042-1048.

65. Knight S, McCubrey RO, Yuan Z, et al. Adverse cardiovascular events in acute coronary syndrome with indications for anticoagulation. *Ther Adv Cardiovasc Dis*. 2016;10(4):231-241.

66. Lamberts M, Gislason GH, Olesen JB, et al. Oral anticoagulation and antiplatelets in atrial fibrillation patients after myocardial infarction and coronary intervention. *J Am Coll Cardiol*. 2013;62(11):981-989.

67. Zannad F, Greenberg B, Cleland JG, et al. Rationale and design of a randomized, double-blind, event-driven, multicentre study comparing the efficacy and safety of oral rivaroxaban with placebo for reducing the risk of death, myocardial infarction or stroke in subjects with heart failure and significant coronary

artery disease following an exacerbation of heart failure: the COMMANDER HF trial. *Eur J Heart Fail.* 2015;17(7):735-742.

68. Janssen Research & Development, LLC, Raritan, NJ, USA; data on file.

69. Miller WL, Grill DE, Borlaug BA. Clinical features, hemodynamics, and outcomes of pulmonary hypertension due to chronic heart failure with reduced ejection fraction: pulmonary hypertension and heart failure. *JACC Heart Fail.* 2013;1:290-299.

70. Lam CS, Roger VL, Rodeheffer RJ, Borlaug BA, Enders FT, Redfield MM. Pulmonary hypertension in heart failure with preserved ejection fraction: a community-based study. *J Am Coll Cardiol.* 2009;53(13):1119-1126.

71. Feitell S, Jacob M. New diagnostic and therapeutic strategies for pulmonary hypertension associated with left heart disease. *Curr Treat Options Cardio Med.* 2016;18:18.

72. Biner S, Siegel RJ, Feldman T, et al; on behalf of the EVEREST investigators. Acute effect of percutaneous MitraClip therapy in patients with haemodynamic decompensation. *Eur J Heart Fail.* 2012;14:939-945.

6. Cardiovascular Implantable Electrophysiologic Devices in the Management of Heart Failure

Introduction

Before the availability of the technology required for development of today's small and reliable cardiovascular implantable electronic devices (CIEDs), physicians tended to think of HF as solely a problem of deranged muscle mechanics and the consequent pathophysiologic responses. However, devices that effectively address the electrophysiologic derangements of HF have pushed cardiologists to expand their thinking and to incorporate the concept that heart disease has electrical as well as mechanical manifestations into their daily clinical practice.

Sudden Death

Sudden cardiac death (SCD) due to ventricular tachycardia/ventricular fibrillation (VT/VF) has garnered steadily growing attention since the introduction of coronary care units almost 50 years ago. In epidemiologic studies prior to the widespread introduction of CIEDs into clinical practice, sudden death largely, attributable to ventricular arrhythmias accounted for approximately half of all the mortality in patients with HF-rEF (**Figure 6.1**).

In a meta-analysis of randomized primary prevention trials, the combined data demonstrated that implantable cardioverter-defibrillator provides a suc-

FIGURE 6.1 — Incidence of Sudden Cardiac Death

Group

- General population
- Patients with high coronary-risk profile
- Patients with previous coronary event
- Patients with ejection fraction <35%, congestive heart failure
- Patients with previous out-of-hospital cardiac arrest
- Patients with previous myocardial infarction, low ejection fraction, and ventricular tachycardia

Incidence of Sudden Death (% of group)

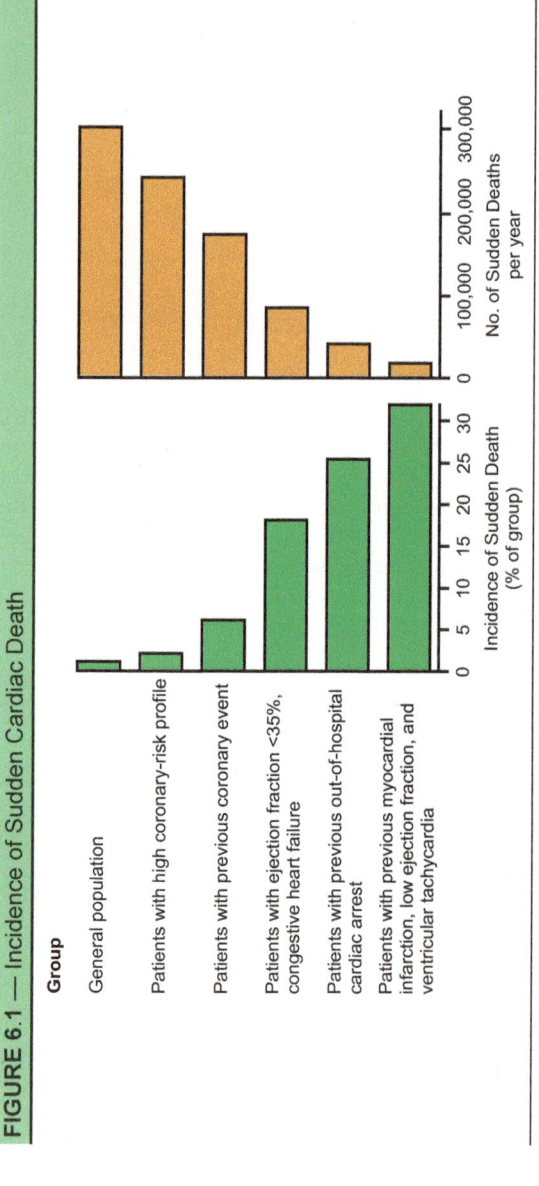

No. of Sudden Deaths per year

Huikuri HV, et al. *N Engl J Med*. 2001;345(20):1473-1482.

cessful management strategy for patients at high risk (**Figure 6.2**).

The current ACC/AHA guidelines reflect the strength of the evidence with a Class 1, Level of Evidence A, recommendation for ICD therapy in the primary prevention of SCD, "to reduce total mortality in selected patients with nonischemic DCM *or* ischemic heart disease at least 40 days post-MI with LVEF of 35% or less and NYHA class II or III symptoms on chronic GDMT, who have reasonable expectation of meaningful survival for more than 1 year."

QRS Widening

Similarly, the association between widening of the QRS complex and a poor prognosis has been extensively documented. For example, in a study of 1418 consecutive patients (average [SD] age 70.5 [10.4] years; 74% male) from a community HF clinic, 485 (34%) had a QRS duration ≥120 ms. The patients with wide QRS were older (72.2 vs 69.3 years), had worse left ventricular systolic function, were on a higher daily dose of diuretic, and were more likely to be on amiodarone (14.4% vs 7.1%) (**Figure 6.3**).[1] In addition, the investigators found a first-year crude incidence of LBBB of 10.4% in patients without LBBB at baseline.

Cardiac resynchronization therapy (CRT) devices offer an effective therapy for left ventricular dyssynchrony associated with QRS widening. A meta-analysis of five landmark randomized clinical trials of CRT that included 3782 patients in sinus rhythm with a median ejection fraction of 24% and median QRS duration of 160 ms (78% LBBB) showed a high probability of benefit from CRT for patients with QRS duration >140 msec (**Figure 6.4**).[2]

In a critical analysis of treatment response to clinical trials, the authors concluded that "The optimal response to treatment, that is, change in outcome, is to be expected among patients at intermediate risk with moderately elevated increases in NT-proBNP" (**Figure 6.5**).[3]

FIGURE 6.2 — Impact of ICD vs Conventional Therapy on Mortality in Trials in Patients With HF-rEF by Etiology

Study or Subcategory	ICD Events	ICD Total	Control Events	Control Total	Weight	Risk Ratio IV, Random, 95% CI	Risk Ratio IV, Random, 95% CI
2.1.1 Ischaemic cardiomyopathy							
01 - MADIT	15	95	39	101	5.5%	0.41 [0.24, 0.69]	
04 - MADIT II	105	742	97	490	24.1%	0.71 [0.56, 0.95]	
08 - SCD-HeFT	120	431	161	453	39.6%	0.78 [0.64, 0.95]	
Subtotal (95% CI)		**1268**		**1044**	**69.3%**	**0.67 [0.51, 0.88]**	
Total events:	240		297				
Heterogeneity: $\tau^2 = 0.03$; $\chi^2 = 5.17$, df = 2 ($P = 0.08$); $I^2 = 61\%$							
Test for overall effect: $Z = 2.88$ ($P = 0.004$)							
2.1.2 Non-ischemic cardiomyopathy							
03 - CAT	13	50	17	54	4.1%	0.83 [0.45, 1.52]	
05 - AMIOVIRT	7	51	9	52	1.8%	0.79 [0.32, 1.97]	
06 - DEFINITE	28	229	40	229	7.6%	0.70 [0.45, 1.09]	
08 - SCD-HeFT	62	398	83	394	17.2%	0.74 [0.55, 1.00]	
Subtotal (95% CI)		**728**		**729**	**30.7%**	**0.74 [0.59, 0.93]**	
Total events:	110		149				
Heterogeneity: $\tau^2 = 0.00$; $\chi^2 = 0.20$, df = 3 ($P = 0.98$); $I^2 = 0\%$							
Test for overall effect: $Z = 2.61$ ($P = 0.009$)							

| **Total (95% CI)** | **1996** | | **1773** | **100.0%** | **0.73 [0.64, 0.82]** |

Total events: 350 446

Heterogeneity: $\tau^2 = 0.00$; $\chi^2 = 5.42$, df = 6 ($P = 0.49$); $I^2 = 0\%$

Test for overall effect: Z = 5.05 ($P < 0.00001$)

0.1 0.2 0.5 1 2 5 10
Favors ICD   Favors control

Theuns DA, et al. *Europace*. 2010;12:1564-1570.

FIGURE 6.3 — Relationship of QRS Duration and LV Dysfunction

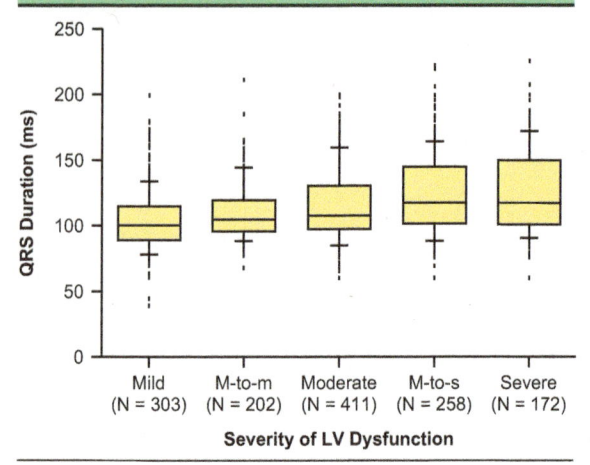

Clark AL, et al. *Eur J Heart Fail*. 2008;10:696-702.

FIGURE 6.4 — Kaplan-Meier Curves Showing Survival in Patients with QRS <120 ms vs ≥120 ms

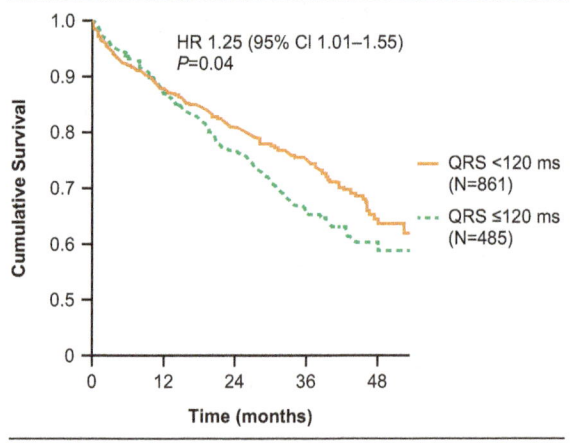

HR 1.25 (95% CI 1.01–1.55)
P=0.04

— QRS <120 ms (N=861)
--- QRS ≤120 ms (N=485)

Clark AL, et al. *Eur J Heart Fail*. 2008;10:696-702.

Dyssynchrony Induced by RV Pacing

In addition to traditional disease-driven indications for CRT, recognition of iatrogenic dyssynchrony associated with right ventricular pacing has widened indications for CRT (**Table 6.1**).[4] Not all patients experience functional deterioration with RV apical pacing. However, patients with impaired left ventricular function appear to be more susceptible to pacing-induced dyssynchrony (**Figure 6.6**).

Upgrading to from RV pacing to CRT may improve LV function and reduce the severity of mitral regurgitation.[4] Clinicians caring for HF patients with conventional pacemakers must be aware of the potential adverse effects of RV apical pacing and consider upgrading these patients to CRT devices.

CRT in Patients With Atrial Fibrillation

A meta-analyses of 23 studies that included a total of 7495 patients receiving CRT compared the outcomes for those with AF, 25.5% of the population, to the outcomes of those with sinus rhythm. Overall, AF patients had an increased risk of nonresponse to CRT, (34.5% vs 26.7%; pooled relative risk [RR] 1.32; 95% CI 1.12, 1.55; $P=0.001$) and also an increased all-cause mortality (10.8% vs 7.1% per year, pooled RR 1.50, 95% CI 1.08, 2.09; $P=0.015$). However, AF patients who underwent AV-nodal ablation (ie, who were essentially 100% paced), had a lower risk of clinical nonresponse (RR 0.40; 95% CI 0.28, 0.58; $P<0.001$) and a reduced risk of death.

A subsequent meta-analysis focused on the impact of AV nodal ablation in conjunction with CRT in the HF-rEF population. This report included six studies; four were retrospective and two were prospective cohort studies. All of the studies reported the effectiveness of biventricular capture using device diagnostics. In those who had AV nodal ablation (AVNA+), biventricular capture was near to complete. In those

FIGURE 6.5 — Effect of CRT vs Control on All-Cause Mortality and All-Cause Mortality Plus Hospitalization

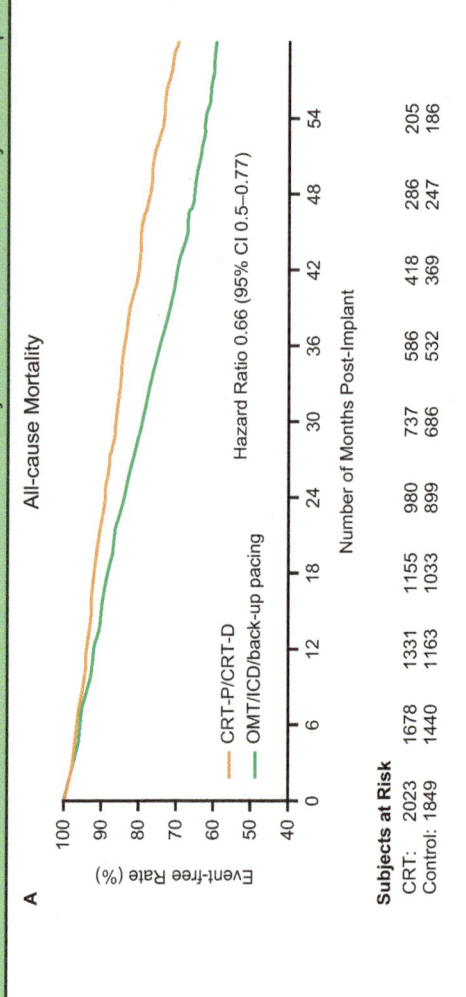

All-cause Mortality

— CRT-P/CRT-D
— OMT/ICD/back-up pacing

Hazard Ratio 0.66 (95% CI 0.5–0.77)

Number of Months Post-Implant

Event-free Rate (%)

Subjects at Risk

	0	6	12	18	24	30	36	42	48	54
CRT:	2023	1678	1331	1155	980	737	586	418	286	205
Control:	1849	1440	1163	1033	899	686	532	369	247	186

B

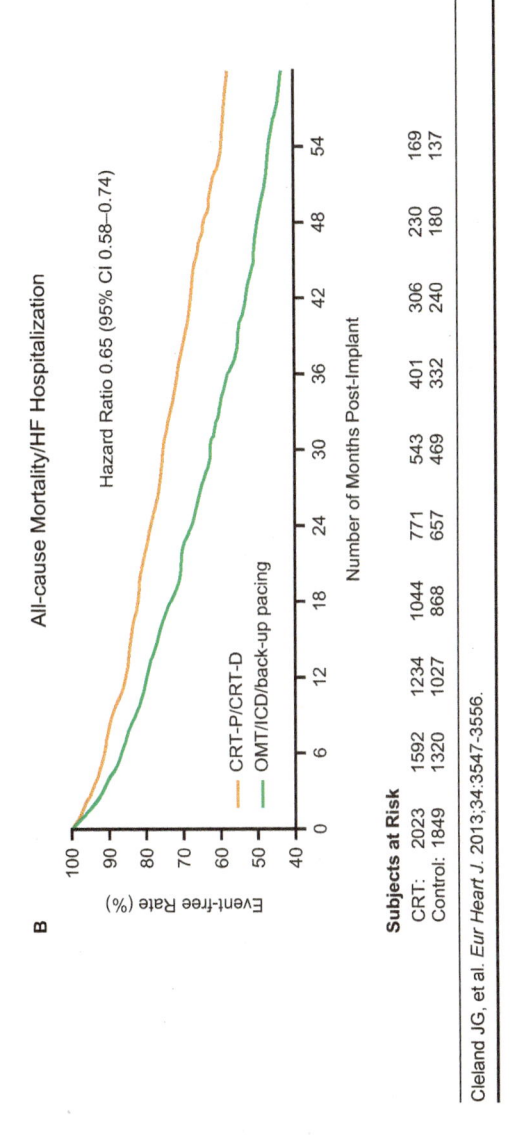

All-cause Mortality/HF Hospitalization

Hazard Ratio 0.65 (95% CI 0.58–0.74)

— CRT-P/CRT-D
— OMT/ICD/back-up pacing

Number of Months Post-Implant

Event-free Rate (%)

Subjects at Risk

	0	6	12	18	24	30	36	42	48	54
CRT:	2023	1592	1234	1044	771	543	401	306	230	169
Control:	1849	1320	1027	868	657	469	332	240	180	137

Cleland JG, et al. *Eur Heart J.* 2013;34:3547-3556.

TABLE 6.1 — Cardiac Effects of Right-Ventricular Pacing

Acute and Long-Term Effects of RV Apical Pacing

Changes in electrical activation and mechanical activation:

Metabolism/Perfusion

- Changes in regional perfusion
- Changes in oxygen demand

Remodeling

- Asymmetric hypertrophy
- Histopathological changes
- Ventricular dilation
- Functional mitral regurgitation

Hemodynamics

- Decreased cardiac output
- Increased LV filling pressures

Mechanical Function

- Changes in myocardial strain
- Interventricular mechanical dyssynchrony
- Intraventricular mechanical dyssynchrony

Tops LF, et al. *J Am Coll Cardiol.* 2009;54(9):764-776.

FIGURE 6.6 — Relationship of LVEF and Extent of Dyssynchrony with RV Pacing

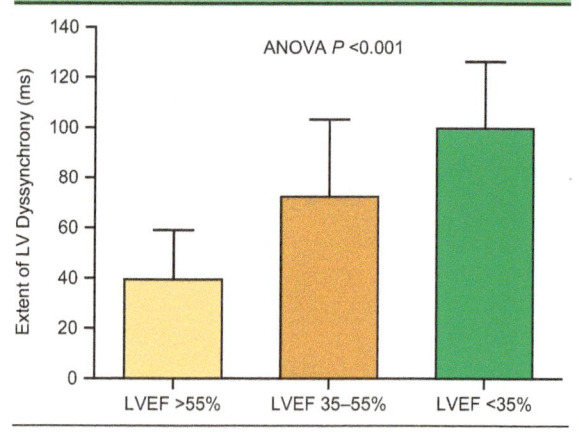

Tops LF, et al. *J Am Coll Cardiol.* 2009;54(9):764-776.

without AV nodal ablation (AVNA−) the percentage of biventricular pacing ranged from 82% to 96.5%. Only three of the studies included in the meta-analysis reported mortality data comparing CRT-AF patients undergoing AVNA with those with pharmacologic rate control; between-study heterogeneity was low and the overall risk ratio for all-cause mortality in AF patients undergoing AVNA was 0.42 (95% CI: 0.26-0.68; $P<0.001$) (**Figure 6.7**).[5]

FIGURE 6.7 — AV Nodal Ablation vs Medical Rate Control for AF Patients Undergoing CRT

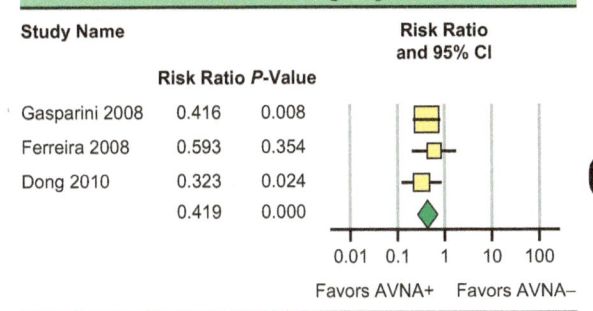

Study Name	Risk Ratio	*P*-Value
Gasparini 2008	0.416	0.008
Ferreira 2008	0.593	0.354
Dong 2010	0.323	0.024
	0.419	0.000

Favors AVNA+   Favors AVNA−

Ganesan AN, et al. *J Am Coll Cardiol.* 2012;59(8):719-726.

The studies supporting AV nodal ablation in conjunction with CRT for patients with AF and wide QRS are primarily observational. However, the available data show that in CRT-AF patients, AV nodal ablation was associated with reduction in all-cause mortality and CV mortality as well as improvements in NYHA functional class compared with pharmacologic rate control.

Although there are realistic concerns about creating pacemaker dependency with AV nodal ablation, given the limited long-term prognosis for HF-rEF patients with AF, the risks seem more than counterbalanced by the potential benefit of CRT in this population.

CIED Therapy and Clinical Management

Effective CIED therapy is now widely used. Based on data derived from a review of 620,291 distinct HF patients identified from commercial claims data, an estimated 24% to 29% of HF-rEF patients in the United States would be expected to have a CIED.[6]

Anticoagulation

In patients with HF and AF, the use of an IEPD does not alter the risk profile for thromboembolic stroke. Nonetheless, in a study of patients with both AF and a CIED who had no contraindications for warfarin, using combined registry and Medicare fee-for-service data, 2049 (79%) of 2586 anticoagulation-eligible patients were discharged without warfarin. At 1-year follow-up, use of anticoagulation was associated with lower mortality, as shown in **Figure 6.8**.[7]

Infection

With increasing use of CIEDs in clinical practice, device-related infection has become a more prominent problem. The infection rate has increased out of proportion to increases in implantation rates, largely due to wider use of complex devices in patients with a greater burden of comorbidity.[8] Consequently, HF clinicians must be alert to the potential for device infection.

In a population-based study of all 5918 consecutive Danish patients who underwent a cardiac implantable electronic device procedure in 1 year (May 2010 to April 2011), 49 (0.8%; 0.6-1.1%) experienced a systemic infection. Systemic infection rates were lowest for new implants at 0.3%, higher for generator replacement, 0.8%, and highest for upgrade/lead revision at 0.9%.[9] A single center study from Canada[10] reported a total of 24 infections among 2417 patients having device surgery (1%). Consistent with the Danish study,

FIGURE 6.8 — Mortality With and Without Anticoagulation in Patients With HF, AF, and an IEPD

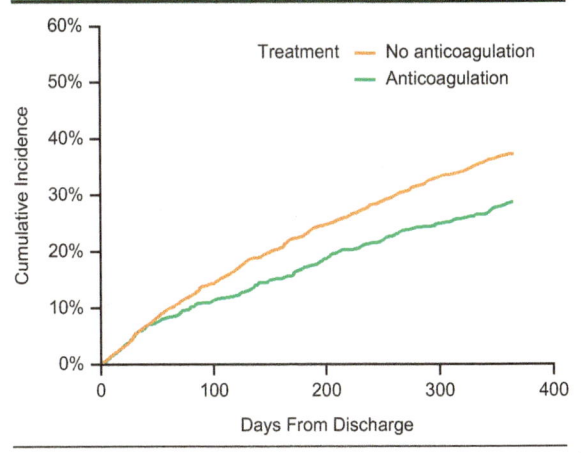

Hess PL, et al. *Clin Cardiol*. 2012;35(11):649-657.

patients who had device infection were more likely to have had a replacement rather than a new implant and had more complex devices.

When device infection is suspected, the application of the traditional modified Duke criteria for diagnosis of endocarditis is limited by the complexity of the lesions seen on echocardiography. In clinical practice, the transesophageal echocardiogram is considered the test of choice for diagnosis of device lead infection or CIED-IE.[11] Recently, 18F-FDG PET/CT has been proposed as a useful diagnostic tool in patients with suspected IE and intracardiac devices.[12]

Figure 6.9 presents the AHA currently recommended approach to device infection.[11]

Summary

The data demonstrating the importance of CIEDs to HF management, both in prevention of SCD and in the therapy of contractile dyssynchrony, strongly

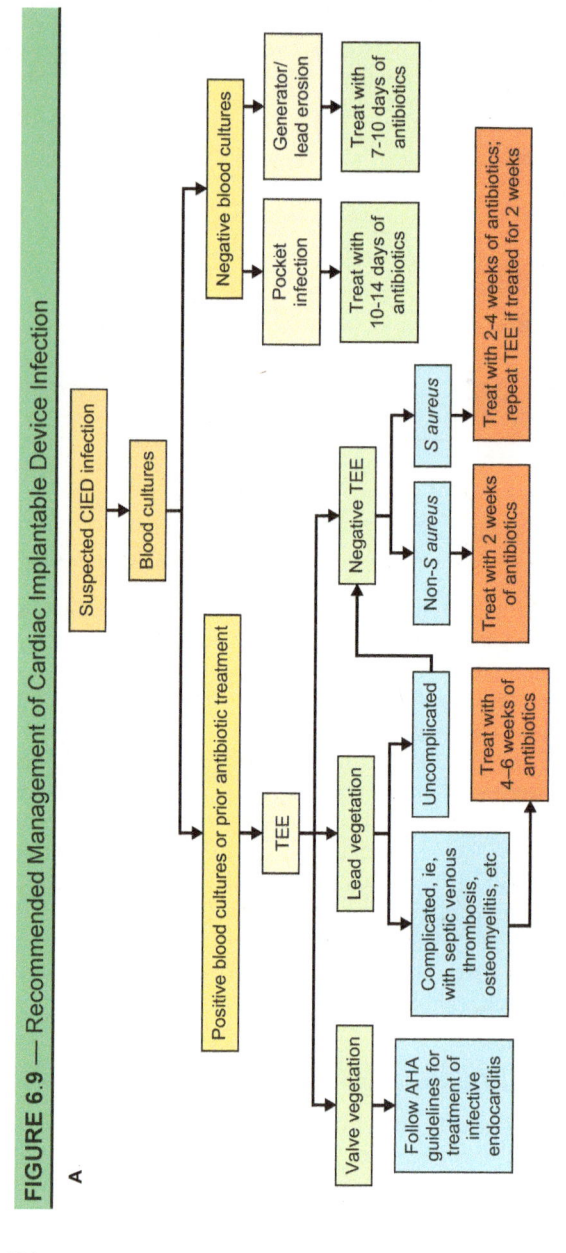

FIGURE 6.9 — Recommended Management of Cardiac Implantable Device Infection

A

B

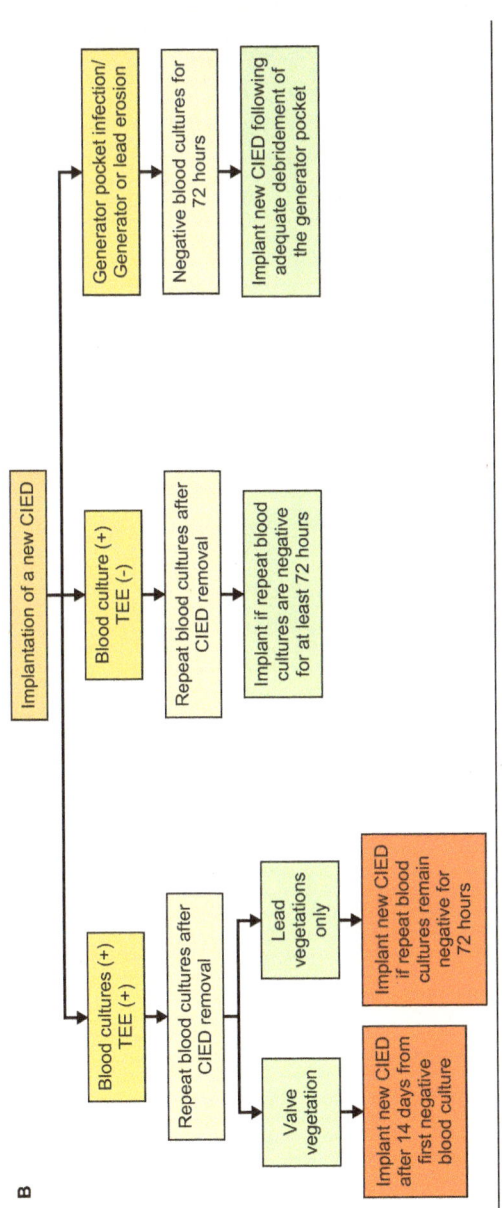

Implantation of a new CIED

- **Blood cultures (+) / TEE (+)**
  - Repeat blood cultures after CIED removal
    - Valve vegetation → Implant new CIED after 14 days from first negative blood culture
    - Lead vegetations only → Implant new CIED if repeat blood cultures remain negative for 72 hours

- **Blood culture (+) / TEE (−)**
  - Repeat blood cultures after CIED removal
  - Implant if repeat blood cultures are negative for at least 72 hours

- **Generator pocket infection / Generator or lead erosion**
  - Negative blood cultures for 72 hours
  - Implant new CIED following adequate debridement of the generator pocket

Baddour LM, et al. *Circulation*. 2010;121:458-477.

support the concept that the HF clinician and the electrophysiologist must be partners in the care of a large subset of the HF population.

Clinicians must constantly search for opportunities to improve patient care by employing appropriate devices, and electrophysiologists must ensure that patients with devices also continue to receive optimal medical management.

REFERENCES

1. Clark AL, Goode K, Cleland JGF. The prevalence and incidence of left bundle branch block in ambulant patients with chronic heart failure. *Eur J Heart Fail.* 2008;10:696-702.

2. Cleland JG, Abraham WT, Linde C, et al. An individual patient meta-analysis of five randomized trials assessing the effects of cardiac resynchronization therapy on morbidity and mortality in patients with symptomatic heart failure. *Eur Heart J.* 2013;34:3547-3556.

3. Cleland JG, Tavazzi L, Daubert JC, Tageldien A, Freemantle N. Cardiac resynchronization therapy: are modern myths preventing appropriate use? *J Am Coll Cardiol.* 2009;53:608-611.

4. Tops LF, Schalij MJ, Bax JJ. The effects of right ventricular apical pacing on ventricular function and dyssynchrony implications for therapy. *J Am Coll Cardiol.* 2009;54(9):764-776.

5. Ganesan AN, Brooks AG, Roberts-Thomson KC, Lau DH, Kalman JM, Sanders P. Role of AV nodal ablation in cardiac resynchronization in patients with coexistent atrial fibrillation and heart failure a systematic review. *J Am Coll Cardiol.* 2012;59:719-726.

6. Mills RM, Zhu V, Cody RJ, Yuan Z. Estimated prevalence of implanted electrophysiologic devices in patients with heart failure. *Am Heart J.* 2015;169:188-189.

7. Hess PL, Greiner MA, Fonarow GC, et al. Outcomes associated with warfarin use in older patients with heart failure and atrial fibrillation and a cardiovascular implantable electronic device: findings from the ADHERE registry linked to Medicare claims. *Clin Cardiol.* 2012;35(11):649-657.

8. Padfield GJ, Steinberg C, Bennett MT, et al. Preventing cardiac implantable electronic device infections. *Heart Rhythm.* 2015;12:2344-2356.

9. Kirkfeldt RE, Johansen JB, Nohr EA, et al. Complications after cardiac implantable electronic device implantations: an analysis of a complete, nationwide cohort in Denmark. *Eur Heart J.* 2014;35(18):1186-1194.

10. Nery P, Fernandes R, Nair G, et al. Device-related infection among patients with pacemakers and implantable defibrillators: incidence, risk factors, and consequences. *J Cardiovascular Electrophysiology.* 2010;21(7):786-790.

11. Baddour LM, Epstein AE, Erickson CC, et al. Update on cardiovascular implantable electronic device infections and their management: a scientific statement from the American Heart Association. *Circulation*. 2010;121:458-477.
12. Sohail MR, Baddour LM. Role of PET imaging in management of implantable electronic device infection. *JACC Cardiovasc Imaging*. 2016;9(3):291-293.

7
Heart Failure With Major Comorbidities

Table 7.1 and **Table 7.2** list the most common comorbidities associated with HF. In a 2011 analysis of almost 5 million Medicare recipients with HF, the vast majority of patients were over the age of 65 and had a median of six comorbid conditions. **Table 7.1** shows data specific to the Medicare population in the United States with chronic HF, whereas **Table 7.2** shows all-comers registry data from several large HF admission registries.

Clinically, patients with diabetes, CKD, and COPD, either alone or in combination, pose the greatest challenges to pharmacologic HF management because the strategies involved in managing both their HF and comorbidities must be modified, and the possibilities of adverse effects are amplified. In addition, we will review recent randomized trials focused on the management of anemia in HF patients and address some important issues in the emerging subspecialty of cardio-oncology.

Heart Failure and Coronary Artery Disease

The 2011 ACC/AHA guidelines list coronary artery disease (CAD) as a comorbidity in approximately 70% of HF patients over the age of 65 years. HF-rEF due to CAD may affect up to 8 million patients in the United States in the coming 2 decades. Even so, current evidence suggests that diagnostic and therapeutic interventions directed toward CAD are underutilized in HF patients.[1]

The Surgical Treatment for Ischemic Heart Failure Extension Study (STICHES) recently reported the 10-year effects of CABG surgery in patients with

TABLE 7.1 — Ten Most Common Co-occurring Chronic Conditions Among Medicare Beneficiaries With Heart Failure[a], 2011

Beneficiaries Age ≥65 y[b] (N = 4,376,150)	N	%	Beneficiaries Age <65 y[c] (N = 571,768)	N	%
Hypertension	3,685,373	84.2	Hypertension	461,235	80.7
Ischemic heart disease	3,145,718	71.9	Ischemic heart disease	365,889	64.0
Hyperlipidemia	2,623,601	60.0	Diabetes	338,687	59.2
Anemia	2,200,674	50.3	Hyperlipidemia	325,498	56.9
Diabetes	2,027,875	46.3	Anemia	284,102	49.7
Arthritis	1,901,447	43.5	Chronic kidney disease	257,015	45.0
Chronic kidney disease	1,851,812	42.3	Depression	207,082	36.2
COPD	1,311,118	30.0	Arthritis	201,964	35.3
Atrial fibrillation	1,247,748	28.5	COPD	191,016	33.4
Alzheimer's disease/dementia	1,207,704	27.6	Asthma	88,816	15.5

[a] N = 4,947,918. [b] Mean number of conditions is 6.1; median is 6. [c] Mean number of conditions is 5.5; median is 5.

Yancy CW, et al. J Am Coll Cardiol. 2013;62(16);e147-e239. *Data source:* Centers for Medicare and Medicaid Services administrative claims data, January-December 2011, from the Chronic Condition Warehouse (CCW), ccwdata.org.

ischemic cardiomyopathy in 1212 patients with LVEF ≤35% who were randomized to optimal medical therapy or optimal medical therapy with CABG. Importantly, 91% of the patients assigned to CABG who underwent surgery received at least one arterial conduit graft. 17.2% of the CABG patients and 19.6% of the medical patients received an implantable cardioverter-defibrillator (with or without CRT). All-cause mortality was lower among patients who were assigned to CABG than those treated medically, 58.9% vs 66.1%. CABG patients had improved survival, a median 7.73 years as compared to medical patients with a median 6.29 years (**Figure 7.1**).[2]

Although HF-rEF due to CAD remains a major problem, STITCHES has provided important data that strongly support surgical revascularization, with arterial conduits whenever possible, in addition to optimal medical and device management for suitable candidates.

Heart Failure and Type 2 Diabetes

Overall, as shown in **Table 7.2**, 40% to 50% of HF patients have T2D as a comorbidity. Patients with type 1 insulin-deficient diabetes (T1D) who develop HF typically have widespread advanced atherosclerotic vascular disease and CKD as well. The authors strongly recommend that these patients should be managed by an experienced clinical team that includes an endocrinologist specializing in care of T1D. **Table 7.3** lists currently approved classes of agents for treatment of T2D.

Concern about the potential adverse effects of oral anti-diabetic agents in T2D patients with HF reflects the fact that thiazolidinediones have been reported to be associated with an increased risk of CV adverse events. Thiazolidinediones, which are insulin sensitizers, have been associated with fluid retention and increased risk of HF in T2D.

TABLE 7.2 — Comorbidities in Patients With Acute HEART Failure From Three Large Registries

	ADHERE Registry		OPTIMIZE-HF Registry		GWTG Registry[b]	
	Reduced (n=25,865) 50%	Preserved (n=26,322) 50%[a]	LVSD (n=20,118) 49%	Preserved (n=21,149) 51%	EF <40% (n=55,083) 50%	EF ≥50% (n=40,354) 36%
	Acute HF, 274 Hospitals, 2001-2004		Acute HF, 259 Hospitals, 2003-2004		Acute HF, 275 Hospitals, 2005-2010	
Age (y)	70±14	74±13	70±14	75±13	70 (58-80)	78 (67-85)
Female	40%	62%	38%	62%	36%	63%
African-American race	22%	17%	21%	15%	25%	16%
Medical History						
COPD or asthma	27%	31%	—	—	27%	33%
Renal insufficiency	26%	26%	—	—	48%	52%
Anemia	—	—	—	—	14%	22%
Diabetes mellitus	40%	45%	24% noninsulin/15% insulin	26% noninsulin/17% insulin	22% oral therapy/18% insulin	24% oral therapy/22% insulin
Obesity (%) or body weight (kg)	—	—	78.5 (65.8-94.0)	78.9 (64.0-97.5)	25%	33%

Laboratory Data

BMI, kg/m^2	—	—	—	—	—	—
Hemoglobin, g/dL	—	—	12.5±2.0	11.9±2.0	12.4 (11-13.8)	11.5 (10.2-12.9)
Creatinine, mg/dL	1.6±1.3	1.7±1.5	1.4 (1.1-1.9)	1.3 (1.0-1.8)	1.3 (1-1.8)	1.3 (1-1.9)

Key: ADHERE, Acute Decompensated Heart Failure National Registry; GWTG, Get With The Guidelines; OPTIMIZE-HF, Organized Program to Initiate Lifesaving Treatment in Hospitalized Patients with Heart Failure.

Values are mean ± SD, median (interquartile range), or percentage.

a A total of 274 hospitals included in the analysis cited.
b Patients with an LVEF between 40% and 49% were excluded from this table.

Modified from Mentz RJ, et al. *J Am Coll Cardiol.* 2014;64(21):2281-2293.

FIGURE 7.1 — Long-Term Endpoints From STICHES: All-Cause Death, Cardiovascular Death, and All-Cause Death or Cardiovascular Hospitalization

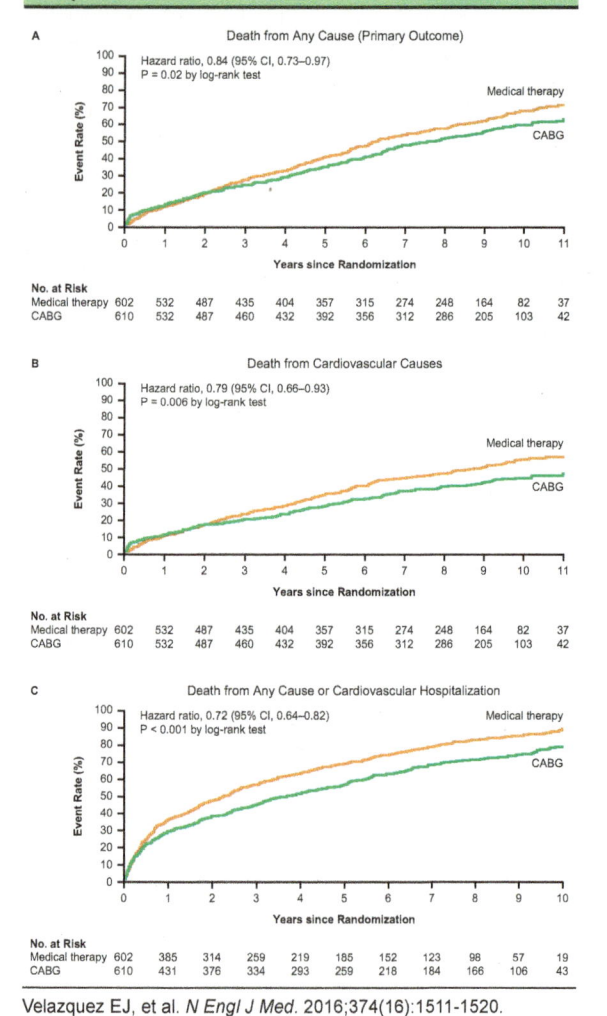

A — Death from Any Cause (Primary Outcome)

Hazard ratio, 0.84 (95% CI, 0.73–0.97)
P = 0.02 by log-rank test

No. at Risk											
Medical therapy	602	532	487	435	404	357	315	274	248	164	82	37
CABG	610	532	487	460	432	392	356	312	286	205	103	42

B — Death from Cardiovascular Causes

Hazard ratio, 0.79 (95% CI, 0.66–0.93)
P = 0.006 by log-rank test

No. at Risk											
Medical therapy	602	532	487	435	404	357	315	274	248	164	82	37
CABG	610	532	487	460	432	392	356	312	286	205	103	42

C — Death from Any Cause or Cardiovascular Hospitalization

Hazard ratio, 0.72 (95% CI, 0.64–0.82)
P < 0.001 by log-rank test

No. at Risk											
Medical therapy	602	385	314	259	219	185	152	123	98	57	19
CABG	610	431	376	334	293	259	218	184	166	106	43

Velazquez EJ, et al. *N Engl J Med.* 2016;374(16):1511-1520.

TABLE 7.3 — Classes of Drugs Approved for T2D

Class of Drug	Drug(s) in Class
Metformin	—
Sulfonylureas	Chlorpropamide
	Glyburide
	Glipizide
	Glimepiride
Meglitinides	Repaglinide
	Nateglinide
Glitazones	Pioglitazone
	Rosiglitazone
Dipeptidyl peptidase 4 (DPP-4) inhibitors or gliptins	Sitagliptin
	Saxagliptin
	Linagliptin
	Alogliptin
Sodium-glucose co-transporter 2 (SGLT2) inhibitors	Canaglifozin
	Dapagliflozin
	Empagliflozin
Bile acid sequestrant	Colesevelam
Dopamine receptor agonist	Bromocriptine mesylate
Alpha glucosidase inhibitors	Acarbose
	Miglitol

DPP-4 inhibition with saxagliptin did not increase or decrease the rate of ischemic events, although the rate of hospitalization for HF was increased.[3] Similarly, a nested case-control study showed a moderate increase in the odds of HF admission with sitagliptin, although this was based on a small number of events.[4,5]

In contrast, a recent large nested case-control study included a total of 1,499,650 patients with a first-ever prescription for a noninsulin antidiabetic drug (biguanides, sulfonylureas, thiazolidinediones, DPP-4 inhibitors, GLP-1 analogues, alpha-glucosidase inhibitors, meglitinides, sodium–glucose cotransporter 2 inhibitors, or combinations of these drugs). The data included over 3.2 million person-years of observation. Patients were divided into two separate cohorts on the basis of the presence or absence of a recorded history of HF at any time before or on the date of study-cohort entry. Incretin-based drugs were defined as dipeptidyl peptidase 4 (DPP-4) inhibitors and glucagon-like peptide 1 (GLP-1) analogues. The authors found that, "As compared with oral antidiabetic drugs used in combination, current treatment with incretin-based drugs was not associated with an increased risk of hospitalization for HF. Similar results were obtained when DPP-4 inhibitors and GLP-1 analogues were considered separately, and the results were consistent across several sensitivity analyses."[6] **Figure 7.2** shows the data for risk of HF hospitalization by study centers.

Metformin has been used for decades with a good record of efficacy and safety in T2D; however, its mechanism of action is not well understood. Although metformin inhibits hepatic glucose output (gluconeogenesis), recent evidence suggests that a decrease in glucose absorption from the gut may also be an important component of its mechanism of action.[7,8]

A review of nine observational cohort studies of metformin treatment included a total of 34,000 patients[9]; no randomized controlled trials were identified. Five of the studies were published in 2010. Overall, as compared with controls (mostly receiving sulfonylurea therapy), metformin was associated with a reduction in mortality, 23% v 37% (pooled adjusted risk estimates: 0.80; 0.74-0.87; I2 = 15%; $P<0.001$). There was no increased risk seen with metformin in HF-rEF patients (mortality pooled adjusted risk estimate: 0.91; 0.72-1.14; I2 = 0%; $P=0.34$), or in those with HF and CKD (pooled adjusted risk estimate: 0.81; 0.64-1.02; $P=0.08$). The authors concluded, "Until trial data become available, metformin should be considered the treatment of choice for patients with diabetes mellitus and HF."

FIGURE 7.2 — Association Between Treatment With Incretin-Based Drugs and the Risk of Hospitalization for Heart Failure Among Patients With and Without a History of Heart Failure

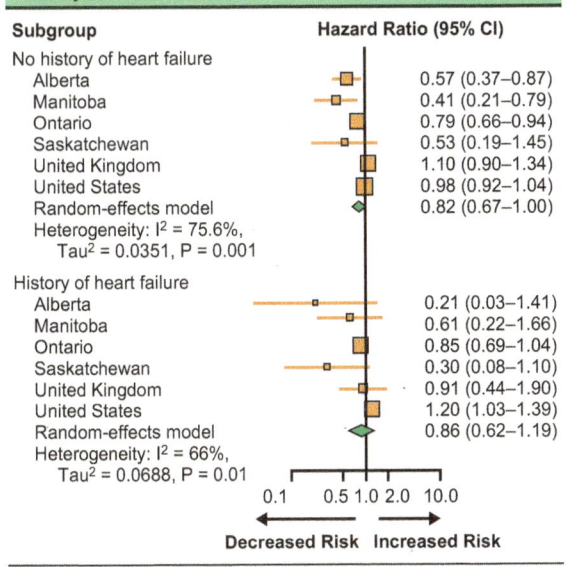

Subgroup	Hazard Ratio (95% CI)
No history of heart failure	
Alberta	0.57 (0.37–0.87)
Manitoba	0.41 (0.21–0.79)
Ontario	0.79 (0.66–0.94)
Saskatchewan	0.53 (0.19–1.45)
United Kingdom	1.10 (0.90–1.34)
United States	0.98 (0.92–1.04)
Random-effects model	0.82 (0.67–1.00)
Heterogeneity: $I^2 = 75.6\%$, $Tau^2 = 0.0351$, $P = 0.001$	
History of heart failure	
Alberta	0.21 (0.03–1.41)
Manitoba	0.61 (0.22–1.66)
Ontario	0.85 (0.69–1.04)
Saskatchewan	0.30 (0.08–1.10)
United Kingdom	0.91 (0.44–1.90)
United States	1.20 (1.03–1.39)
Random-effects model	0.86 (0.62–1.19)
Heterogeneity: $I^2 = 66\%$, $Tau^2 = 0.0688$, $P = 0.01$	

0.1   0.5 1.0 2.0   10.0

Decreased Risk   Increased Risk

Filion KB, et al. *N Engl J Med*. 2016;374:1145-1154.

However, the advent of sodium-glucose cotransporter-2 (SGLT2) inhibitors for the management of T2D has now raised the possibility that a new class of oral agents for T2D may actually reduce CV events. SGLT2 inhibitors cause competitive, reversible, selective inhibition of the SGLT2 transporter in the proximal tubule of the kidney. This leads to suppression of reabsorption of sodium and glucose in the proximal tubules, which increases glucose excretion in urine. Both glucose balance and caloric balance thus become negative, and both blood glucose level and insulin secretion are reduced[10,11] (**Figure 7.3**).

A systematic review and meta-analysis that included six regulatory submissions (37,525 participants) and 57 published trials (33,385 participants)

FIGURE 7.3 — Mechanism of Action of SGLT2 Inhibitors

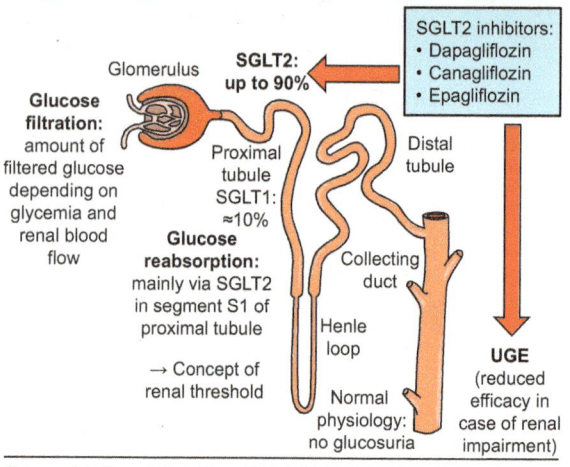

Scheen AJ. *Expert Opin Drug Metab Toxicol.* 2014;10(5):647-663.

provided data for seven different SGLT2 inhibitors.[12] Overall SGLT2 inhibitors protected against the risk of major adverse CV events (relative risk 0.84 [95% CI 0.75-0.95]; $P=0.006$), CV death (0.63 [0.51-0.77]; $P<0.0001$), HF (0.65 [0.50-0.85]; $P=0.002$), and death from any cause (0.71 [0.61-0.83]; $P<0.0001$). Data for HF were available only for empagliflozin, which had a strong protective effect (0.65 [0.50-0.85]). There was an adverse effect on nonfatal stroke (1.30 [1.00-1.68]; $P=0.049$). These data suggest net protection of SGLT2 inhibitors against CV outcomes and death. With regard to the efficacy endpoints, the results were driven by empagliflozin, the only SGLT2 inhibitor that has reported a dedicated long-term CV safety trial. However, there was no evidence that the different drugs acted differently. A separate network meta-analysis reached a similar conclusion.[13]

Figure 7.4 summarizes the efficacy data from the review and meta-analysis. **Figure 7.5** shows CV outcomes and death in the EMPA-REG OUTCOME trial.

Although generally well tolerated, SGLT2 inhibitors have significant adverse effects, as detailed in **Figure 7.6**.

The most prominent adverse effects are urogenital infections, most likely due to the increase in glycosuria associated with these drugs. There are a number of CV outcomes trials currently underway with SGLT2 inhibitors (**Table 7.4**).

Although the optimal management strategy for patients with coexisting HF and T2D continues to evolve, based on currently available data, the expert consensus appears to favor the use of either metformin or an SGLT2 inhibitor as a primary agent, and the combination of metformin and an SGLT2 inhibitor when more than one agent is required. Because of the potential for osmotic diuresis with use of SGLT2 inhibitors, a cautious reduction of loop diuretic dose and careful monitoring of fluid and electrolyte status will be required when initiating these agents in HF patients.

Heart Failure With COPD

■ Prevalence of COPD in the HF Population

About 20% to 30% of HF-rEF patients also have a diagnosis of COPD and an estimated 20% or more of COPD patients have HF-rEF.[14,15] Figures for HF-pEF are more uncertain but likely similar. In one small study, HF-pEF was present in one fifth of patients with exacerbated COPD.[16]

■ β-Blockers for HF in Patients With COPD

The ESC HF guidelines succinctly outline the major problems clinicians encounter in caring for patients with co-existing HF and COPD. First, because pulmonary function is often abnormal on the basis of HF alone, the diagnosis of COPD or asthma may be difficult, especially in patients with HF-pEF. **Figure 7.7** offers suggestions for using B-type natriuretic peptide levels in the evaluation of HF during a COPD exacerbation, and **Figure 7.8** offers guidance on the

FIGURE 7.4 — Efficacy Data, Systematic Review, and Network Meta-analysis

	SGLT2 Inhibitor (n/N)	Control (n/N)		Relative Risk (95% CI)
MACE				
Canagliflozin	104/6396	62/3403		1.02 (0.74-1.42)
Dapagliflozin	73/5936	62/3403		0.67 (0.48-0.94)
Empagliflozin	490/4687	282/2333		0.86 (0.75-0.99)
Ipragliflozin	7/628	10/368		0.41 (0.16-1.07)
(I^2 = 43%)				0.84 (0.75-0.95)
MACE plus				
Canagliflozin	130/6395	71/3327		0.95 (0.72-1.27)
Dapagliflozin	97/5936	81/3403		0.69 (0.51-0.92)
Empagliflozin	621/7082	359/3547		0.87 (0.77-0.98)
(I^2 = 24%)				0.85 (0.77-0.95)
Cardiovascular death				
Canagliflozin	21/6396	16/3327		0.68 (0.36-1.31)
Empagliflozin	172/4687	137/2333		0.62 (0.50-0.78)
(I^2 = 0%)				0.63 (0.51-0.77)
Non-fatal MI				
Canagliflozin	45/6396	27/3327		0.87 (0.54-1.39)
Empagliflozin	213/4687	121/2333		0.88 (0.70-1.09)
(I^2 = 0%)				0.88 (0.72-1.07)

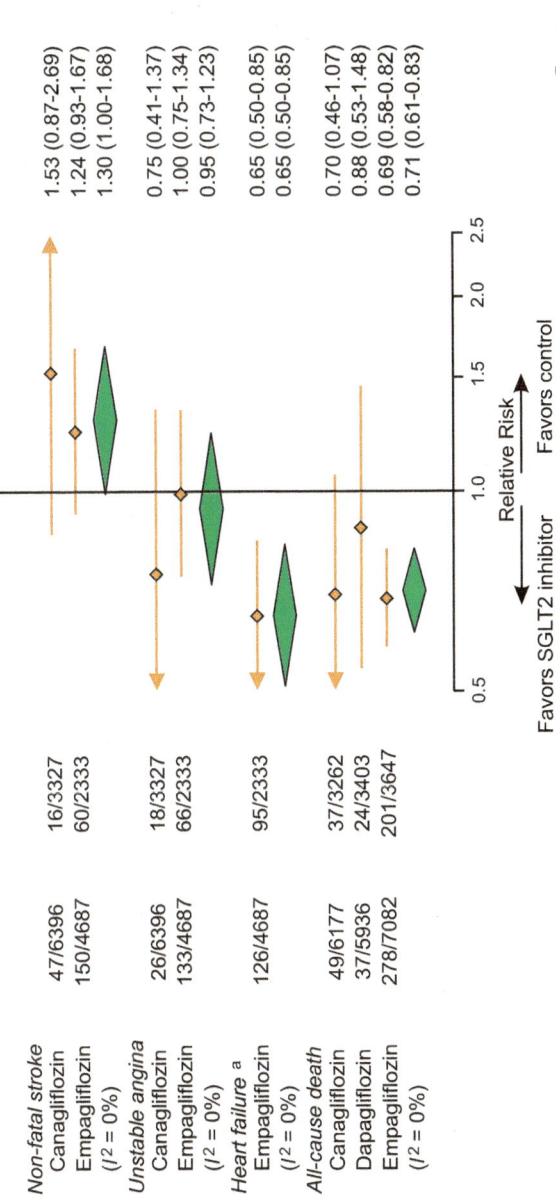

Non-fatal stroke				
Canagliflozin	47/6396	16/3327		1.53 (0.87-2.69)
Empagliflozin	150/4687	60/2333		1.24 (0.93-1.67)
($I^2 = 0\%$)				1.30 (1.00-1.68)
Unstable angina				
Canagliflozin	26/6396	18/3327		0.75 (0.41-1.37)
Empagliflozin	133/4687	66/2333		1.00 (0.75-1.34)
($I^2 = 0\%$)				0.95 (0.73-1.23)
Heart failure [a]				
Empagliflozin	126/4687	95/2333		0.65 (0.50-0.85)
($I^2 = 0\%$)				0.65 (0.50-0.85)
All-cause death				
Canagliflozin	49/6177	37/3262		0.70 (0.46-1.07)
Dapagliflozin	37/5936	24/3403		0.88 (0.53-1.48)
Empagliflozin	278/7082	201/3647		0.69 (0.58-0.82)
($I^2 = 0\%$)				0.71 (0.61-0.83)

Favors SGLT2 inhibitor ← Relative Risk → Favors control

Continued

FIGURE 7.4 — Continued

Key: MACE, major adverse cardiovascular events (cardiovascular death, non-fatal myocardial infarction, or non-fatal stroke); MACE plus, MACE and admission to hospital for unstable angina; SGLT2, sodium-glucose cotransporter-2.

Estimates for each drug were derived directly from regulatory documents or fixed-effects meta-analysis of effect estimates from multiple sources. Summary effects for all compounds were obtained from fixed-effects meta-analysis.

[a] Data available only for empagliflozin.

Modified from Wu JHY, et al. *Lancet Diabetes Endocrinol.* 2016;pii:S2213-8587(16)00052-8.

interpretation of echo and radionuclide ventricular function data in patients with stable COPD.

Second, the recommended therapies for the two conditions often seem to conflict, at least on first glance.[17] COPD is often associated with delayed diagnosis of CHF and is the most commonly listed reason for the failure to follow guideline recommendations for β-blockade in HF-rEF despite extensive safety data with these agents in patients with moderate to severe COPD.[18]

Table 7.5 shows the effects of HF-approved β-blockers on lung function in COPD patients.

A review of 22 studies, 11 of single-dose treatment and 11 of treatment for 2 days to 16 weeks, found that cardioselective β-blockers did not change FEV_1 or respiratory symptoms compared to placebo in COPD patients. In addition, cardioselective β-blockers did not impair the FEV_1 treatment response to $β_2$-agonists.[19]

Ivabradine for Heart Rate Reduction in HF-rEF With COPD

Nonetheless, some patients with coexisting HF-rEF and COPD may not tolerate recommended doses of β-blockers. In this situation, ivabradine may have additive value. A post hoc analysis of data from the SHIFT trial demonstrated that the treatment effect of ivabradine was maintained with a variety of comorbidities, including COPD.[20] In a specific subgroup analysis from SHIFT that focused on COPD in SHIFT, 11% of patients in the trial had a diagnosis of COPD. **Table 7.6** shows the baseline characteristics of those subjects with and without COPD.

HF medications were similar in the two groups, except for β-blockade (69% vs 92% at randomization). After 28 days, the mean reduction in placebo corrected heart rate in patients on ivabradine was similar in the COPD and non-COPD groups. **Figure 7.9** shows Kaplan-Meier plots for the cumulative composite endpoint in patients with and without COPD for ivabradine and placebo.

FIGURE 7.5 — CV Outcomes and Death in the EMPA-REG OUTCOME Trial

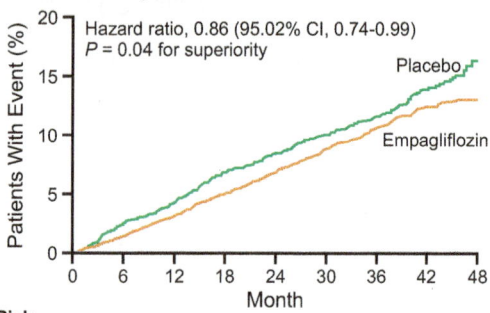

A. Primary Outcome

Hazard ratio, 0.86 (95.02% CI, 0.74-0.99)
$P = 0.04$ for superiority

No. at Risk
Empagliflozin	4687	4580	4455	4328	3851	2821	2359	1534	370
Placebo		2333	2256	2194	2112	1875	1380	1161	741	166

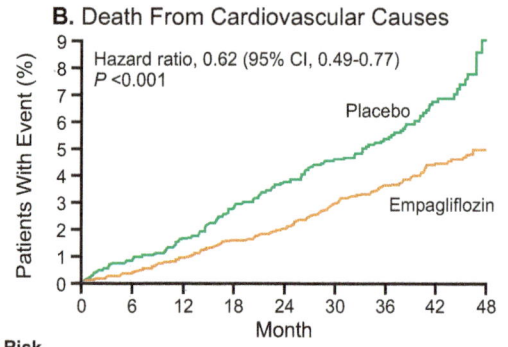

B. Death From Cardiovascular Causes

Hazard ratio, 0.62 (95% CI, 0.49-0.77)
$P < 0.001$

No. at Risk
Empagliflozin	4687	4651	4608	4556	4128	3079	2617	1722	414
Placebo		2333	2303	2280	2243	2012	1503	1281	825	177

Continued

Comparing the subjects with and without COPD, the primary composite endpoint and both its components, all-cause mortality and all-cause hospitalization, occurred significantly more often in the COPD group than in non-COPD patients. Although the treatment effects did not achieve statistical significance in this subgroup analysis, the relative risk of the primary composite endpoint decreased similarly in both groups, and there was no significant difference in

FIGURE 7.5 — *Continued*

C. Death From Any Cause

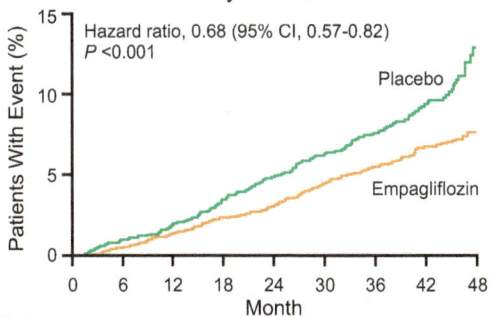

Hazard ratio, 0.68 (95% CI, 0.57-0.82)
$P < 0.001$

No. at Risk
Empagliflozin 4687 4651 4608 4556 4128 3079 2617 1722 414
Placebo   2333 2303 2280 2243 2012 1503 1281 825 177

D. Hospitalization for Heart Failure

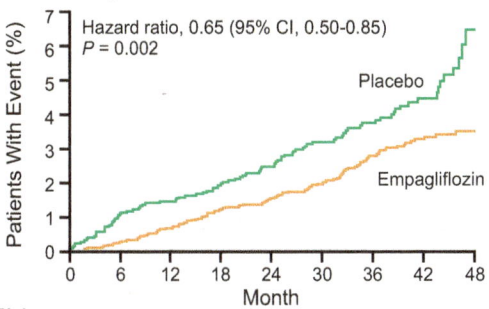

Hazard ratio, 0.65 (95% CI, 0.50-0.85)
$P = 0.002$

No. at Risk
Empagliflozin 4687 4614 4523 4427 3988 2950 2487 1634 395
Placebo   2333 2271 2226 2173 1932 1424 1202 775 168

Zinman B, et al. *N Engl J Med*. 2015;373:2117-2128.

the impact of ivabradine in both groups (*P* value for interaction = 0.82) Overall, the COPD patients had more frequent adverse events than non-COPD patients (84% vs 74%), but adverse event rates did not differ significantly comparing the ivabradine vs placebo arms within either the COPD or non-COPD groups.[21]

In summary, HF-rEF patients with coexisting COPD should be managed with careful attention to

FIGURE 7.6 — Adverse Effects of SGLT2 Inhibitors

	Drugs With Data	SGLT2 Inhibitors (n/N)	Control (n/N)		Relative Risk (95% CI)	I^2 (%)
Data from regulatory submissions						
Urinary tract infection	6	1419/19835	690/10847		1.15 (1.06-1.26)	0
Genital infection	6	1243/19835	143/10847		4.75 (4.00-5.63)	59%[a]
Cancer	6	253/25071	112/12454		1.07 (0.85-1.34)	0
Bone fracture	5	301/19120	161/10383		0.99 (0.82-1.21)	29%
Volume depletion	6	505/19835	159/10847		1.53 (1.27-1.83)	40%
Thromboembolism	3	26/13375	6/6976		1.54 (0.63-3.79)	0
Hypoglycemia	6	2283/18147	1308/9364		1.00 (0.94-1.07)	67%[a]
Acidosis	1	1/1630	0/311		0.57 (0.02-14.10)	NA
Kidney disease	4	145/20973	661/11709		1.21 (0.91-1.62)	10%
Data from scientific reports						
Urinary tract infection	6	1852/17096	972/8965		1.02 (0.95-1.10)	45%[a]
Genital infection	6	1419/19702	279/10094		2.88 (2.48-3.34)	79%[a]
Cancer	3	13/1865	14/1290		0.72 (0.34-1.54)	0
Bone fracture	4	254/8469	142/4914		0.96 (0.78-1.18)	21%

Volume depletion	4	438/14402	184/7782	1.16 (0.98-1.38)	0
Thromboembolism	1	30/4687	20/2333	0.75 (0.42-1.31)	0
Hypoglycemia	7	3204/19260	2093/10289	0.95 (0.91-1.00)	89%[a]
Acidosis	1	4/4687	1/2333	1.99 (0.22-17.80)	NA
Kidney disease	2	292/7075	171/3955	0.83 (0.69-1.00)	6%

Favors SGLT2 inhibitor ← → Favors control

Relative Risk

[a] P heterogeneity <0.05.

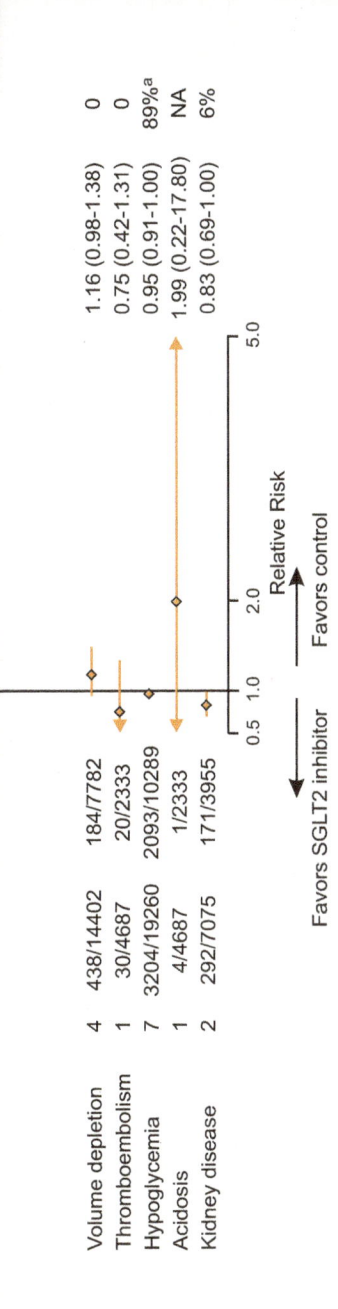

Modified from Wu JHY, et al. *Lancet Diabetes Endocrinol.* 2016;pii:S2213-8587(16)00052-8.

TABLE 7.4 — Currently Ongoing Cardiovascular Outcomes Trials With SGLT2 Inhibitors

Trial	N	Drug	Population	Primary Outcome
Canvas	4330	Canagliflozin vs placebo	T2D with history of atherosclerosis	CV death, nonfatal MI, stroke
Canvas-R	>5800	Canagliflozin	T2D with history or risk of CVD	Progression of albuminuria
Declare-TIMI 58	17,150	Dapagliflozin vs placebo	T2D + CVD or CVD risk	CV death, MI, stroke
Credence	4200	Empagliflozin vs placebo	T2D, stage 2 or 3 CKD on maximum ACE/ARB	ESKD, renal and vascular outcomes of canagliflozin vs placebo
Vertis	3900	Ertugliflozin vs placebo	T2D + CVD	CV death, MI, stroke

FIGURE 7.7 — Evaluation of Heart Failure During COPD Exacerbation Using B-Type Natriuretic Peptide Levels

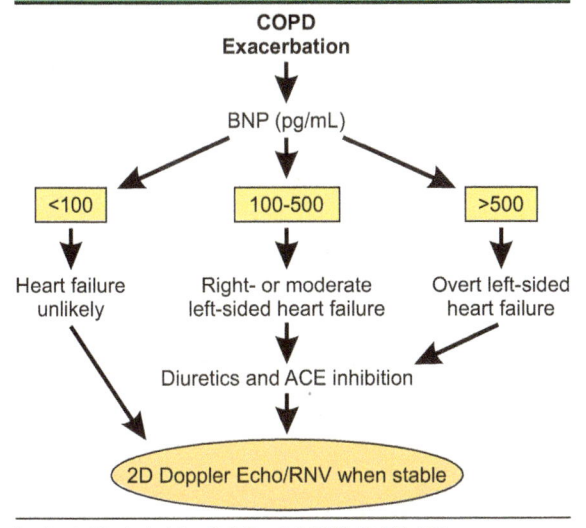

```
           COPD
        Exacerbation
             ↓
         BNP (pg/mL)
       ↙     ↓      ↘
    <100   100-500   >500
```

<100	100-500	>500
Heart failure unlikely	Right- or moderate left-sided heart failure	Overt left-sided heart failure

Diuretics and ACE inhibition

2D Doppler Echo/RNV when stable

Le Jemtel T, et al. *J Am Coll Cardiol.* 2007;49:171-180.

---

fluid and electrolyte balance, and with early intervention for exacerbations of respiratory disease. Also, the ACC/AHA guidelines advocate influenza and pneumococcal immunization. Administering influenza A vaccine to elderly patients with HF during the 1991-1992 influenza epidemic reduced the rate of HF hospitalization by 37%.[22]

Although there are few randomized trial data, chronic therapy with long-acting anticholinergic agents is recommended for COPD patients with HF rather than use of inhaled β agonists. HF should be managed with a guideline directed drug strategy that includes β-blockers as tolerated; cardioselective agents are probably preferable at least on theoretical grounds. Ivabradine appears to be both effective and safe in these patients and should be used for heart rate reduction as described in the prescribing information.

FIGURE 7.8 — Use of 2D and Doppler Echo and Radionuclide Ventriculography in the Cardiac Evaluation of Patients With Stable COPD

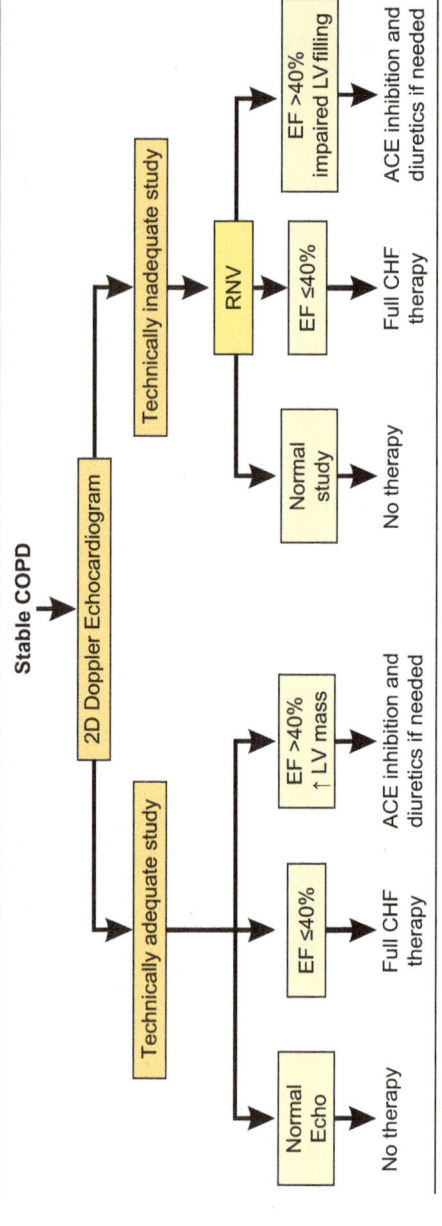

Le Jemtel T, et al. *J Am Coll Cardiol.* 2007;49:171-180.

TABLE 7.5 — β-Blockers for HF and Their Effects on Lung Function and Symptoms in COPD Patients

	Adrenergic Receptor-Blocking Activity	Doses in Heart Failure	Doses Used in Referenced Trials	Long-Term FEV$_1$ Treatment Effect in Airway Disease — Irreversible	Long-Term FEV$_1$ Treatment Effect in Airway Disease — Reversible	Respiratory Symptoms
Bisoprolol	β-1	1.25–10 mg daily	20 mg daily	NA	NA	None
Metoprolol (Toprol-XL)	β-1	12.5–200 mg daily	200 mg daily	NA	NA	1/6 patients
			100 mg twice daily	NA	Excluded	None
			100 mg twice daily	NA	Not specified	None
			50 mg three times daily	↓ (reversed with β-agonist), NS	Not specified	None
			100 mg twice daily	↓ (reversed with β-agonist)	Not specified	None
Carvedilol	β-1	3.125–25 mg twice daily	29 ± 19 mg daily	NA	Excluded	1/31 patients
	β-2		12.5–25 mg twice daily	NA	Not specified	13/89 patients
	α-1					

Key: **NA**, not applicable; **NS**, not significant.

Le Jemtel TH, et al. *J Am Coll Cardiol.* 2007;49(2):171-180.

TABLE 7.6 — Baseline Characteristics of SHIFT Subjects With and Without COPD

	COPD			Non-COPD			P value		
								COPD vs Non-COPD	
	IVA n=358	PBO n=372	All n=730	IVA n=2883	Placebo n=2892	All n=5775	IVA	PBO	All
Demographic Characteristics									
Age (y)	65.3±9.5	64.9±9.8	65.1±9.7	60.7±11.3	60.0±11.6	60.4±11.5	<0.001	<0.001	<0.001
Male	291 (81%)	305 (82%)	596 (82%)	2171 (75%)	2203 (76%)	4374 (76%)	0.012	0.012	<0.001
Caucasian	340 (95%)	358 (96%)	698 (96%)	2539 (88%)	2534 (88%)	5073 (88%)	<0.001	<0.001	<0.001
Current smokers	96 (27%)	111 (30%)	207 (28%)	445 (15%)	466 (16%)	911 (16%)	<0.001	<0.001	<0.001
BMI (kg/m²)	28.1±5.5	28.0±5.5	2.80±5.5	28.0±5.0	27.9±5.0	28.0±5.0	0.81	0.92	0.81
Cardiovascular Parameters									
Resting rate (bpm)	81.7±10.1	83.4±11.7	82.5±11.0	79.5±9.4	79.7±9.4	79.6±9.4	<0.001	<0.001	<0.001
Systolic BP (mm Hg)	123.8±17.6	123.7±16.3	123.7±16.9	121.7±15.9	121.1±15.8	121.4±15.8	<0.024	<0.001	<0.001
Diastolic BP (mm Hg)	74.8±10.2	76.0±9.6	75.4±9.9	75.9±9.5	75.5±9.4	75.7±9.4	<0.042	0.40	0.40
LVEF (%)	27.8±5.5	28.7±5.2	28.3±5.4	29.2±5.1	29.0±5.2	29.1±5.1	<0.001	0.25	<0.001
eGFR (mL/min/1.73 m²)	70.3±21.3	72.3±23.1	71.3±22.2	74.9±23.0	75.0±23.0	75.0±23.0	<0.001	0.032	<0.001
Serum creatinine (μmol/L)	101.5±27.7	100.5±30.1	101.0±29.0	96.1±26.3	96.2±25.7	96.1±26.0	<0.001	0.004	<0.001

Hemoglobin (g/L)	140.3±15.4	142.0±15.0	141.2±15.2	141.2±14.7	141.8±14.9	141.5±14.8	0.29	0.74	0.63
Medical History									
Ischemic HF	243 (68%)	242 (65%)	485 (66%)	1972 (68%)	1961 (68%)	3933 (68%)	0.84	0.29	0.36
NYHA Class III/IV HF	201 (56%)	236 (64%)	437 (60%)	1454 (51%)	1443 (50%)	2897 (50%)	0.042	<0.001	<0.001
History of MI	191 (53%)	192 (52%)	383 (52%)	1638 (57%)	1645 (57%)	3283 (57%)	0.21	0.054	0.024
History of hypertension	248 (69%)	264 (71%)	512 (70%)	1914 (66%)	1888 (65%)	3802 (66%)	0.28	0.029	0.021
History of diabetes	112 (31%)	124 (33%)	236 (32%)	861 (30%)	882 (30%)	1743 (30%)	0.58	0.27	0.24
History of stroke	31 (9%)	40 (11%)	71 (10%)	197 (7%)	255 (9%)	452 (8%)	0.20	0.220	0.075
Atrial fibrillation/flutter	39 (11%)	41 (11%)	80 (11%)	224 (8%)	218 (8%)	442 (8%)	0.041	0.019	0.002
CAD	263 (74%)	264 (71%)	527 (72%)	2098 (73%)	2107 (73%)	4205 (73%)	0.78	0.44	0.72
Treatment at Randomization									
β-blocker	242 (68%)	264 (71%)	506 (69%)	2655 (92%)	2659 (92%)	5314 (92%)	<0.001	<0.001	<0.001
β-blocker dose[a]									
• ≥50% of target dose	99 (41.4%)	129 (50.0%)	228 (45.9%)	1482 (56.9%)	1471 (56.3%)	2935 (56.6%)			<0.001
• Target dose	34 (14.2%)	42 (16.3%)	76 (5.3%)	709 (27.2%)	703 (26.9%)	1412 (27.1%)			<0.001

Continued

TABLE 7.6 — Continued

	COPD			Non-COPD			P value COPD vs Non-COPD		
	IVA n=358	Placebo n=372	All n=730	IVA n=2883	PBO n=2892	All n=5775	IVA	PBO	All
Demographic Characteristics
Inhaled drugs for COPD	190 (53%)	181 (49%)	371 (51%)	97 (3%)	115 (4%)	212 (4%)	<0.001	0.001	<0.001
Oral β₂ agonists	49 (14%)	62 (17%)	111 (15%)	17 (<1%)	36 (1%)	53 (<1%)	<0.001	<0.001	<0.001
ACE inhibitor	285 (80%)	287 (77%)	572 (78%)	2280 (79%)	2264 (78%)	4544 (79%)	0.82	0.62	0.84
Diuretics	324 (91%)	327 (88%)	651 (89%)	2395 (83%)	2368 (82%)	4763 (82%)	<0.001	0.004	<0.001
Ivabradine	—	—	358 (49%)	—	—	2883 (50%)	—	—	0.65

Key: IVA, ivabradine; PBO, placebo.

[a] Target dosages according to guidelines in the management of heart failure; percentages calculated for patients with relevant daily dose details.

Tavazzi L, et al. *Int J Cardiol.* 2013;170:182-188.

FIGURE 7.9 — Ivabradine vs Placebo: K-M Curves for the Occurrence of the Primary Composite Endpoint in SHIFT for Patients With and Without COPD

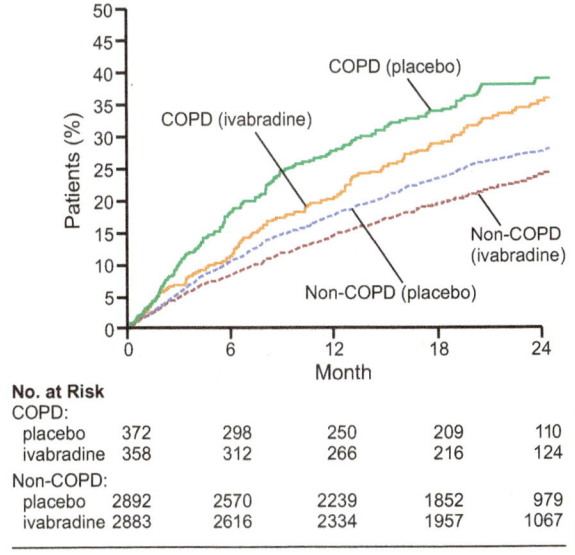

No. at Risk					
COPD:					
placebo	372	298	250	209	110
ivabradine	358	312	266	216	124
Non-COPD:					
placebo	2892	2570	2239	1852	979
ivabradine	2883	2616	2334	1957	1067

Tavazzi L, et al. *Int J Cardio.* 2013;170(2):182-188.

Heart Failure in Patients With CKD

■ Definition and Pathophysiology

Chronic kidney disease is defined primarily on the basis of estimates of glomerular filtration rate using serum creatinine, age, sex, and race as key variables. The details of the choice of estimating equations are beyond the scope of this discussion; however, all of the equations require that patients must be clinically stable when the serum creatinine is measured. In a careful study comparing the estimating equations in 110 HF-rEF patients (age, 57 ± 11.7 years; left ventricular ejection fraction, 0.27 ± 0.09; NYHA class, 2.5 ± 0.9), the MDRD formula was the most precise and had the best prognostic performance.[23]

Table 7.7 shows the prevalence of CKD in the general population and in HF-rEF patients.

In addition to estimates of GFR, measurement of urinary albumin excretion with the albumin/creatinine ratio on a morning spot urine sample is also important for the identification of kidney disease. Microalbuminuria is defined as a ratio between 3 and 30 mg/mmol and macroalbuminuria as a ratio above 30 mg/mmol.[24] In a subset of 2743 North American patients from the Candesartan in Heart Failure: Assessment of Reduction in Mortality and Morbidity (CHARM) Programme, 58% had a normal UACR, 30% had micro albuminuria, and 11% had macro albuminuria.[25] In this HF population, which included both HF-pEF and HF-rEF, an elevated UACR was associated with a substantially increased risk of adverse clinical outcomes and increased mortality. After adjustment for other risk factors in a multivariable model, both microalbuminuria and macroalbuminuria "remained strong independent predictors, with a 60% to 80% adjusted increase in the risk of death and a 30% to 70% increase in the adjusted risk of admission for HF." **Figure 7.10** shows Kaplan-Meier plots for death and HF admission stratified by albuminuria status for these patients.

As shown in **Figure 7.11**, both HF and CKD contribute to a broad-based negative feedback cycle in patients with coexisting disease.

■ Prevalence of Coexisting CKD in the Heart Failure Population

In an analysis of ADHERE data from October of 2001 to July of 2004, data required to estimate GFR (abbreviated MDRD study equation: serum creatinine, age, sex, and race) were available for 118,465 HF admissions. The analysis did not stratify the data by ejection fraction and also may have included some patients who had more than one admission to a registry hospital during the study period. This may have led to modest over-representation particularly of the more severe stages of CKD (Stage 4 and Stage 5). However,

TABLE 7.7 — Prevalence of CKD in the General Population and in HF-rEF Patients

CKD Stage	Description	GFR, mL/min/1.73 m^2	Prevalence in the General Population (%)	Prevalence in HF-rEF (%)
1	Kidney damage with normal GFR	≥90	3.3	2.8
2	Kidney damage with mild reduced GFR	60-89	3.0	10.6
3	Moderate renal dysfunction	30-59	4.3	45.5
4	Severe renal dysfunction	15-29	0.2	7.8
5	End-stage renal disease	<15	0.2	1.3

Prevalence of CKD in HF is provided for HF patients with reduced ejection fraction (HF-rEF). Kidney damage is defined as structural kidney disease and/or persistent elevated urinary albumin excretion. Data on the prevalence of CKD in HF patients with preserved EF are not available, but the GFR distribution is similar.

Waldum-Grevbo B. *Cardiology*. 2015;131(2):130-138.

FIGURE 7.10 — K-M Plots for Cardiovascular Death or Admission for Chronic Heart Failure and All-Cause Mortality, Stratified by Albuminuria Status from CHARM

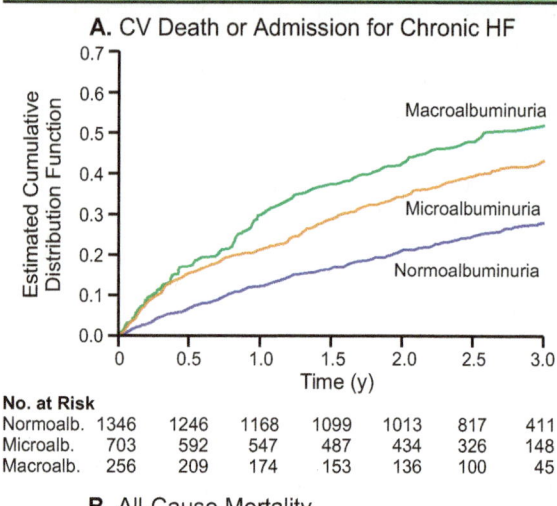

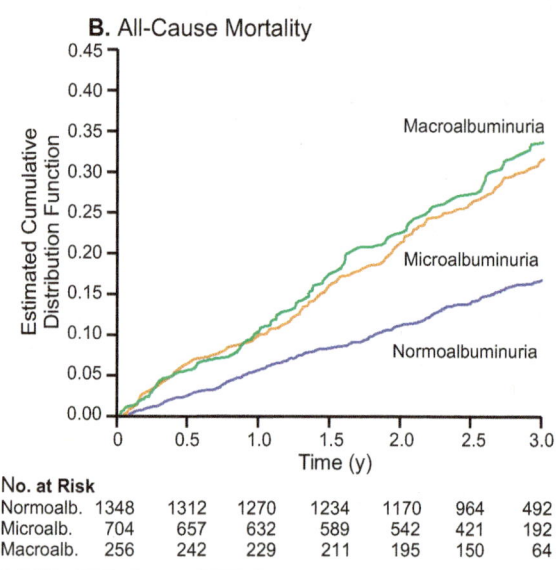

A. CV Death or Admission for Chronic HF

No. at Risk

Normoalb.	1346	1246	1168	1099	1013	817	411
Microalb.	703	592	547	487	434	326	148
Macroalb.	256	209	174	153	136	100	45

B. All-Cause Mortality

No. at Risk

Normoalb.	1348	1312	1270	1234	1170	964	492
Microalb.	704	657	632	589	542	421	192
Macroalb.	256	242	229	211	195	150	64

Jackson CE, et al; CHARM Investigators and Committees. *Lancet*. 2009;374(9689):543-550.

FIGURE 7.11 — Multiple Processes Contribute to Negative Feedback Cycles in Patients With Both HF and CKD

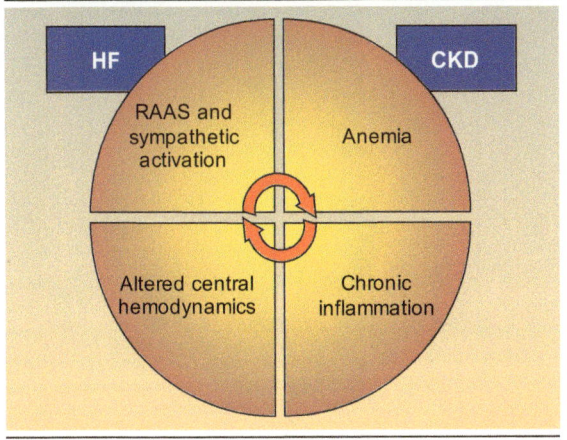

- HF
  - RAAS and sympathetic activation
  - Altered central hemodynamics
- CKD
  - Anemia
  - Chronic inflammation

Adapted from Mentz RJ, et al. *J Am Coll Cardiol.* 2014;64(21):2281-2293.

using National Kidney Foundation classification, more than half the admissions were associated with significant renal dysfunction.[26]

Figure 7.12 shows the prevalence and severity of renal dysfunction in over 118,000 hospital admissions for HF.

■ Impact of CKD in HF-rEF

The SOLVD Prevention and Treatment trials studied enalapril in patients with asymptomatic (prevention, $n=4228$) and symptomatic (treatment, $n=2569$) HF. Inclusion required an LVEF ≤35% and patients with creatinine values >2.0 mg/dL were excluded. Despite these limitations, a retrospective analysis showed, "a consistent and independent association of moderate renal insufficiency with an increased risk for all-cause mortality." This association held both active and placebo arms, and for patients with and without hypertension, with and without ischemic LV dysfunc-

FIGURE 7.12 — Prevalence and Severity of Renal Dysfunction in Over 118,000 Hospital Admissions for Heart Failure

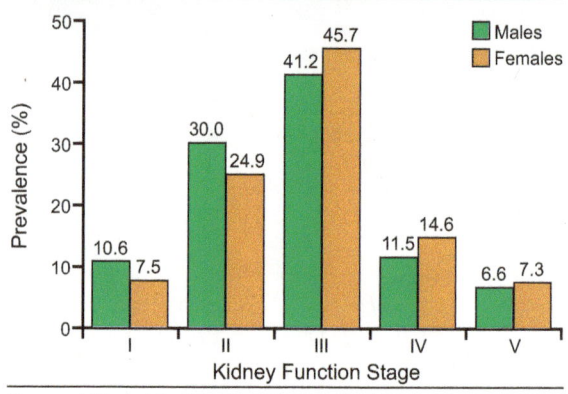

Kidney Function Stage	Males	Females
I	10.6	7.5
II	30.0	24.9
III	41.2	45.7
IV	11.5	14.6
V	6.6	7.3

Heywood JT, et al; for the ADHERE Scientific Advisory Committee and Investigators. *J Card Fail.* 2007;13:422-430.

tion, and with and without diabetes. The investigators concluded, "It is reasonable to consider the hypothesis that moderate renal insufficiency may be causally related to a greater rate of progression of left ventricular systolic dysfunction and increased mortality risk."[27]

■ Impact of CKD in HF-pEF

In the DIG Trial, which included 7788 ambulatory chronic HF patients in normal sinus rhythm, 49% of the patients with HF-rEF had CKD compared to 45% of the HF-pEF patients. Mortality due to all causes occurred in 757 patients without CKD during 7,216 years of follow up (1049/10,000 person years) and 882 patients with CKD during 6877 years (1282/10,000 person years) of follow up (HR = 1.22, 95% CI = 1.09-1.36; $P<0.0001$). In a propensity-matched analysis, although CKD was associated with increased mortality in both groups, the impact of CKD was greater in the HF-pEF patients[28] (**Figure 7.13**).

The Candesartan in Heart Failure: Assessment of Reduction in Mortality and Morbidity (CHARM)-

FIGURE 7.13 — Kaplan-Meier Plot of All-Cause Mortality in a Propensity-Matched Analysis of the DIG Trial

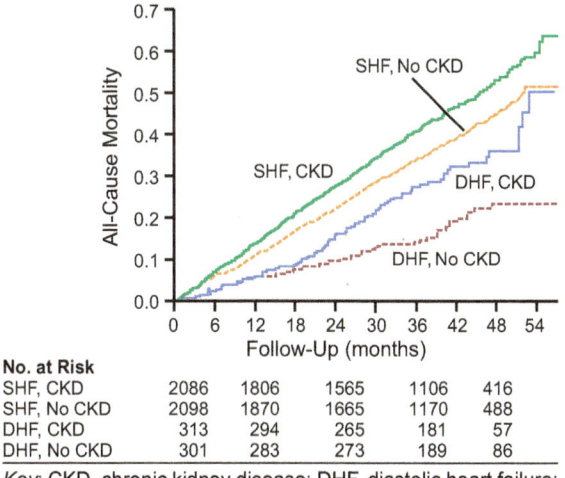

No. at Risk					
SHF, CKD	2086	1806	1565	1106	416
SHF, No CKD	2098	1870	1665	1170	488
DHF, CKD	313	294	265	181	57
DHF, No CKD	301	283	273	189	86

Key: CKD, chronic kidney disease; DHF, diastolic heart failure; SHF, systolic heart failure.

This graph shows the impact of CKD in patients with HF-rEF (SHF) and with HF-pEF (DHF).

Ahmed A, et al. *Am J Cardiol*. 2007;99(3)393-398.

Overall program evaluated the use of candesartan in three different HF populations: LVEF higher than 40% (CHARM-Preserved), LVEF ≥40% who were treated with an ACE inhibitor (CHARM-Added), or those with LVEF ≥40% or lower and not treated with an ACE inhibitor because of previous intolerance (CHARM-Alternative). Patients with serum creatinine >3.0 mg/dL were excluded. An estimated glomerular filtration rate (eGFR) at baseline was calculated (modified MDRD equation) in 2680 patients with sufficient data.

Figure 7.14 shows Kaplan-Meier plots demonstrating the impact of renal dysfunction on the incidence of CV death or HF hospitalization for the study populations with HF-rEF and HF-pEF, stratified by renal function.

FIGURE 7.14 — Kaplan-Meier Plots Illustrating the Impact of Renal Dysfunction on the Incidence of Cardiovascular Death or Heart Failure Hospitalization for the Study Populations With HF-rEF and HF-pEF, Stratified by Renal Function

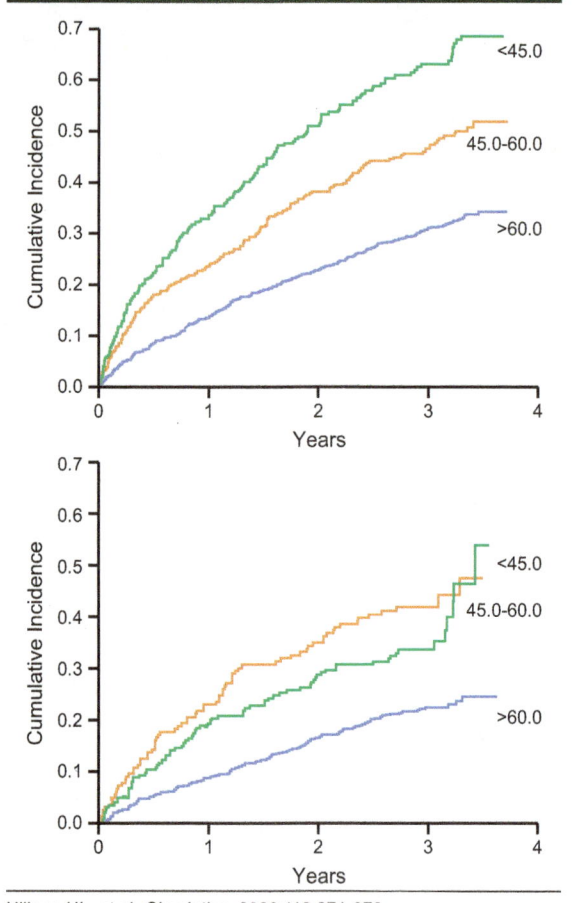

Hillege HL, et al. *Circulation*. 2006;113:671-678.

The CHARM data show that renal function was strongly associated with outcome in both HF-rEF and HF-pEF patients. In addition, the investigators noted that, "risk from renal insufficiency persists even after adjustment for all other known covariates, including LVEF. Moreover, no evidence for interaction was observed among renal function, treatment allocation, and primary outcome."[29]

Management Principles for Patients With HF and CKD

Table 7.8 summarizes the key management principles for patients with coexisting HF and CKD.[24]

Anemia in Heart Failure

In a recent observational study of 4456 patients referred for suspected HF with a median age of 73 years, 40% female, and 40% with reduced ejection fraction, 28% had anemia (defined as hemoglobin <12 g/dL in women and <13 g/dL in men). Overall, both anemia and iron deficiency were common, and associated with higher all-cause mortality which was largely driven by cardiovascular deaths.[30]

The RED-HF Trial (Reduction of Events by Darbepoetin Alfa in Heart Failure) was a randomized double-blind trial of treatment of 2278 HF-rEF patients and mild-to-moderate anemia with an erythropoiesis-stimulating agent, darbepoetin alfa. Active treatment led to "an early and sustained increase" in hemoglobin; however, there was no reduction in death or hospitalization for worsening heart failure and there was a significant increase in thromboembolic events with darbepoetin.[31]

In contrast, the FAIR-HF (Ferinject Assessment in Patients with Iron Deficiency and Chronic Heart Failure) study enrolled 459 patients with chronic HF-rEF who met criteria for iron deficiency as defined by a ferritin level <100 μg/L, or between 100 and 299 μg/L if the transferrin saturation was <20%, and

TABLE 7.8 — Key Management Principles for Patients With Coexisting HF and CKD

- Fragility:
  - Small changes in drug doses or fluid balance have large effects
- Hyperkalemia:
  - CKD patients are more prone to drug-induced or procedure-induced hyperkalemia
- Unnecessary reduction of RAAS inhibition:
  - In CKD, serum creatinine levels are highly volume sensitive
  - Restoration of fluid balance is preferable to interruption of RAAS blockade
- GDMT target doses may be impacted by reduced renal function:
  - Both tubular and glomerular function play a role in drug handling.
- With ACEi or ARB initiation, expect initial elevation of serum creatinine by 20% (within 2 months):
  - Patients experiencing an initial modest increase in creatinine are the ones who may benefit most from treatment
- Carvedilol, bisoprolol, and metoprolol are not dependent on renal elimination:
  - No firm data are available for HF patients with severe renal dysfunction; however, it seems likely that β-blockers improve outcome in these patients
- MRAs have a significant treatment benefit in HF patients with moderate renal dysfunction

a hemoglobin level of 95 to 135 g/L.[32] The patients were randomized to receive 200 mg of intravenous iron (ferric carboxymaltose) or saline (placebo). Patients were treated weekly until iron repletion was achieved (the correction phase), then every 4 weeks during the maintenance phase, which started at week 8 or week 12, depending on the required iron-repletion dose. The primary end points were the self-reported Patient Global Assessment and NYHA functional class, both at week 24. The authors reported that "Treatment with ferric carboxymaltose for 24 weeks in patients who had chronic heart failure and iron deficiency with or without anemia improved symptoms, functional capacity, and the quality of life."

Similarly, CONFIRM-HF (Ferric Carboxymaltose Evaluation on Performance in Patients With Iron Deficiency in Combination With Chronic Heart Failure) was a double-blind, placebo-controlled trial that enrolled 304 ambulatory HF-rEF, elevated natriuretic peptides, and iron deficiency defined as ferritin <100 ng/mL or 100-300 ng/mL if transferrin saturation <20%. Patients were randomized to treatment with intravenous iron as ferric carboxymaltose or to saline placebo for 52 weeks. The primary end point was the change in 6-minute-walk-test distance from baseline to Week 24. The patients assigned to intravenous iron had a sustained improvement in functional capacity, improved quality of life, and a reduced risk of hospitalization, as shown in **Figure 7.15**.[33] In both FAIR-HF and CONFIRM-HF the safety profile of ferric carboxymaltose was satisfactory; "as studied in FAIR-HF and CONFIRM-HF, a low risk of adverse effects is observed and only few injections are needed to treat ID (in CONFIRM-HF over 75% of the patients required a maximum of two injections of FCM to correct and maintain iron therapy)." [33]

In summary, iron deficiency with or without anemia is associated with poor outcomes in heart failure. Randomized controlled trials using new formulations of intravenous iron have demonstrated improvement in functional capacity and favorable safety profiles in HF-rEF patients. Iron repletion should be considered for HF-rEF patients with laboratory findings consistent with iron deficiency, whether or not anemia is present. **Figure 7.16** shows a suggested algorithm for the diagnosis of iron deficiency in HF-rEF, and **Figure 7.17** shows a suggested treatment algorithm.[34] To date, no data are available regarding iron deficiency and/or repletion outcomes in HF-pEF patients.

FIGURE 7.15 — 6-Minute Walk Test: Fatigue and Quality of Life Score Over Time

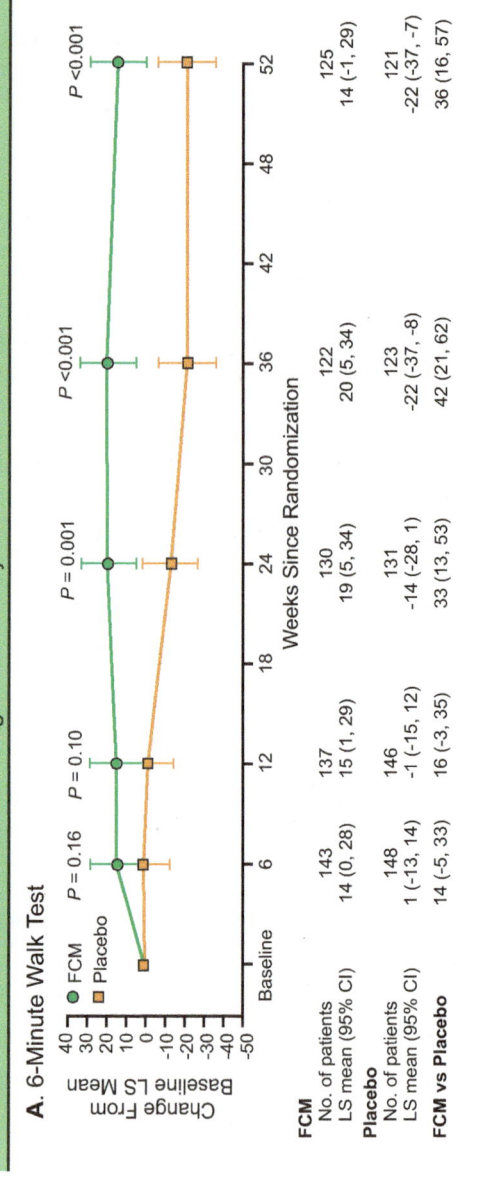

A. 6-Minute Walk Test

	Baseline	6	12	24	36	52
		$P=0.16$	$P=0.10$	$P=0.001$	$P<0.001$	$P<0.001$
FCM						
No. of patients		143	137	130	122	125
LS mean (95% CI)		14 (0, 28)	15 (1, 29)	19 (5, 34)	20 (5, 34)	14 (-1, 29)
Placebo						
No. of patients		148	146	131	123	121
LS mean (95% CI)		1 (-13, 14)	-1 (-15, 12)	-14 (-28, 1)	-22 (-37, -8)	-22 (-37, -7)
FCM vs Placebo		14 (-5, 33)	16 (-3, 35)	33 (13, 53)	42 (21, 62)	36 (16, 57)

Weeks Since Randomization

B. Fatigue

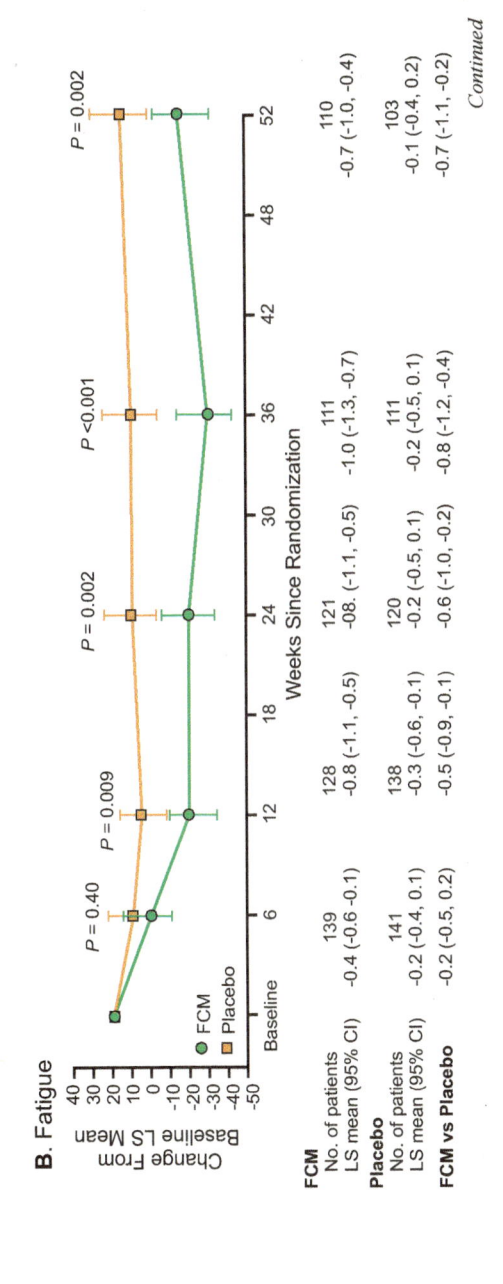

	Baseline	6	12	18	24	30	36	42	48	52
		P = 0.40	P = 0.009		P = 0.002		P <0.001			P = 0.002

FCM
No. of patients: 139, 128, 121, 111, 110
LS mean (95% CI): -0.4 (-0.6, -0.1), -0.8 (-1.1, -0.5), -08. (-1.1, -0.5), -1.0 (-1.3, -0.7), -0.7 (-1.0, -0.4)

Placebo
No. of patients: 141, 138, 120, 111, 103
LS mean (95% CI): -0.2 (-0.4, 0.1), -0.3 (-0.6, -0.1), -0.2 (-0.5, 0.1), -0.2 (-0.5, 0.1), -0.1 (-0.4, 0.2)

FCM vs Placebo: -0.2 (-0.5, 0.2), -0.5 (-0.9, -0.1), -0.6 (-1.0, -0.2), -0.8 (-1.2, -0.4), -0.7 (-1.1, -0.2)

Continued

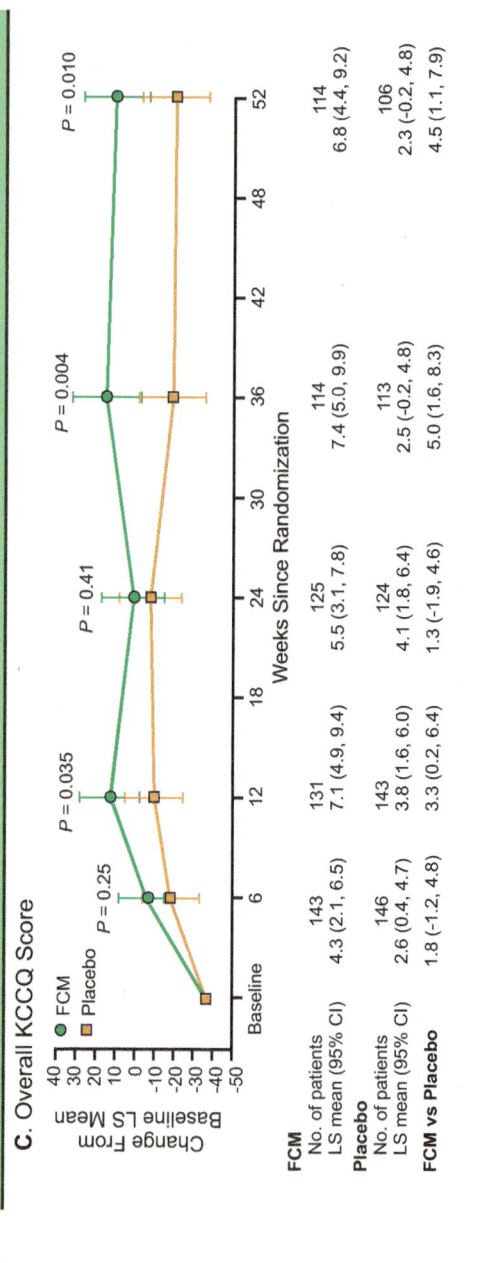

FIGURE 7.15 — Continued

C. Overall KCCQ Score

	Baseline	6	12	24	36	52
		$P = 0.25$	$P = 0.035$	$P = 0.41$	$P = 0.004$	$P = 0.010$

FCM
- No. of patients: 143, 131, 125, 114, 114
- LS mean (95% CI): 4.3 (2.1, 6.5), 7.1 (4.9, 9.4), 5.5 (3.1, 7.8), 7.4 (5.0, 9.9), 6.8 (4.4, 9.2)

Placebo
- No. of patients: 146, 143, 124, 113, 106
- LS mean (95% CI): 2.6 (0.4, 4.7), 3.8 (1.6, 6.0), 4.1 (1.8, 6.4), 2.5 (-0.2, 4.8), 2.3 (-0.2, 4.8)

FCM vs Placebo: 1.8 (-1.2, 4.8), 3.3 (0.2, 6.4), 1.3 (-1.9, 4.6), 5.0 (1.6, 8.3), 4.5 (1.1, 7.9)

Y-axis: Change From Baseline LS Mean (-50 to 40)
X-axis: Weeks Since Randomization

D. EQ-5D VAS

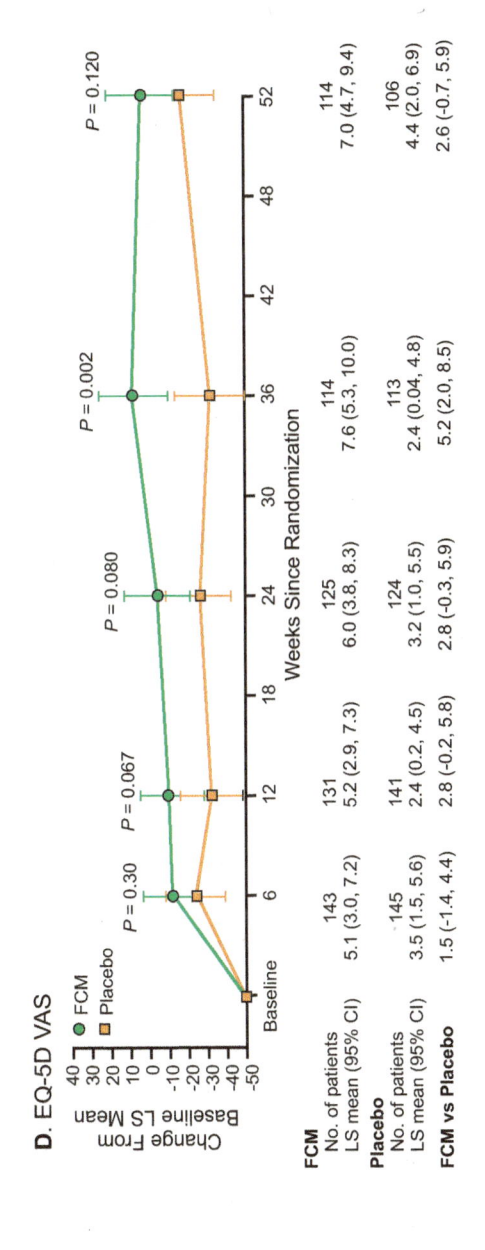

	6	12	24	36	52
P =	0.30	0.067	0.080	0.002	0.120

FCM
No. of patients: 143, 131, 125, 114, 114
LS mean (95% CI): 5.1 (3.0, 7.2), 5.2 (2.9, 7.3), 6.0 (3.8, 8.3), 7.6 (5.3, 10.0), 7.0 (4.7, 9.4)

Placebo
No. of patients: 145, 141, 124, 113, 106
LS mean (95% CI): 3.5 (1.5, 5.6), 2.4 (0.2, 4.5), 3.2 (1.0, 5.5), 2.4 (0.04, 4.8), 4.4 (2.0, 6.9)

FCM vs Placebo: 1.5 (−1.4, 4.4), 2.8 (−0.2, 5.8), 2.8 (−0.3, 5.9), 5.2 (2.0, 8.5), 2.6 (−0.7, 5.9)

Continued

FIGURE 7.15 — *Continued*

Key: FCM, ferric carboxymaltose.

Shown are data across the study period using a repeat measures model for the changes (least squares mean with the 95% CIs on the 6MWT (A), fatigue score (assessed using a 10-point visual analogue fatigue scale, ranging from 1 for no fatigue to 10 for very severe fatigue) (B), Kansas City Cardiomyopathy questionnaire (KCCQ) score (on which the overall score ranges from 0 to 100, with a higher score indicating a better QoL) (C), and the European Quality of Life-5 Dimensions (EQ-5D) Visual Analogue Scale (on which the score ranges from 0 to 100, with higher scores indicating better health) (D).

Ponikowski P, et al; CONFIRM-HF Investigators. *Eur Heart J.* 2015;36(11):657-668.

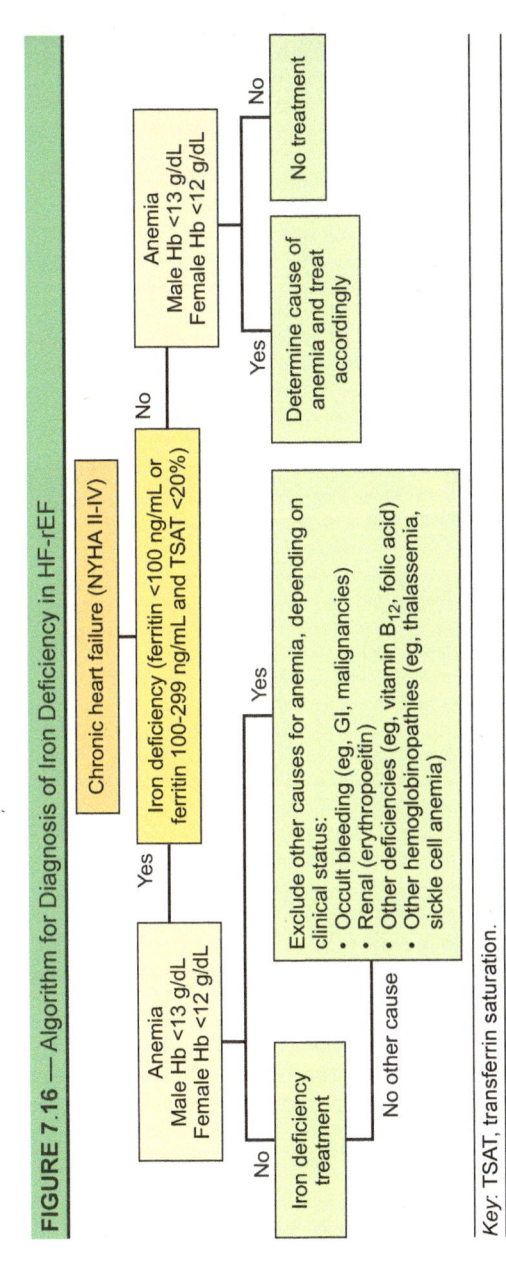

FIGURE 7.16 — Algorithm for Diagnosis of Iron Deficiency in HF-rEF

```
                    Anemia
                  Male Hb <13 g/dL
                  Female Hb <12 g/dL
                   /            \
                 Yes            No
                  |              |
        Chronic heart failure (NYHA II-IV)
                  |
        Iron deficiency (ferritin <100 ng/mL or
        ferritin 100-299 ng/mL and TSAT <20%)
           /                      \
         Yes                       No
          |                         |
  Exclude other causes        Anemia
  for anemia, depending       Male Hb <13 g/dL
  on clinical status:         Female Hb <12 g/dL
  • Occult bleeding            /         \
    (eg, GI, malignancies)    Yes         No
  • Renal (erythropoeitin)     |           |
  • Other deficiencies    Determine    No treatment
    (eg, vitamin B₁₂,     cause of
    folic acid)           anemia and
  • Other hemoglobinopathies treat
    (eg, thalassemia,      accordingly
    sickle cell anemia)
          |
      No other cause
          |
   Iron deficiency
      treatment
```

Key: TSAT, transferrin saturation.

McDonagh T, Macdougall IC. *Eur J Heart Fail.* 2015;17(3):248-262.

FIGURE 7.17 — Treatment Algorithm for Iron Deficiency in HF-rEF

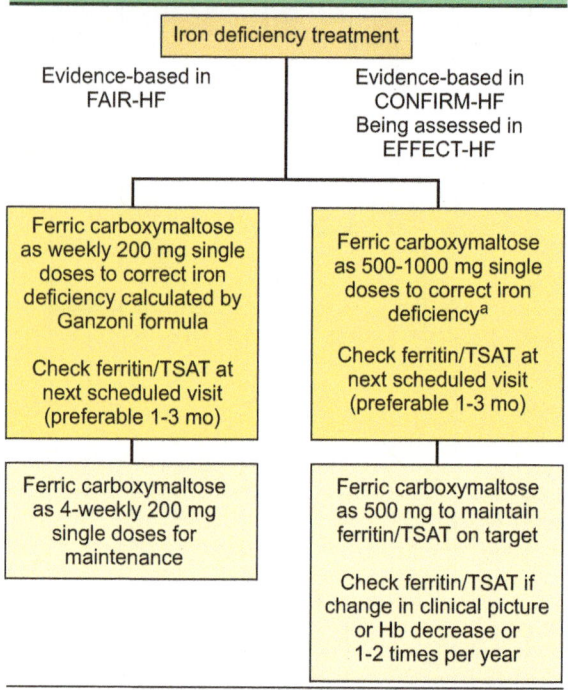

Iron deficiency treatment

Evidence-based in FAIR-HF

- Ferric carboxymaltose as weekly 200 mg single doses to correct iron deficiency calculated by Ganzoni formula

  Check ferritin/TSAT at next scheduled visit (preferable 1-3 mo)

- Ferric carboxymaltose as 4-weekly 200 mg single doses for maintenance

Evidence-based in CONFIRM-HF Being assessed in EFFECT-HF

- Ferric carboxymaltose as 500-1000 mg single doses to correct iron deficiency[a]

  Check ferritin/TSAT at next scheduled visit (preferable 1-3 mo)

- Ferric carboxymaltose as 500 mg to maintain ferritin/TSAT on target

  Check ferritin/TSAT if change in clinical picture or Hb decrease or 1-2 times per year

[a] See summary of product characteristics for ferric carboxymaltose.

McDonagh T, Macdougall IC. *Eur J Heart Fail.* 2015;17(3):248-262.

Heart Failure in Patients With Cancer (Cardio-oncology)

A substantial increase in the population of patients with coexisting cancer and heart disease, particularly HF, represents an unanticipated consequence of the striking improvement in cancer therapies over the past quarter century. As shown in **Figure 7.18**, anticancer agents have multiple, diverse adverse cardiac effects.

Chemotherapeutic agents, such as anthracyclines, antimetabolites, and cyclophosphamide, can induce permanent myocardial cell injury by multiple mechanisms and also by long-term cardiac remodeling. Signaling inhibitors such as human epidermal growth factor receptor 2 (HER2/erbB2) and angiogenesis inhibitors predominantly affect cardiac metabolism and contractile proteins and are associated with transient contractile dysfunction.[35]

Table 7.9 lists a number of important anticancer drugs and their CV effects.

Table 7.10 explains the frequency, mechanism, and reversibility associated with a variety of cancer therapies.

The newer signaling inhibitor agents may be associated with cardiotoxicity; fortunately, their effects may be more reversible than those of the anthracyclines. However, it is important for cardiologists to be aware of and recognize the risk factors and prevention strategies for patients receiving these agents. **Table 7.11** summarizes the key facts about anti-HER2 and VEGF cardiotoxicity.

In addition to HF, a number of anticancer drugs may cause QT-prolongation. This can be particularly important in the setting of diarrhea- and vomiting-induced electrolyte disturbances, and with concomitant medications (anti-emetics) that may further prolong the QT interval. One of the most important of the QT-prolonging agents, arsenic trioxide, may prolong the QT interval in up to 40% of treated patients, with a significant risk of Torsades de Pontes (TdP). Several of the newer signaling inhibitors may also prolong the QT interval, however, TdP is infrequent with their use.

Table 7.12 outlines CV risk assessment, monitoring, and management recommendations for patients who are at risk for cancer-related heart disease and HF.

Finally, radiation therapy directed at the chest in the treatment of breast cancer and lymphoma may lead to widespread cardiac and vascular injury, including the pericardium, valves, and the coronary circulation from the epicardial conduit vessels to the microvascular level. An expert consensus statement from the

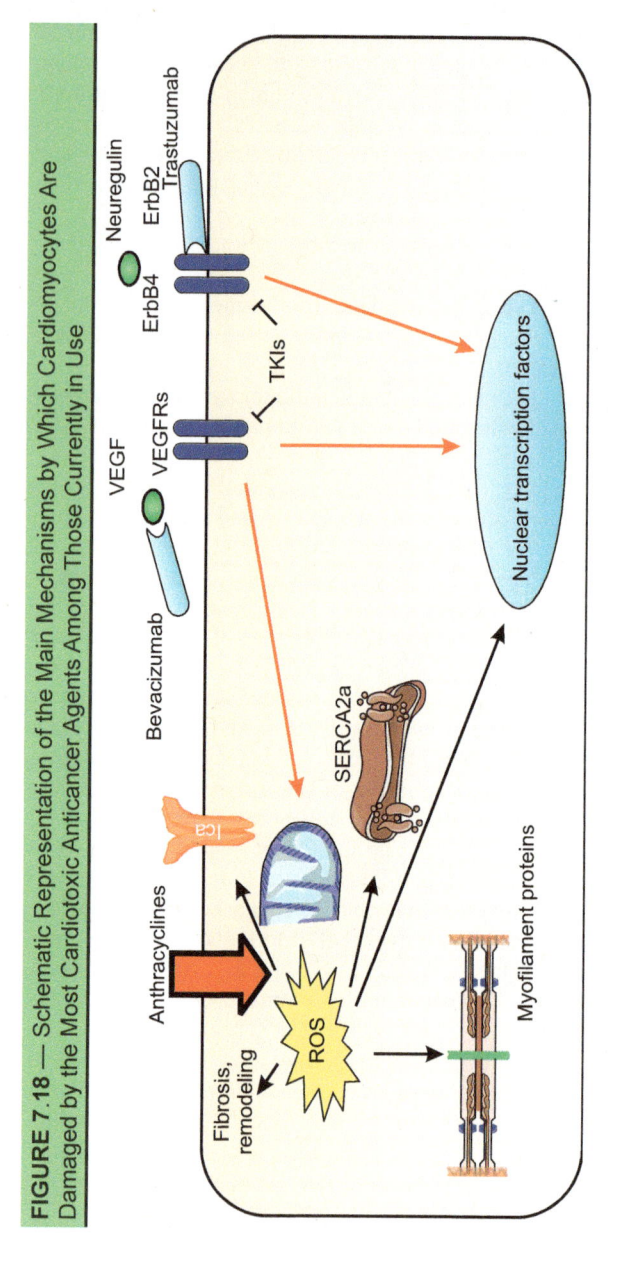

FIGURE 7.18 — Schematic Representation of the Main Mechanisms by Which Cardiomyocytes Are Damaged by the Most Cardiotoxic Anticancer Agents Among Those Currently in Use

Anthracyclines induce a DNA damage response and reactive oxygen species (ROS) production; these two initial events result in a cascade of secondary alterations affecting mitochondrial integrity and function, intracellular calcium dynamics, and contractile proteins. By blocking the activity of tyrosine kinase receptors, such as vascular endothelial growth factor receptor (VEGFR) or ErbB2/ErbB4, bevacizumab, trastuzumab, and tyrosine kinase inhibitors (TKIs) alter mitochondria and modulate gene expression. SERCA2a: sarcoendoplasmic reticulum calcium ATPase. Red arrows indicate physiologic, homeostatic effects. Black arrows indicate deleterious effects.

Modified from Molinaro M, et al. *Biomed Res Int*. 2015;2015:138148. http://dx.doi.org/10.1155/2015/138148.

TABLE 7.9 — Systemic Anticancer Drugs With Important Cardiovascular Effects

	Class/Drug		Selected Indications	Important CV Side Effects
Cytostatic chemotherapeutics	**Anthracyclines/Analogues**			
	Doxorubicin		Lymphoma	Cardiac dysfunction/HF
	Daunorubicin		Leukemia	
	Epirubicin		Breast cancer	
			Ovarian cancer	
			Sarcoma	
	Mitoxantrone		Leukemia	
			Multiple sclerosis	
	Pyrimidine Analogues			
	Fluorouracil (5-FU)		Colorectal cancer	Coronary spasms/ischemia
	Capecitabine		Breast cancer	
	Alkylating Agents			
	Cyclophosphamide		Breast cancer	Myocarditis (rare)
	Cisplatin		Genitourinary cancer	Thrombosis
	Antimicrotubule Agents			
	Paclitaxel		Breast cancer	Bradycardia
			Colorectal cancer	

Signaling inhibitors

Anti-HER2

Trastuzumab	Breast cancer	Cardiac dysfunction
Lapatinib	Gastric cancer	

Angiogenesis Inhibitors/Anti-VEGF

Bevacizumab	Gastrointestinal cancer	Hypertension
Sunitinib	Renal cell carcinoma	Endovascular damage
Sorafenib	Hepatocellular carcinoma	

BCR-ABL Inhibitors

Imatinib	Leukemia	Edema, cardiac dysfunction (rare)
Dasatinib	Gastric cancer	QTc prolongation
Nilotinib		

Hermann J, et al. *Mayo Clin Proc.* 2014;89(9):1287-1306.

TABLE 7.10 — Frequency, Mechanism, and Reversibility of Important Anticancer Agents

Cardiac Response	Drug	Frequency	Mechanism	Reversibility
Contractile dysfunction/heart failure	Anthracyclines	Cumulative dose-related	Myocyte death	Minimal
	Cyclophosphamide	Rare	Myocarditis	Partial
	Cisplatin	Rare	Unknown	Unknown
	Trastuzumab	Variable[a]	Contractile protein dysfunction	High
	Lapatinib			Reported
	Bevacizumab	Low	Hypertension?	Reported
	Sunitinib	Low	Mitochondrial dysfunction	Partial
	Sorafenib	Rare		Unknown
	Imatinib	Rare	Mitochondrial dysfunction	High
Arterial hypertension	*All angiogenesis inhibitors*	Moderate, dose-dependent	Endothelial dysfunction	Unknown
Myocardial ischemia	Pyrimidine analogues	Moderate	Direct vasospasm	High, unless infarction

Thromboembolism	Cisplatin	Moderate	Endothelial dysfunction	Variable
	All angiogenesis inhibitors	Moderate	Endothelial dysfunction	Variable
Arrhythmia/ QT prolongation	Arsenic trioxide	Moderate	HERG K + blockage	High
	Lapatinib	Rare	HERG K + blockage	Unknown
	Sunitinib	Rare	HERG K + blockage	Unknown
	Nolitinib	Rare	HERG K + blockage	Unknown
	Dasatinib	Rare	HERG K + blockage	Unknown

a Frequency in combination with anthracyclines.

Herrmann J, et al. *Mayo Clin Proc.* 2014;89(9):1287-1306.

TABLE 7.11 — Cardiotoxicity Related to Anti-HER2 and VEGF: Frequency, Mechanism, and Reversibility of Important Anticancer Agents

Anti-HER2 and VEGF Cardiotoxicity

- Contractile dysfunction related to contractile element and mitochondrial dysfunction
- Mostly reversible
- Risk factors:
  - Anthracycline-related (when used with anthracyclines, all anthracycline risk factors apply)
  - Lower pre-trastuzumab LV ejection fraction
  - Higher age
  - Pre-existing heart disease
- Prevention:
  - Decreased anthracyclinc burden
  - Increased time between anthracyclin and trastuzumab?

Herrmann J, et al. *Mayo Clin Proc.* 2014;89(9):1287-1306.

European Association of Cardiovascular Imaging and the American Society of Echocardiography recommends echocardiographic surveillance starting 5 years after treatment in high-risk patients and 10 years in all other patients.[36] High-risk patients should also receive a functional noninvasive stress test within 5 to 10 years of completion of chest radiation therapy. Of note, radiation therapy to the chest increases the technical complexity of cardiac surgery and risk of postoperative wound complications.

REFERENCES

1. Young JB, Stehlik J. Where's Waldo? Ischemic heart disease in new onset-heart failure, or finding Wald0. *J Am Coll Cardiol.* 2016. In press.

2. Velazquez EJ, Lee KL, Jones RH, et al. Coronary-artery bypass surgery in patients with ischemic myopathy. *N Engl J Med.* 2016;374:1511-1520.

3. Mentz RJ, Kelly JP, von Lueder TG, et al. Noncardiac comorbidities in heart failure with reduced versus preserved ejection fraction. *J Am Coll Cardiol.* 2014;64:2281-2293.

4. Weir DL, McAlister FA, Senthilselvan A Minhas-Sandu JK, Eurich DT. Sitagliptin use in patients with diabetes and heart failure: a population-based retrospective cohort study. *J Am Coll Cardiol HF.* 2014;2:573-582.

5. Bhatt DL, Cavender MA. Do dipeptidyl peptidase-4 inhibitors increase the risk of heart failure? *J Am Coll Cardiol HF.* 2014;2:583-585.

6. Filion KB, Azoulay L, Platt RW, et al. A multicenter observational study of incretin-based drugs and heart failure. *N Engl J Med.* 2016;374:1145-1154.

7. An H, He L. Current understanding of metformin effect on the control of hyperglycemia in diabetes. *J Endocrinol.* 2016;228:R97-R106.

8. Song R. Mechanism of metformin: a tale of two sites. *Diabetes Care.* 2016;39(2):187-189.

9. Eurich DT, Weir DL, Majumdar SR, et al. Comparative safety and effectiveness of metformin in patients with diabetes mellitus and heart failure: systematic review of observational studies involving 34000 Patients. *Circ Heart Fail.* 2013;6:395-402.

10. Kimura G. Importance of inhibiting sodium-glucose cotransporter and its compelling indication in type 2 diabetes: pathophysiological hypothesis. *J Am Soc Hypertens.* 2016;10:271-278

11. Triplitt C, Cornell S. Canagliflozin treatment in patients with type 2 diabetes mellitus. *Clin Med Insights Endocrinol Diabetes.* 2015;8:73-81.

12. Wu JHY, Foote C, Blomster J, et al. Effects of sodium-glucose cotransporter-2 inhibitors on cardiovascular events, death, and major safety outcomes in adults with type 2 diabetes: a systematic review and meta-analysis. *Lancet Diabetes Endocrinol.* 2016;4(5):411-419.

TABLE 7.12 — Assessment, Monitoring, and Management Recommendations for Patients at Risk of Cardiotoxicity (Stage A)

1—Risk Assessment (tests: TTE with strain, EKG, cTn)

Medication-Related Risk (risk score)		Patient-Related Risk Factors
High (4)	Anthracyclines, cyclophosphamide, ifosfamide, clofarabine, herceptin	• Cardiomyopathy or heart failure • CAD or equivalent (including PAD) • Hypertension • Diabetes mellitus • Prior or concurrent anthracycline • Prior to concurrent chest radiation • Age <15 or >65 years • Female gender
Intermediate (2)	Docetaxel, pertuzumab, sunitinib, sorafinib	
Low (1)	Bevacizumab, dasatinib, imatinib, lapatinib	
Rare (0)	Etoposide, rituximab, thalidomide	

Overall Risk by Cardiotoxicity Risk Score (CRS)

Risk categories by drug-related risk score plus number of patient-related risk factors):
CRS >6: very high, 5-6: high, 3-4: intermediate, 1-2: low, 0: very low

2—Monitoring Recommendations	
Very high cardiotoxicity risk	TTE with strain before every (other) cycle, end, 3-6 months, and 1 year, optional EKG, cTn with TTE during chemotherapy
High cardiotoxicity risk	TTE with strain every 3 cycles, end, 3-6 months, and 1 year after chemotherapy, optional EKG, cTn with TTE during chemotherapy
Intermediate cardiotoxicity risk	TTE with strain, mid-term, end, and 3-6 months after chemotherapy, optional EKG, cTn mid-term of chemotherapy
Low cardiotoxicity risk	Optional TTE with strain ± EKG, cTn at end of chemotherapy
Very low cardiotoxicity risk	None
3—Management Recommendations (apply as preventive measures before/with abnormalities during/after chemotherapy)	
Very high cardiotoxicity	Initiate ACEi/ARB, carvedilol, and statins, starting at lowest dose and start chemotherapy in 1 week from initiation to allow steady state, uptitrate as tolerated
High cardiotoxicity risk	Initiate ACEi/ARB ± carvedilol ± statins
Intermediate cardiotoxicity risk	Discuss risk and benefit of medications
Low cardiotoxicity risk	None, monitoring only
Very low cardiotoxicity risk	None, monitoring only

13. Shyangdan DS, Uthman OA, Waugh N. SGLT-2 receptor inhibitors for treating patients with type 2 diabetes mellitus: a systematic review and network meta-analysis. *BMJ Open.* 2016;6(2):e009417.

14. Jaiswal A, Chichra A, Nguyen VQ, et al. Challenges in the management of patients with chronic obstructive pulmonary disease and heart failure with reduced ejection fraction. *Curr Heart Fail Rep.* 2016;13:30-36.

15. Hawkins NM, Petrie MC, Jhund PS, et al. Heart failure and chronic obstructive pulmonary disease: diagnostic pitfalls and epidemiology. *Eur J Heart Fail.* 2009;11(2):130-139.

16. Marcun R, Stankovic I, Vidakovic R, et al. Prognostic implications of heart failure with preserved ejection fraction in patients with an exacerbation of chronic obstructive pulmonary disease. *Intern Emerg Med.* 2016;11(4):519-527.

17. Task Force for the Diagnosis and Treatment of Acute and Chronic Heart Failure 2012 of the European Society of Cardiology. ESC Guidelines for the diagnosis and treatment of acute and chronic heart failure 2012. *Eur Heart J.* 2012;33:1787-1847.

18. Le Jemtel TH, Padeletti M, Jelic S. Diagnostic and therapeutic challenges in patients with coexistent chronic obstructive pulmonary disease and chronic heart failure. *J Am Coll Cardiol.* 2007;49:171-180.

19. Salpeter S, Ormiston T, Salpeter E. Cardioselective beta-blockers for chronic obstructive pulmonary disease. *Cochrane Database Syst Rev.* 2005;(4):CD003566.

20. Böhm M, Robertson M, Ford I, et al. Influence of cardiovascular and noncardiovascular co-morbidities on outcomes and treatment effect of heart rate reduction with ivabradine in stable heart failure (from the SHIFT Trial). *Am J Cardiol.* 2015;116(12):1890-1897.

21. Tavazzi L, Swedberg K, Komajda M, et al. Clinical profiles and outcomes in patients with chronic heart failure and chronic obstructive pulmonary disease: an efficacy and safety analysis of SHIFT study. *Int J Cardiol.* 2013;170:182-188.

22. Hawkins NM, Petrie MC, Jhund PS, Chalmers GW, Dunn FG, McMurray JJ. Heart failure and chronic obstructive pulmonary disease: diagnostic pitfalls and epidemiology. *Eur J Heart Fail.* 2009;11(2):130-139.

23. Smilde TD, van Veldhuisen DJ, Navis G, Voors AA, Hillege HL. Drawbacks and prognostic value of formulas estimating renal function in patients with chronic heart failure and systolic dysfunction. *Circulation.* 2006;114:1572-1580.

24. Waldum-Grevbo B. What physicians need to know about renal function in outpatients with heart failure. *Cardiology.* 2015;131(2):130-138.

25. Jackson CE, Solomon SD, Gerstein HC, et al. Albuminuria in chronic heart failure: prevalence and prognostic importance. *Lancet.* 2009;374:543-550.

26. Heywood JT, Fonarow GC, Costanzo MR, et al, for the ADHERE Scientific Advisory Committee and Investigators. High prevalence of renal dysfunction and its impact on outcome in 118,465 patients hospitalized with acute decompensated heart failure: a report from the ADHERE database. *J Card Fail.* 2007;13:422-430.

27. Dries DL, Exner DV, Domanski MJ, et al. The prognostic implications of renal insufficiency in asymptomatic and symptomatic patients with left ventricular systolic dysfunction. *J Am Coll Cardiol.* 2000;35:681-689.

28. Ahmed A, Rich MW, Sanders PW, et al. Chronic kidney disease associated mortality in diastolic versus systolic heart failure: a propensity matched study. *Am J Cardiol.* 2007;99:393-398.

29. Hillege HL, Nitsch D, Pfeffer MA, et al, for the Candesartan in Heart Failure: Assessment of Reduction in Mortality and Morbidity (CHARM) Investigators. Renal function as a predictor of outcome in a broad spectrum of patients with heart failure. *Circulation.* 2006;113:671-678.

30. Cleland JGF, Zhang J, Pellicori P, et al. Prevalence and outcomes of anemia and hematinic deficiencies in patients with chronic heart failure. *JAMA Cardiol.* 2016;1(5):539-547.

31. Swedberg K, Young JB, Anand IS, et al. Treatment of anemia with darbepoetin alfa in systolic heart failure. *N Engl J Med.* 2013;368:1210-1219.

32. Anker SD, Comin CJ, Filippatos G, et al. Ferric carboxymaltose in patients with heart failure and iron deficiency. *N Engl J Med.* 2009;361:2436-2448.

33. Ponikowski P, van Veldhuisen DJ, Comin-Colet J, et al. Beneficial effects of long-term intravenous iron therapy with ferric carboxymaltose in patients with symptomatic heart failure and iron deficiency. *Eur Heart J.* 2015;36:657-668.

34. McDonagn T, Macdougall IC. Iron therapy for the treatment of iron deficiency in chronic heart failure: intravenous or oral? *Eur J Heart Fail.* 2015;17:248-262.

35. Suter TM, Ewer MS. Cancer drugs and the heart: importance and management. *Eur Heart J.* 2013;34:1102-1111.

36. Lancellotti P, Nkomo VT, Badano LP, et al. Expert consensus for multi-modality imaging evaluation of cardiovascular complications of radiotherapy in adults: a report from the European Association of Cardiovascular Imaging and the American Society of Echocardiography. *J Am Soc Echocardiogr.* 2013;26:1013-1032.

8 Interventions for Heart Failure

Aortic Stenosis

The prevalence of significant valvular heart disease increases with age in the general population and exceeds 10% in those over age 75 years.[1] In the over-75 age group, some 2% to 3% of individuals have aortic stenosis, and approximately one third of the symptomatic patients do not undergo surgical aortic valve replacement.[2]

In a 5-year follow-up of 2150 medically managed Medicare patients with aortic stenosis who had a hospitalization for HF, the mean duration of survival was 1.8 ± 1.6 years.[3] **Figure 8.1** shows the survival rates for the entire study population and for the high-risk and non–high-risk subjects separately.

The development and rapid improvement of transcatheter aortic valve replacement (TAVR) techniques now offers an alternative to surgical aortic valve replacement in such patients. A systematic review of functional status and quality of life after TAVR[4] that included 60 observational studies and two randomized trials found overall improvement in NYHA functional class that was sustained at 2 years post-procedure. **Figure 8.2** shows a Forrest plot of the data from the studies included in the review.

Despite substantial variability among the studies, there was evidence for efficacy in that TAVR was associated with improvement in symptoms, physical functioning, and disease-specific measures of quality of life. On the other hand, in this population with multiple comorbidities, improvement in more general health measures were smaller and less consistent.

In a meta-analysis of complications of TAVR that included 49 studies with a total of 16,063 patients, the

FIGURE 8.1 — Survival Rates After Heart Failure Hospitalization in Medically Managed Medicare Patients with Aortic Stenosis

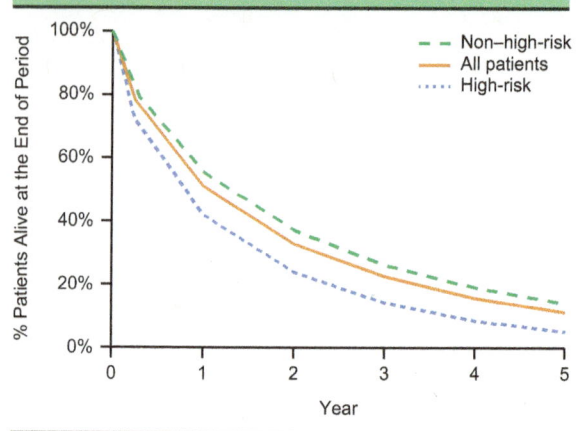

Clark, MA, et al. *Circ Cardiovasc Qual Outcomes.* 2012;5:697-704.

most common complications were heart block in 13% of patients, vascular access complications in 10%, and renal failure with 4.9% requiring dialysis. Overall 30-day and 1-year survival after TAVR were 91.9% (95% CI, 91.1% to 92.8%) and 79.2% (CI, 76.9% to 81.4%), respectively.[5]

Currently, there are two TAVR systems approved for use in the United States. The Edwards Sapien (Sapien, Sapien XT, and Sapien 3) transcatheter valve system is approved for "relief of aortic stenosis in patients with symptomatic heart disease due to severe native calcific aortic stenosis who are judged by a heart team, including a cardiac surgeon, to be at high or greater risk for open surgical therapy (ie, Society of Thoracic Surgeons operative risk score ≥8% or at a ≥15% risk of mortality at 30 days)." The Medtronic Evolut R System is FDA approved for "patients with severe aortic stenosis who are at high or extreme risk for surgery and for those with a failed surgical bioprosthesis."

In summary, TAVR has become an important option for older patients with HF due to stenotic aortic valve disease. Primary care physicians and HF cardiologists should actively consider the possibility of intervention for hemodynamically significant aortic stenosis for older patients who would not have been candidates for surgical aortic valve replacement in the past. **Figure 8.3** presents a schematic for decision-making in patients considered for TAVR.[6]

Mitral Regurgitation

As noted above, valvular heart disease has become an important problem in our ageing population. Mitral regurgitation (MR) affects nearly 10% of persons aged 75 or older.[7] Until very recently, effective treatment of mitral regurgitation required surgical valve repair or replacement. However, up to 50% of patients were managed non-operatively due to advanced age, LV dysfunction, or comorbidities that precluded surgery.

Importantly, mitral regurgitation may either be a cause of HF, as occurs with MR as a primary valve abnormality due to degenerative processes such as leaflet prolapse or flail leaflet associated with chordal rupture, or MR may be functional, occurring secondary to HF of various etiologies due to ventricular remodeling with impairment of leaflet coaptation from LV dilatation, subsequent leaflet tethering and/or annular dilatation.[8]

Current guidelines support surgical repair of degenerative mitral regurgitation in symptomatic patients and those with LV dilatation or dysfunction (class I), with a class IIa recommendation for those with new onset atrial fibrillation or pulmonary hypertension. Intervention for functional mitral regurgitation is more controversial, reflecting in part the advanced age and greater surgical risks associated with surgical repair in this setting. However, a substantial number of patients with MR of either etiology are not considered for surgical intervention.[8,9]

FIGURE 8.2 — Changes in NYHA Class After TAVR, After SAVR, and with Conservative Treatment

A. Mean change in NYHA class from baseline to 6–11 months

Author (Year)	Baseline Sample Size	Baseline Mean NYHA Class	Baseline SD NYHA Class	Follow-Up Sample Size	Follow-Up Mean NYHA Class	Follow-Up SD NYHA Class		Mean NYHA Class Change (95% CI)
TAVR								
Akin (2012)	11	3.20	0.80	8	1.34	0.70		−1.9 (−2.5, −1.2)
Attias (2010)	83	3.41	0.54	66	1.80	0.87		−1.5 (−1.7, −1.3)
Bagur (2011)	64	3.00	0.00	64	1.55	0.53		−1.5 (−1.6, −1.3)
Bedogni (2011)	25	3.16	0.37	21	1.19	0.39		−2.0 (−2.2, −1.8)
Bekeredjian (2010)	80	3.10	0.60	80	1.40	0.60		−1.7 (−1.9, −1.5)
Bleiziffer (2012)	227	3.42	0.63	159	1.69	0.67		−1.7 (−1.8, −1.6)
Chodor (2010)	11	3.09	0.29	10	2.10	0.30		−1.0 (−1.2, −0.8)
D'Onofrio (2011)	504	3.16	0.91	428	1.81	0.88		−1.4 (−1.5, −1.2)
Georgiadou (2011)	36	3.03	0.69	28	1.21	0.41		−1.8 (−2.1, −1.6)
Gilard (2012)	3132	2.88	0.63	1207	1.67	0.68		−1.2 (−1.3, −1.2)
Goncalves (2013)	74	2.99	0.42	53	1.49	0.66		−1.5 (−1.7, −1.3)
Himbert (2009)	75	3.36	0.58	61	1.77	0.61		−1.6 (−1.8, −1.4)
Himbert (2012)	15	3.27	0.44	13	1.81	0.88		−1.5 (−1.9, −1.0)
Kodali (2011)	55	3.22	0.65	38	1.76	0.84		−1.5 (−1.7, −1.2)
Latib (2012)	18	3.17	0.90	17	1.50	0.50		−1.7 (−2.1, −1.2)

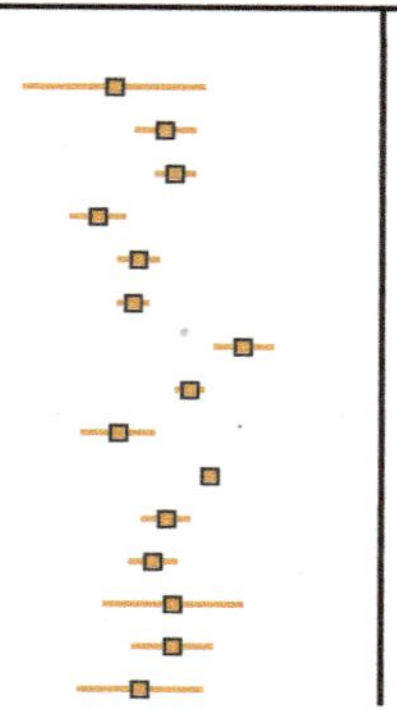

Study	N	Mean	SD	N	Mean	SD		Effect (95% CI)
Lefevre (2010)	130	3.00	0.61	95	1.60	0.71		−1.4 (−1.6, −1.2)
Osten (2010)	46	3.28	0.45	26	1.27	0.44		−2.0 (−2.2, −1.8)
Puls (2012)	180	3.15	0.50	128	1.59	0.79		−1.6 (−1.7, −1.4)
Schoenenberger (2013)	119	2.58	1.12	106	1.80	0.87		−0.8 (−1.0, −0.6)
Schueler (2012)	44	2.90	0.60	44	1.77	0.65		−1.1 (−1.3, −0.9)
Seiffert (2012)	11	3.10	0.57	8	2.25	1.05		−0.8 (−1.6, −0.1)
Stortecky (2012)	62	2.63	0.79	56	1.39	0.56		−1.2 (−1.5, −1.0)
Thielmann (2009)	39	3.28	0.55	19	1.21	0.52		−2.1 (−2.4, −1.8)
Treede (2010)	31	2.68	0.53	16	1.38	0.60		−1.3 (−1.6, −1.0)
Tzikas (2010)	96	3.15	0.91	68	2.06	1.03		−1.1 (−1.4, −0.8)
Ussia (2011)	79	2.80	0.60	70	1.60	0.50		−1.2 (−1.4, −1.0)
Ussia (2011)	143	2.73	0.61	124	1.50	0.59		−1.2 (−1.4, −1.1)
Webb (2007)	50	3.16	0.58	35	1.54	0.55		−1.6 (−1.8, −1.4)
Yamamoto (2012)	136	2.73	0.62	114	1.73	0.74		−1.0 (−1.1, −0.9)
Stortechky (2011)	40	2.70	0.80	36	1.50	0.70		−1.2 (−1.5, −0.9)
PARTNER Cohort A	348	3.47	0.60	296	1.80	0.76		−1.7 (−1.8, −1.6)
PARTNER Cohort B	179	3.36	0.62	125	1.84	0.70		−1.5 (−1.7, −1.4)
SAVR								
Stortechky (2011)	40	2.80	0.90	36	1.30	0.70		−1.5 (−1.8, −1.2)
PARTNER Cohort A	349	3.45	0.61	267	1.74	0.74		−1.7 (−1.8, −1.6)
Conservative Treatment								
PARTNER Cohort B ST	179	3.39	0.60	106	2.90	0.82		−0.5 (−0.7, −0.3)

Mean Change in NYHA Class (Follow-up − Baseline)

Continued

FIGURE 8.2 — Continued

B. Mean change in NYHA class from baseline to 12–23 months

Author (Year)	Baseline Sample Size	Baseline Mean NYHA Class	Baseline SD NYHA Class	Follow-Up Sample Size	Follow-Up Mean NYHA Class	Follow-Up SD NYHA Class	Mean NYHA Class Change (95% CI)
TAVR							
Bleiziffer (2012)	227	3.42	0.63	157	1.75	0.62	−1.7 (−1.8, −1.5)
De Brito (2012)	35	3.06	0.67	31	1.45	0.61	−1.6 (−1.9, −1.3)
Dvir (2012)	202	3.33	0.58	81	1.51	0.67	−1.8 (−2.0, −1.6)
Gilard (2012)	3132	2.88	0.63	402	1.67	0.66	−1.2 (−1.3, −1.1)
Gotzmann (2011)	51	3.08	0.44	51	2.01	1.00	−1.1 (−1.3, −0.8)
Grimaldi (2012)	145	2.80	0.58	124	1.50	0.70	−1.3 (−1.4, −1.2)
Gurvitch (2010)	70	3.11	0.49	57	1.42	0.62	−1.7 (−1.9, −1.5)
Kalavrouziotis (2011)	35	3.39	0.68	31	1.55	0.56	−1.8 (−2.1, −1.6)
Kodali (2011)	55	3.22	0.65	28	1.43	0.68	−1.8 (−2.1, −1.5)
Krane (2012)	186	3.05	0.42	106	2.04	0.74	−1.0 (−1.2, −0.9)
Lefevre (2010)	130	3.00	0.61	82	1.71	0.75	−1.3 (−1.5, −1.1)
Munoz-Garcia (2012)	133	3.23	0.65	80	1.34	0.52	−1.9 (−2.1, −1.7)
Osten (2010)	46	3.28	0.45	14	1.14	0.35	−2.1 (−2.4, −1.9)
Pasic (2011)	14	3.43	0.50	12	1.50	0.50	−1.9 (−2.3, −1.6)
Thielmann (2009)	39	3.28	0.55	10	1.30	0.64	−2.0 (−2.4, −1.5)

Study	N	Baseline	SD	N	Follow-up	SD	Mean Change (95% CI)
Thomas (2011)	1038	2.80	0.82	771	2.03	1.02	−0.8 (−0.9, −0.7)
Ussia (2010)	110	2.76	1.09	106	1.45	0.60	−1.3 (−1.5, −1.1)
Ussia (2011)	143	2.73	0.61	119	1.54	0.61	−1.2 (−1.3, −1.1)
Ussia (2012)	181	2.78	0.63	139	1.48	0.60	−1.3 (−1.4, −1.2)
Webb (2007)	50	3.16	0.58	17	1.76	0.73	−1.4 (−1.8, −1.0)
Webb (2009)	144	3.11	0.65	99	1.97	0.97	−1.2 (−1.4, −1.0)
Wilbring (2012)	7	3.00	0.00	7	2.00	0.54	−1.0 (−1.4, −0.6)
Ye (2010)	71	3.23	0.86	36	1.83	0.90	−1.4 (−1.8, −1.0)
Dvir (2013)	100	3.34	0.51	39	1.85	0.80	−1.5 (−1.8, −1.2)
Wenaweser (2011)	257	2.61	0.78	213	1.38	0.64	−1.2 (−1.3, −1.1)
PARTNER Cohort A	348	3.47	0.60	264	1.70	0.77	−1.8 (−1.9, −1.7)
PARTNER Cohort B	179	3.36	0.62	124	1.89	0.85	−1.5 (−1.6, −1.3)
SAVR							
Dvir (2013)	61	2.98	0.74	30	2.10	1.01	−0.9 (−1.3, −0.5)
Wenaweser (2011)	107	2.33	0.81	87	1.39	0.63	−0.9 (−1.1, −0.7)
PARTNER Cohort A	349	3.45	0.61	262	1.72	0.78	−1.7 (−1.8, −1.6)
Conservative Treatment							
Dvir (2013) ST	27	3.59	0.62	12	3.00	0.58	−0.6 (−1.0, −0.2)
Dvir (2013) MT	155	2.88	0.78	70	2.90	0.94	0.0 (−0.2, 0.3)
Wenaweser (2011) MT	77	2.64	0.79	35	2.71	0.81	0.1 (−0.3, 0.4)
PARTNER Cohort B ST	179	3.39	0.60	85	2.73	0.73	−0.7 (−0.8, −0.5)

Mean Change in NYHA Class (Follow-up − Baseline)

Kim CA, et al. *Ann Intern Med*. 2014;160:243-254.

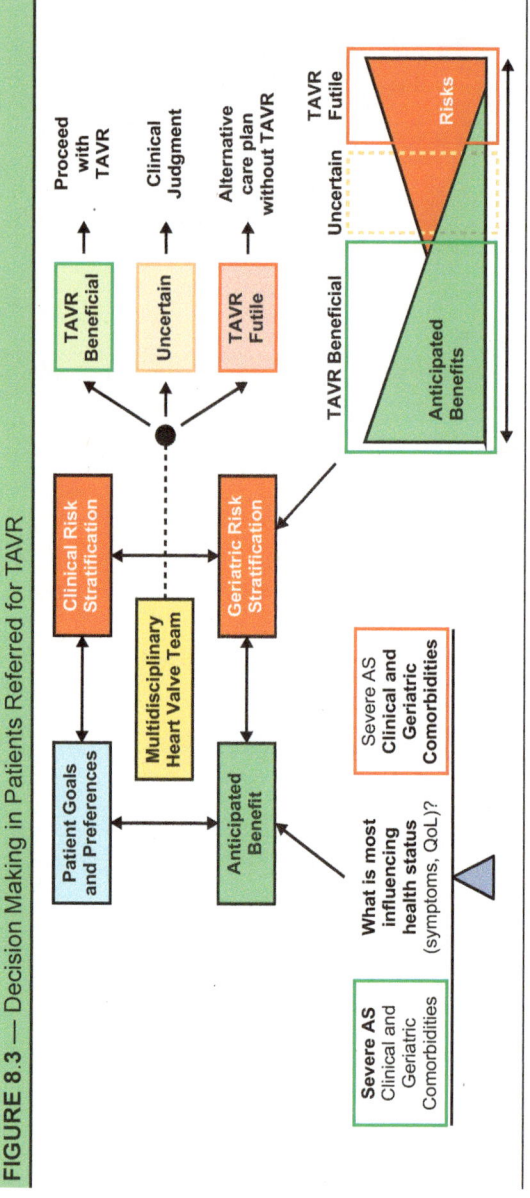

FIGURE 8.3 — Decision Making in Patients Referred for TAVR

Lindman BR, et al. *JACC Cardiovasc Interv.* 2014;7:707-716.

A catheter-based approach to mitral valve repair for MR that mimics the Alfieri central stitch surgical procedure, was first performed successfully in 2003.[10] Subsequently, the MitraClip (Abbot Vascular, Abbot Park, Illinois) system has been used in more than 16,000 patients and has been the subject of numerous reports.[8] **Figure 8.4** shows the approach.

The EVEREST II trial, a multicenter, randomized controlled trial, compared percutaneous repair versus surgery (either replacement or repair) in patients with symptomatic severe MR (≥3+) who were suitable candidates for surgical treatment.[11] The initial 1-year results showed significant improvement in

FIGURE 8.4 — MitraClip Implantation

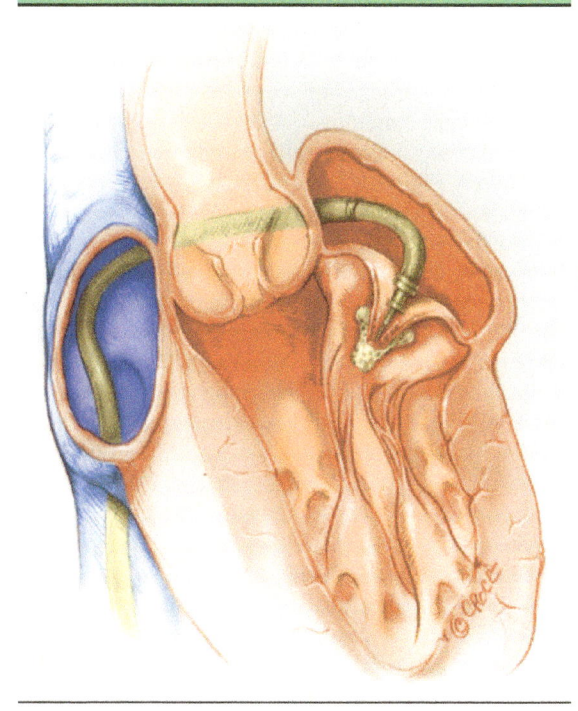

Wan B, et al. Ann *Cardiothorac Surg*. 2013;2(6):683-692.

LV dimensions and volumes, as well as improvement in NYHA class and quality of life. The 5-year results of EVEREST II showed no difference in mortality between the treatment groups; 20.8% and 26.8%, ($P=0.4$) for percutaneous repair and surgery, respectively. There was a low rate of crossover to MV surgery in the percutaneous repair patient after the first 6 months. Adverse events between 1 and 5 years were uncommon in both groups.[12]

A recent meta-analysis comparing outcomes for the MitraClip device and for surgery[13] included four publications: one randomized controlled trial (RCT) and three prospective observational studies. Compared to surgical patients, the MitraClip patients were older, had lower ejection fraction, and higher EuroSCORE risk. The MitraClip group had significantly more patients with post procedural MR severity graded >2 (17.2% vs 0.4%; $P<0.0001$), but mortality was similar in both groups at both 30 days (1.7% vs 3.5%; $P=0.54$) and 12 months (7.4% vs 7.3%; $P=0.66$), as were neurologic events and reoperations for failed procedures. **Figure 8.5** shows the 1-year results from the meta-analysis.

Of particular importance to HF management, data now accumulating from both clinical trials and observational registries support MR reduction with the MitraClip as a treatment option for patients with severely reduced LV function (EF <30%). In a European study of 51 CRT nonresponders with a mean LVEF of 27%, percutaneous valve repair improved NYHA functional class and reduced LV volumes in approximately 70% of the patients.[14] Uncontrolled observational reports evaluating the MitraClip in patients at high-risk for surgical repair who had MR associated with NYHA III-IV symptoms and markedly reduced ejection fraction have shown improvement in NYHA Class and 6-minute walk test performance, and reduction in NT-proBNP levels.[15,16]

At this time, there are no data demonstrating improvement in survival with the procedure. Safety

FIGURE 8.5 — Meta-analysis of 1 Year Events for MitraClip vs Surgery

Study or Subgroup	MitraClip Events	MitraClip Total	Surgery Events	Surgery Total	Weight	Odds Ratio M-H, Random, 95% CI
Feldman	11	181	5	89	46.5%	1.09 [0.37, 3.23]
Paranskaya	2	24	0	26	5.8%	5.89 [0.27, 129.15]
Taramasso	6	52	10	91	47.7%	1.06 [0.36, 3.10]
Total (95% CI)		**257**		**206**	**100.0%**	**1.18 [0.56, 2.48]**
Total events	19		15			

Heterogeneity: Tau^2 = 0.00; Chi^2 = 1.11, df = 2 (P = 0.57); I^2 = 0%
Test for overall effect: Z = 0.44 (P = 0.66)

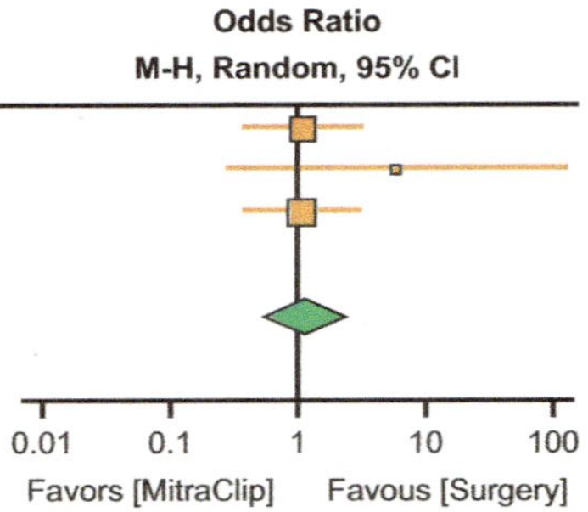

Wan B, et al. *Ann Cardiothorac Surg.* 2013;2:683-692.

data across the board have been reassuring and indicate that a "learning curve" with steadily decreasing procedure times and complications exists. In a meta-analysis of 16 studies that included 2980 patients receiving the MitraClip, the acute procedural success rate was 91% with a mortality of 0.1%. Thirty-day mortality was 4.2% and increased to approximately 16% at long-term follow-up at 310 days. Blood transfusion was the most common adverse procedural event.[17]

Table 8.1 lists the complications associated with the MitraClip procedure.

TABLE 8.1 — Complications of the MitraClip Procedure

Complications Associated With Percutaneous Valve Implantation

- Partial clip detachment
- Thrombus formation on the catheter
- Chordae tendineae entrapment by the MitraClip
- Pericardial effusion or tamponade
- Persistent atrial septal defect
- Cardiac arrhythmias
- Air embolism

Based on current evidence, surgery is the standard treatment for MR in eligible patients. However, the available data suggest that percutaneous mitral valve repair is associated with similar mortality rates and symptomatic improvement.

Left Atrial Appendage Closure

As noted in *Chapter 5*, atrial fibrillation occurs in 30% to 40% of HF patients. Because age and heart failure are major components of the accepted stroke-risk scoring systems ($CHADS_2$ and CHADS-Vasc), chronic oral anticoagulation for prevention of thromboembolic stroke is generally appropriate for heart failure patients. However, a large subset of HF patients have absolute or relative contraindications to chronic anticoagulation or refuse anticoagulant prophylaxis. As a result, only 50% to 60% of the eligible patients actually receive chronic oral anticoagulation.[18]

In patients with chronic AF, the left atrial appendage (LAA) is felt to be the origin of 80% to 85% of thromboembolic strokes, and a number of percutaneously delivered LAA occlusion devices have been developed. Currently, the Watchman Left Atrial Appendage Closure Device is FDA approved to reduce the risk of thromboembolism from the left atrial appendage in patients with non-valvular atrial fibrillation who:

- Are at increased risk for stroke and systemic embolism based on CHADS2 or CHA2DS2-VASc scores and are recommended for anticoagulation therapy
- Are deemed by their physicians to be suitable for warfarin; and
- Have an appropriate rationale to seek a non-pharmacologic alternative to warfarin, taking into account the safety and effectiveness of the device compared to warfarin. **Figure 8.6** shows the device and implantation approach.

A long-term prospective single-center analysis that included 102 consecutive patients who underwent implantation of the (second-generation) Watchman device between June 2006 and August 2010 provided important efficacy data. The mean follow-up was 3.0 ± 1.6 years. In this series, 96% of patients had successful implantations and 9 of 102 had procedure-related adverse events. (Three had pericardiocentesis; another four had pericardial effusions treated conservatively. One patient had a rash, and one had a minor post-procedural femoral bleed.) The annual rate of ischemic stroke was 0.7%, and of combined ischemic stroke and TIA was 1.4%. Eighty-nine of 96 patients were free of any stroke or TIA.[19] **Figure 8.7** below shows the Kaplan Meier curves for cumulative event rates in this series.

FIGURE 8.6 — The Watchman Left Atrial Appendage Closure Device

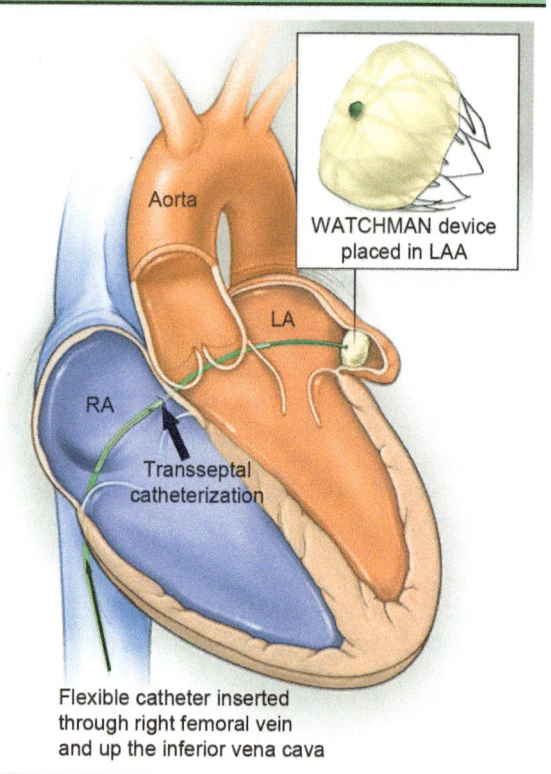

The device is a self-expanding nitinol structure that is delivered percutaneously with femoral venous access and transseptal technique to the LAA. The device is positioned with the use of angiography and TEE. Implantation is performed in either a cardiac catheterization or electrophysiology laboratory with the patient under general anesthesia or conscious sedation.

Maisel WH. *N Engl J Med*. 2009;360(25):2601-2603.

A pooled patient-level analysis of the two randomized clinical trials comparing WATCHMAN with long-term warfarin in atrial fibrillation addressed bleeding rates. Overall, there were 1114 patients (732 assigned to device and 382 to warfarin). The mean age was

72.9±8.5 years, and the mean CHA_2DS_2-VASc score was 3.7±1.4. Major bleeding from randomization to the end of follow-up was similar in the WATCHMAN compared to warfarin groups; 3.5 and 3.6 events/100 patient-years. However, 48% of the bleeding events in the device group occurred during the periprocedural phase, within 7 days after randomization. The LAA closure device group had a significantly reduced rate of major bleeding compared with long-term warfarin beyond 7 days post-randomization (1.8 events vs 3.6 events per 100 patient-years; RR: 0.49; 95% CI: 0.32-0.75; $P=0.001$), and particularly beyond 6 months post-randomization when the device group had discontinued antithrombotics.[20] **Figure 8.8** shows Kaplan Meier curves for major bleeding over various periods of follow-up.

In summary, HF patients with atrial fibrillation who are not candidates for stroke prophylaxis with chronic oral anticoagulation should be considered for LAA closure device placement.

Implantable Hemodynamic Monitoring

Currently, more than 1 million HF hospitalizations per year cost Medicare more than $17 billion annually. These staggering numbers and a growing realization that recurrent hospitalizations are associated with poor outcomes have prompted widespread interest in attempts to decrease hospitalization. However, outpatient monitoring programs based on intensive weight surveillance and/or monitoring of vital signs via telemetry have not proven effective.[21]

The COMPASS-HF (Chronicle Offers Management to Patients with Advanced Signs and Symptoms of Heart Failure) trial,[22] using an implantable hemodynamic monitoring device that required an RV sensing lead, demonstrated a reduction in the risk of first hospitalization although the overall outcome was neutral. COMPASS-HF, however, provided two critical insights that paved the way for future success with ambulatory hemodynamic monitoring. First, the

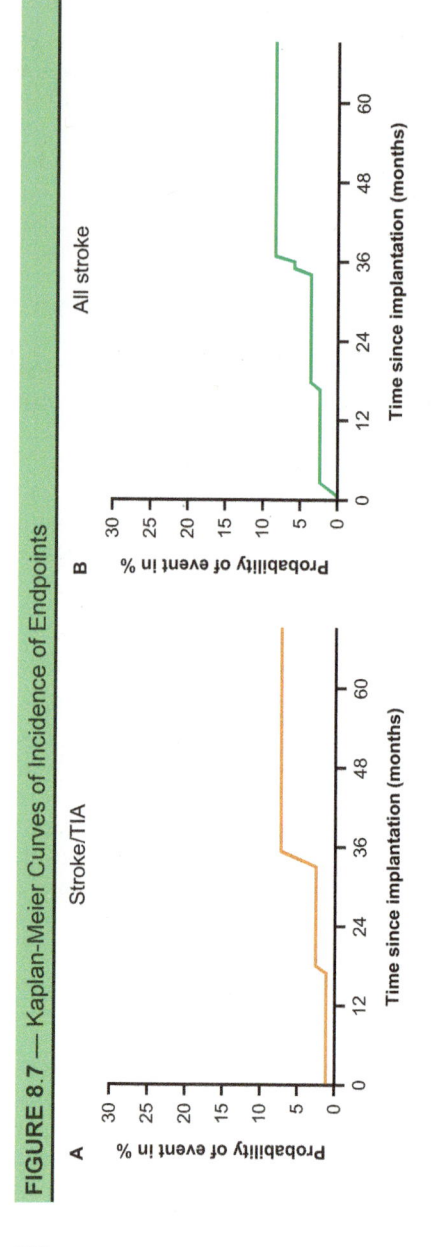

FIGURE 8.7 — Kaplan-Meier Curves of Incidence of Endpoints

A. Stroke/TIA

B. All stroke

All-cause mortality/all stroke

All-cause mortality

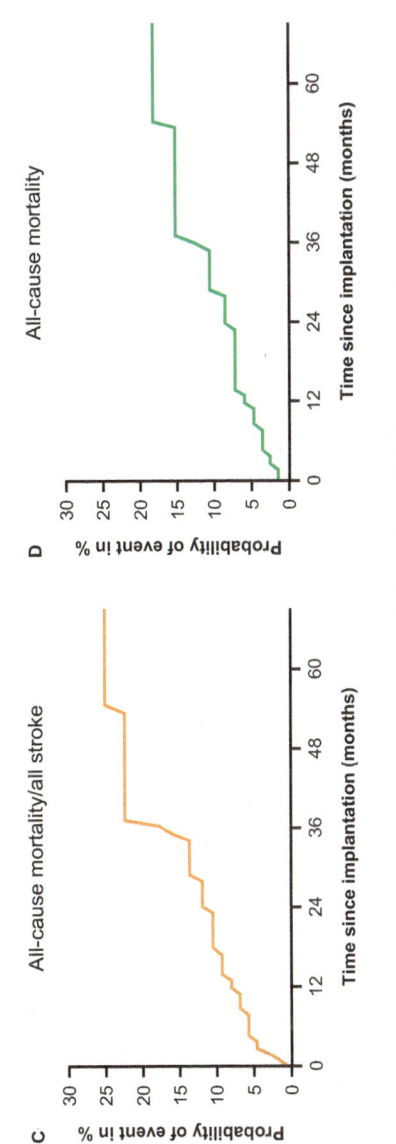

Time (months)	0	12	24	36	48	60
Patients at risk	96	80	65	40	34	18

Incidence of stroke and transient ischemic attack (TIA) *(A)*, hemorrhagic and ischemic stroke *(B)*, all-cause mortality and all-cause stroke *(C)*, and all-cause mortality *(D)* for all patients with successful Watchman implantation are illustrated over time.

Wiebe J, et al. *J Am Coll Cardiol Interv*. 2015;8(15):1915-1921.

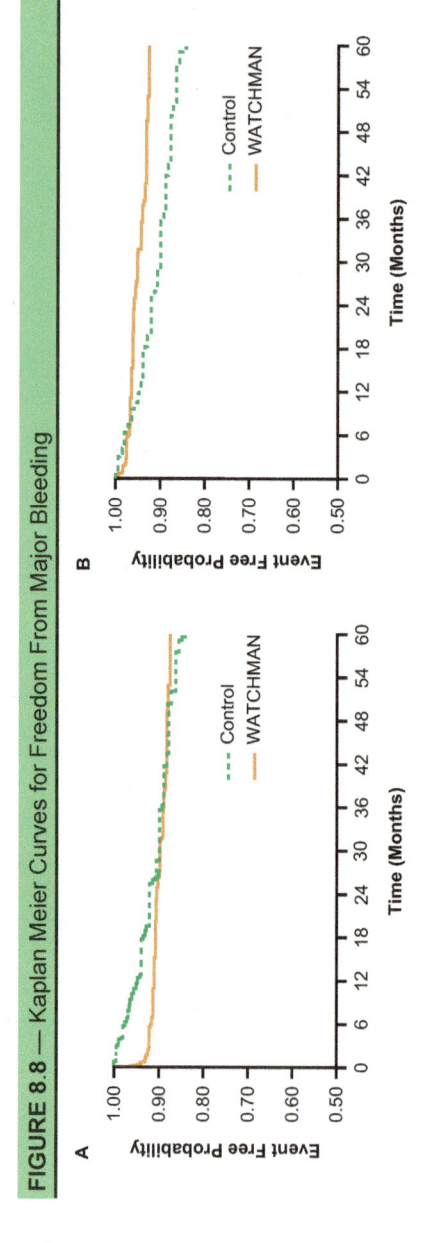

FIGURE 8.8 — Kaplan Meier Curves for Freedom From Major Bleeding

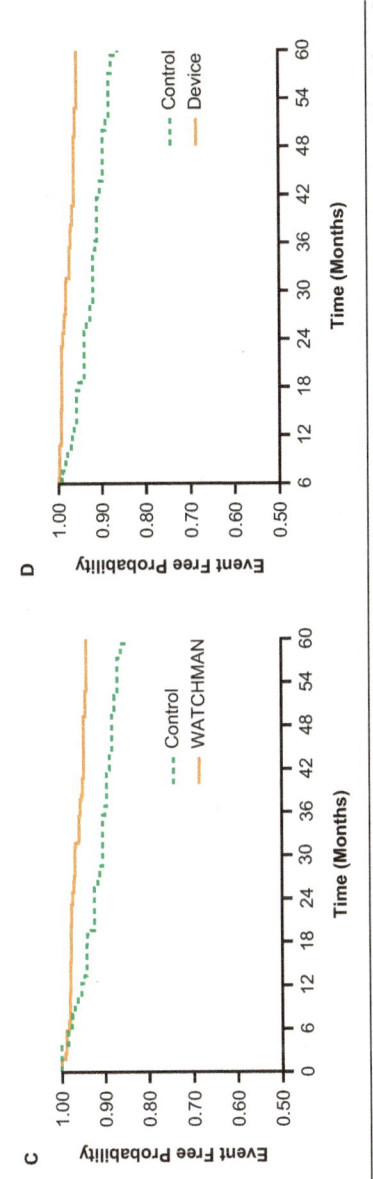

Freedom from first major bleed from randomization to the end of follow-up (P=0.97) (A). Freedom from first major bleed from 8 days post-randomization to the end of follow-up (the post-procedural period) (P=0.002) (B). Freedom from first major bleed from 45 days post-randomization to the end of follow-up (HR: 0.38; 95% CI: 0.33 to 0.44; P<0.001) (C). Freedom from first major bleed from 6 months post-randomization to the end of follow-up (HR: 0.28; 95% CI: 0.23 to 0.35; P<0.001) (D).

Price MJ, et al. *J Am Coll Cardiovasc Interv.* 2015;8(15):1925-1932.

data clearly confirmed that ambulatory HF patients showed increases in filling pressures 2 to 3 weeks before a clinical HF event. Second, the trial clarified that the monitoring system could only provide data; hemodynamic goals for therapy and a protocol-driven response to changes in filling pressures would be required for the monitoring system data to meaningfully impact therapy.

The CardioMEMS Heart Sensor Allows Monitoring of Pressure to Improve Outcomes in NYHA Class III Heart Failure Patients (CHAMPION) trial enrolled 550 patients with New York Heart Association (NYHA) class III HF, irrespective of the left ventricular ejection fraction, and a previous hospital admission for HF.[23] CHAMPION, which employed a wireless, totally implantable sensor, was a single blind trial undertaken to demonstrate that an implantable hemodynamic monitoring system could reduce hospitalization rates in patients with HF. The trial incorporated the critical concept that the success of implantable hemodynamic monitoring depends on the premise that elevated filling pressures can be modified with adjustments of medical therapy. The goal of treatment in the trial was to achieve a PA mean pressure <25 mm Hg and a PA-diastolic pressure ≤20 mm Hg.

The primary efficacy endpoint was the rate of heart-failure-related hospitalizations at 6 months. The safety endpoints assessed at 6 months were freedom from device-related or system-related complications (DSRC) and freedom from pressure-sensor failures. At 6 months, the active treatment group ($N=270$) had 84 heart-failure–related hospitalizations while the control group ($N=280$) had 120 (rate 0.32 vs 0.44, HR 0.72, 95% CI 0.60-0.85, $P=0.0002$).

The specific interventions that were employed in the CHAMPION Trial have been reported in detail.[24] **Figure 8.9** shows the treatment algorithm for trends in PA pressure. As shown in **Figure 8.10**, the active treatment group had many more medication changes than the controls across all drug classes. Importantly, decreases in diuretic dose were strikingly more frequent in the active PA-pressure monitoring group, as shown in **Figure 8.11**.

As noted in the report of specific interventions, PA-pressure guided management in patients with HF-rEF facilitated higher dosing of neurohormonal antagonists. The detailed analysis of pharmacologic management in CHAMPION underscores the importance of having specified hemodynamic targets for therapeutic interventions and guiding such interventions following a specified algorithm.

This approach is essential to effectively translating the strategy used in the CHAMPION trial into clinical practice. The CardioMEMS HF System (St Jude Medical) was FDA approved in 2014 for wirelessly measuring and monitoring PA pressure and heart rate in New York Heart Association (NYHA) Class III HF patients who have been hospitalized for HF in the previous year.

In summary, despite the advanced age and frailty of most patients with HF, important new interventions for both aortic and mitral valve dysfunction and for chronic hemodynamic monitoring offer opportunities to improve both functional status and clinical outcomes for many individuals.

Mechanical Circulatory Support

The clinical realization that patients with HF-rEF can be successfully managed with mechanical support of left ventricular function reflects three issues, two of which are rapidly changing. First, the option for cardiac transplantation has always been strictly limited by donor availability. Second, the 2001 REMATCH study[25] documented for the first time that left ventricular mechanical support was a viable option for prolonged management of many patients. Third, progressive technical improvements in left ventricular assist devices (LVADs), particularly the introduction of axial flow pumps, have made the devices clinically

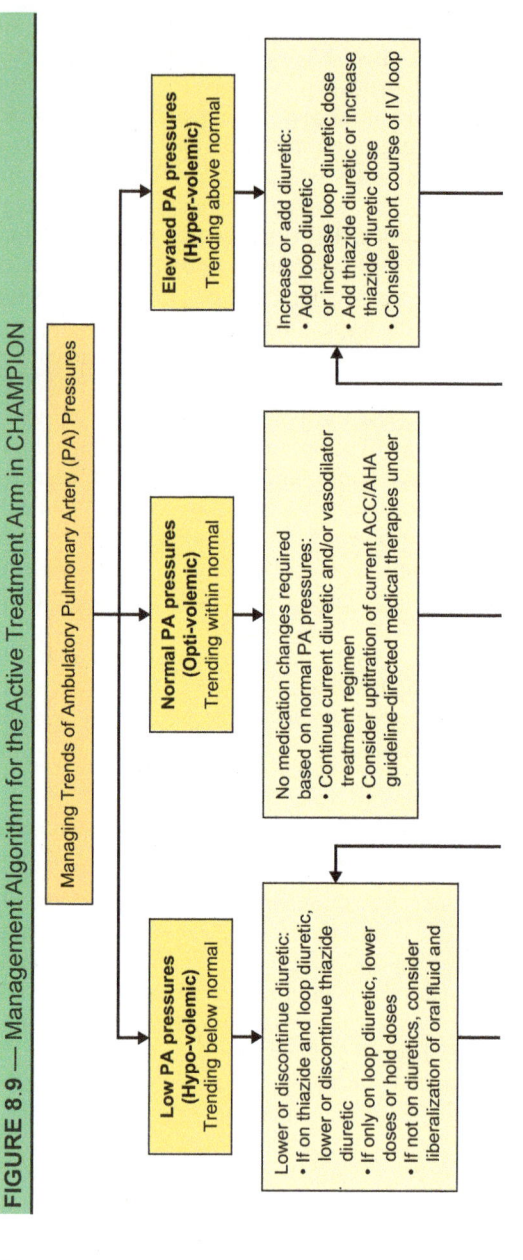

FIGURE 8.9 — Management Algorithm for the Active Treatment Arm in CHAMPION

Managing Trends of Ambulatory Pulmonary Artery (PA) Pressures

Low PA pressures (Hypo-volemic) Trending below normal

Lower or discontinue diuretic:
- If on thiazide and loop diuretic, lower or discontinue thiazide diuretic
- If only on loop diuretic, lower doses or hold doses
- If not on diuretics, consider liberalization of oral fluid and

Normal PA pressures (Opti-volemic) Trending within normal

No medication changes required based on normal PA pressures:
- Continue current diuretic and/or vasodilator treatment regimen
- Consider uptitration of current ACC/AHA guideline-directed medical therapies under

Elevated PA pressures (Hyper-volemic) Trending above normal

Increase or add diuretic:
- Add loop diuretic or increase loop diuretic dose
- Add thiazide diuretic or increase thiazide diuretic dose
- Consider short course of IV loop

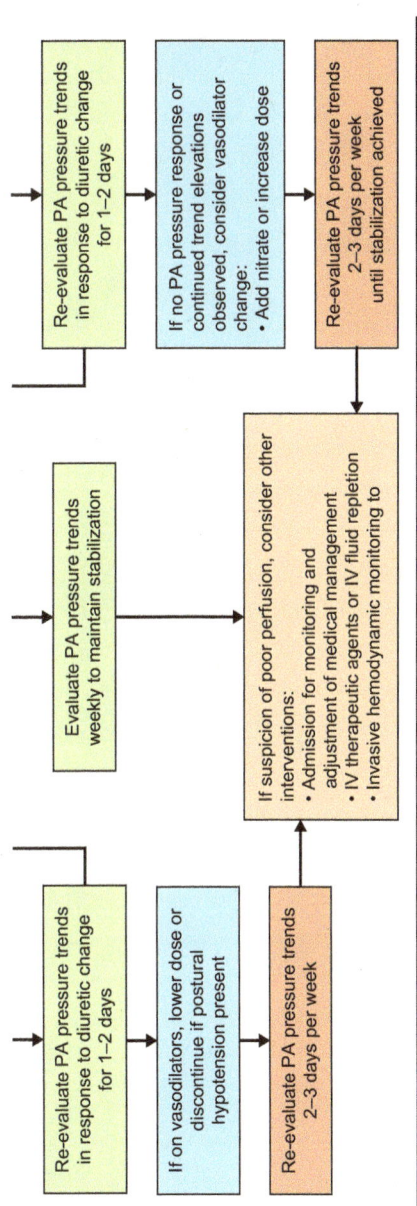

```
┌─────────────────────────┐      ┌─────────────────────────┐      ┌─────────────────────────┐
│ Re-evaluate PA pressure │      │   Evaluate PA pressure  │      │ Re-evaluate PA pressure │
│ trends in response to   │      │   trends weekly to      │      │ trends in response to   │
│ diuretic change for     │      │   maintain stabilization│      │ diuretic change for     │
│ 1–2 days                │      │                         │      │ 1–2 days                │
└───────────┬─────────────┘      └───────────┬─────────────┘      └───────────┬─────────────┘
            │                                │                                │
┌───────────▼─────────────┐                  │                    ┌───────────▼─────────────┐
│ If on vasodilators,     │                  │                    │ If no PA pressure       │
│ lower dose or           │                  │                    │ response or continued   │
│ discontinue if postural │                  │                    │ trend elevations        │
│ hypotension present     │                  │                    │ observed, consider      │
└───────────┬─────────────┘                  │                    │ vasodilator change:     │
            │                                │                    │  • Add nitrate or       │
┌───────────▼─────────────┐                  │                    │    increase dose        │
│ Re-evaluate PA pressure │                  │                    └───────────┬─────────────┘
│ trends 2–3 days per     │                  │                                │
│ week                    │                  │                    ┌───────────▼─────────────┐
└─────────────────────────┘                  │                    │ Re-evaluate PA pressure │
                                             │                    │ trends 2–3 days per     │
                                             │                    │ week until stabilization│
                                             │                    │ achieved                │
                                             │                    └─────────────────────────┘
                                 ┌───────────▼─────────────────────────────────┐
                                 │ If suspicion of poor perfusion, consider    │
                                 │ other interventions:                        │
                                 │  • Admission for monitoring and adjustment  │
                                 │    of medical management                    │
                                 │  • IV therapeutic agents or IV fluid        │
                                 │    repletion                                │
                                 │  • Invasive hemodynamic monitoring to       │
                                 └─────────────────────────────────────────────┘
```

The PA pressure treatment guidelines for the CHAMPION trial used a treatment algorithm in response to patient hemodynamic trend data. The low PA pressure and elevated PA pressure algorithms implemented change protocols for diuretic and/or vasodilator therapies to achieve hemodynamic stabilization. In the presence of normal PA pressures, continuation of existing patient treatment regimens with consideration for further uptitration of guideline-directed medical therapy was recommended.

, ostanzo MR, et al *JACC Heart Fail*. 2016;4(5):333-344.

FIGURE 8.10 — Changes in Medication Overall and by Class of Agent in Active vs Control Groups in CHAMPION

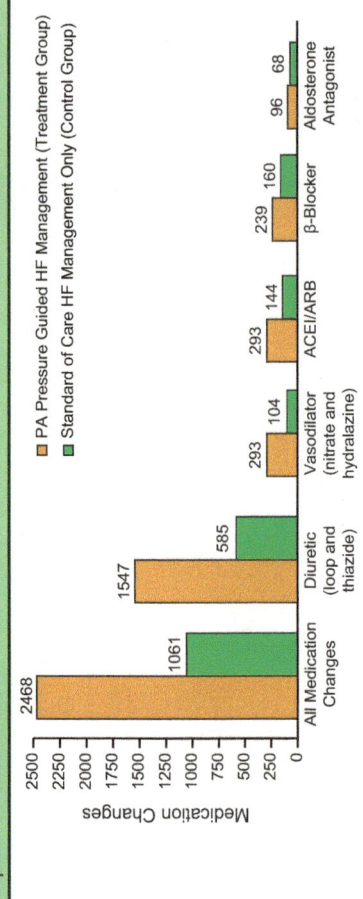

Total HF medication changes occurring during the 6-month follow-up period were compared between the active monitoring group (PA pressure-guided HF management added to standard of care management of patient clinical signs and symptoms) (*orange bars*) and the blind therapy group (HF management including only standard assessment of weights and patient-reported symptoms) (*green bars*). In addition, medication changes by HF drug class were compared between groups.

Costanzo MR, et al. *JACC Heart Fail.* 2016;4(5):333-344.

FIGURE 8.11 — Increases and Decreases in Medication Dose in the Active and Control Groups in CHAMPION

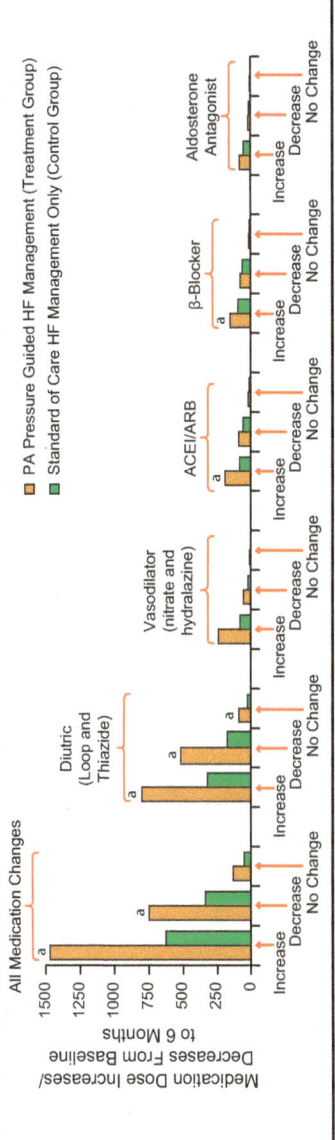

No Change represents instances where a medication was changed (eg, dose frequency, route, etc) that resulted in no net daily dose equivalent change. Increases and decreases in all classes of HF medications during the 6-month follow-up period were compared between the active monitoring group *(orange bars)* and the blind therapy group *(green bars)*. The greater number of medication decreases in the active monitoring group is entirely caused by a greater number of reductions in diuretic doses.

[a] $P<0.05$ PA Pressure Guided HF Management vs Standard of Care HF Management.

Costanzo MR, et al. *JACC Heart Fail.* 2016;4(5):333-344.

acceptable in terms of cost, size, efficacy, and durability. **Figure 8.12** shows the HeartMate II device used in the ROADMAP Study.

The Interagency Registry for Mechanically Assisted Circulatory Support classification for advanced heart failure, shown in **Table 8.2**, provides a clinically useful approach for describing LVAD candidates.

The ROADMAP Study (Risk Assessment and Comparative Effectiveness of Left Ventricular Assist Device [LVAD] and Medical Management [ROADMAP]; NCT01452802), published in 2015[26] was a prospective, multicenter observational study of 200 patients with INTERMACS profiles 4, 5, and 6 who had one or more hospitalizations for HF-rEF in the last 12 months and a 6MWD <300 m. All patients had NYHA functional class IIIB/IV symptoms, were not dependent on intravenous inotropic support, and met the US FDA–approved indications for HeartMate II LVAD destination therapy. Patients who met entry criteria elected to continue optimal medical management (OMM) or to undergo LVAD implantation.

The primary composite endpoint was survival on original therapy with improvement in 6MWD ≥75 m at 12 months. "Of the 103 OMM patients, 18 died, 18 received a delayed LVAD at least 1 month after enrollment (including one patient receiving a total artificial heart), and nine patients withdrew from the study before reaching an outcome, leaving 58 patients alive on original OMM therapy at 12 months." In contrast, "For the 97 patients in the LVAD arm, 17 died, three received a heart transplant (two urgent and one elective), and three withdrew from the study within 30 days of enrollment before receiving an LVAD, leaving 74 patients on LVAD support at 12 months." The LVAD patients experienced greater improvements in functional status and quality of life; however, they experienced substantially more adverse events (AEs). Bleeding was the most common LVAD AE. Taken together, surgical and nonsurgical bleeding accounted

FIGURE 8.12 — The HeartMate II LVAD

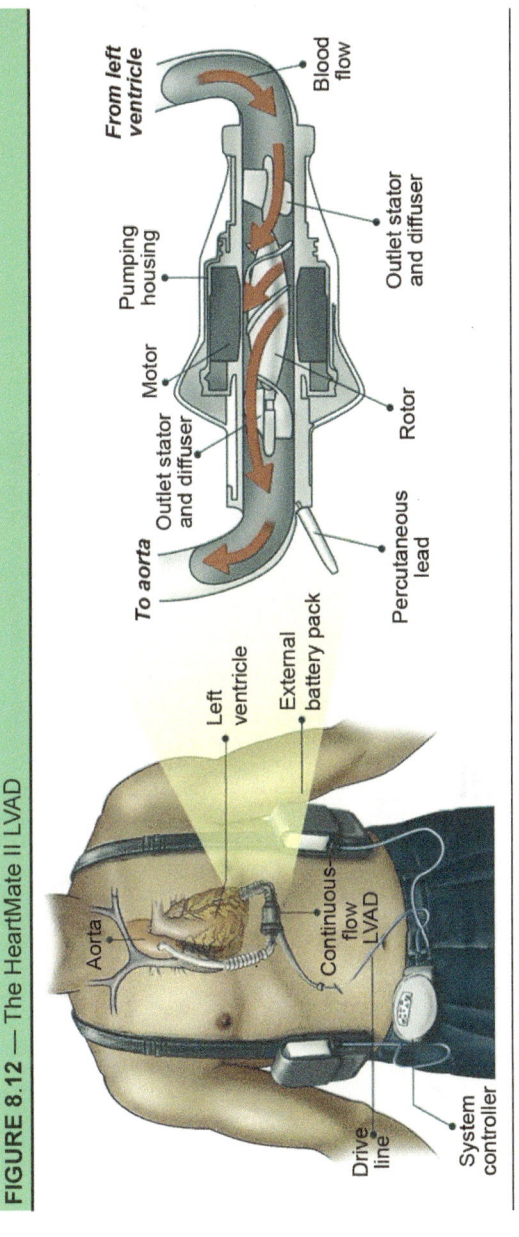

Sajgalik P, et al. *Mayo Clin Proc.* 2016;91:927-940.

TABLE 8.2 — INTERMACS (Interagency Registry for Mechanically Assisted Circulatory Support) Stages for Classifying Patients with Advanced Heart Failure

INTERMACS Level	NYHA Class	Description	Device	1-y Survival With LVAD Therapy
1. Cardiogenic shock "Crash and burn"	IV	Hemodynamic instability in spite of increasing doses of catecholamines and/or mechanical circulatory support with critical hypoperfusion of target organs (severe cardiogenic shock).	ECLS, ECMO, percutaneous support devices	52.6±5.6%
2. Progressive decline despite inotropic support "Sliding on inotropes"	IV	Intravenous inotropic support with acceptable blood pressure but rapid deterioration of renal function, nutritional state, or signs of congestion.	ECLS, ECMO, LVAD	63.1±3.1%
3. Stable but inotrope dependent "Dependent stability"	IV	Hemodynamic stability with low or intermediate doses of inotropics, but necessary due to hypotension, worsening of symptoms, or progressive renal failure.	LVAD	78.4±2.5%
4. Resting symptoms "Frequent flyer"	IV ambulatory	Temporary cessation of inotropic treatment is possible, but patient presents with frequent symptom recurrences and typically with fluid overload.	LVAD	78.7±3.0%

5. Exertion intolerant "Housebound"	IV ambulatory	Complete cessation of physical activity, stable at rest, but frequently with moderate fluid retention and some level of renal dysfunction.	LVAD	93.0±3.9%
6. Exertion limited "Walking wounded"	III	Minor limitation on physical activity and absence of congestion while at rest. Easily fatigued by light activity.	LVAD/Discuss LVAD as option	—
7. "Placeholder"	III	Patient in NYHA Class III with no current or recent unstable fluid balance.	Discuss LVAD as option	—

[a] Kaplan-Meier estimates with standard error of the mean for 1 year survival with LVAD therapy. Patients were censored at time of last contact, recovery or heart transplantation. Due to small numbers outcomes for INTERMACS levels 5, 6, 7 were combined.

Ponikowski P, et al. *Eur Heart J.* 2016;37:2129-2200.

for 65% of LVAD AEs. Worsening HF accounted for 82% of OMM events. **Figure 8.13** shows the overall outcomes from ROADMAP.

As shown in **Table 8.3**, the 2016 ESC Guidelines include long-term LVAD therapy among the current indications for mechanical circulatory assist devices. **Table 8.4** shows the 2016 ESC guideline patient eligibility criteria for LVAD implantation.

Based on current guidelines, chronic LVAD therapy should be considered as an option for NYHA III HF-rEF patients who have recurrent hospitalizations or severe exercise intolerance despite OMM, keeping in mind that patients with higher BMI and severe diabetes tend to have poorer outcomes.[27] However, the guidelines emphasize that despite technological improvements, adverse events including bleeding, thromboembolism, and pump thrombosis, as well as driveline infections and device failure, continue to impact LVAD patients. Because these events require highly specialized management, mechanical cardiac support is only an option at centers with appropriately trained physicians and surgeons and an outpatient LVAD clinic with trained nursing staff. A recent review from the Mayo Clinic addresses these issues in detail.[28]

REFERENCES

1. Gottdiener JS, Scott CG, Enriquez-Sarano M, et al. Burden of valvular heart diseases: a population-based study. *Lancet*. 2006;368:1005-1011.

2. Bach DS, Siao D, Girard SE, Duvernoy C, McCallister BD Jr, Gualano SK. Evaluation of patients with severe symptomatic aortic stenosis who do not undergo aortic valve replacement: the potential role of subjectively overestimated operative risk. *Circ Cardiovasc Qual Outcomes*. 2009;2:533-539.

3. Clark MA, Arnold SV, Duhay FG, et al. Five-year clinical and economic outcomes among patients with medically managed severe aortic stenosis: results from a Medicare claims analysis. *Circ Cardiovasc Qual Outcomes*. 2012;5(5):697-704.

4. Kim CA, Rasania SP, Afilalo J, Popma JJ, Lipsitz LA, Kim DH. Functional status and quality of life after transcatheter aortic valve replacement: a systematic review. *Ann Intern Med*. 2014;160:243-254.

5. Khatri PJ, Webb JG, Rodés-Cabau J, et al. Adverse effects associated with transcatheter aortic valve implantation: a meta-analysis of contemporary studies. *Ann Intern Med*. 2013;158:35-46.

6. Lindman BR, Alexander KP, O'Gara PT, Afilalo J. Futility, benefit, and transcatheter aortic valve replacement. *JACC Cardiovasc Interv*. 2014;7:707-716.

7. Nkomo VT, Gardin JM, Skelton TN, Gottdiener JS, Scott CG, Enriquez-Sarano M. Burden of valvular heart diseases: a population-based study. *Lancet*. 2006;368:1005-1011.

8. Beigel R, Wunderlich NC, Kar S, Siegel RJ. The evolution of percutaneous mitral valve repair therapy. *J Am Coll Cardiol*. 2014;64:2688-2700.

9. Fama NP, Ross HJ, Verma S. Mitral Clip–looking back and moving forward. *Curr Opin Cardiol*. 2016;31:169-175.

10. Condado JA, Acquatella H, Rodriguez L, et al. Percutaneous edge-to-edge mitral valve repair: 2-year follow-up in the first human case. *Catheter Cardiovasc Interv*. 2006;67:323-325.

11. Feldman T, Foster E, Glower DD, et al. Percutaneous repair or surgery for mitral regurgitation. *N Engl J Med*. 2011;364:1395-1406.

12. Feldman T, Kar S, Elmariah S, et al. Randomized comparison of percutaneous repair and surgery for mitral eegurgitation: 5-year results of EVEREST II. *J Am Coll Cardiol*. 2015;66:2844-2854.

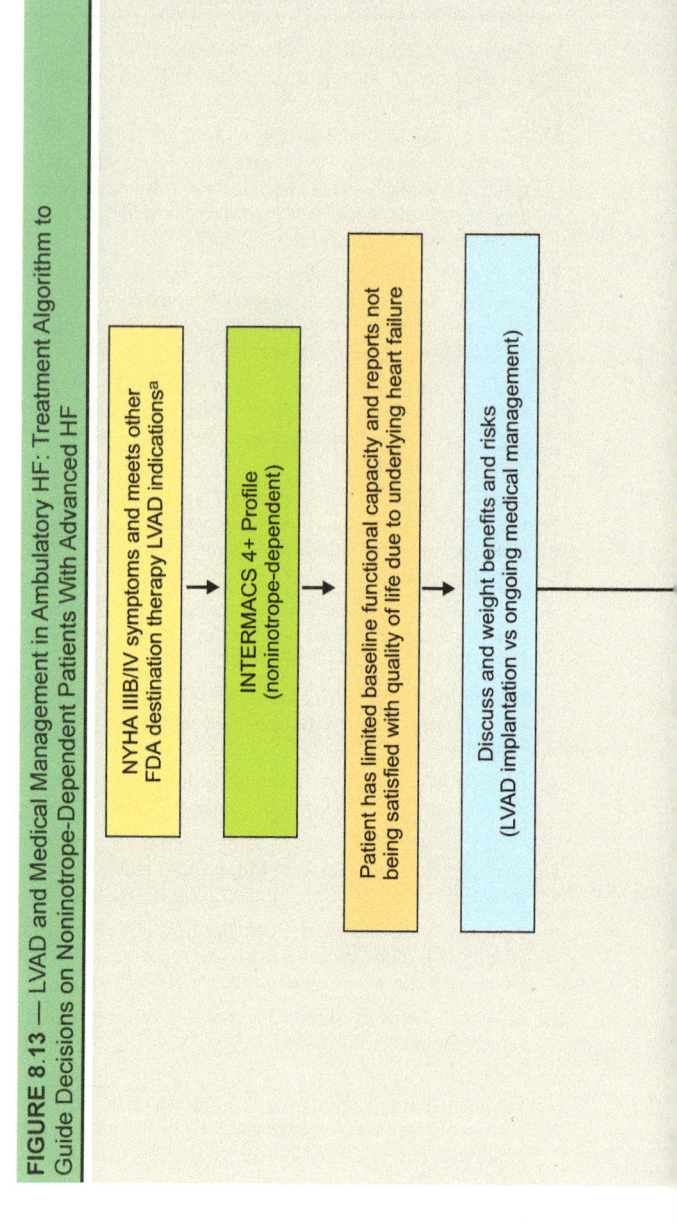

FIGURE 8.13 — LVAD and Medical Management in Ambulatory HF: Treatment Algorithm to Guide Decisions on Noninotrope-Dependent Patients With Advanced HF

NYHA IIIB/IV symptoms and meets other FDA destination therapy LVAD indications[a]

→

INTERMACS 4+ Profile (noninotrope-dependent)

→

Patient has limited baseline functional capacity and reports not being satisfied with quality of life due to underlying heart failure

→

Discuss and weight benefits and risks (LVAD implantation vs ongoing medical management)

ROADMAP Results[b]

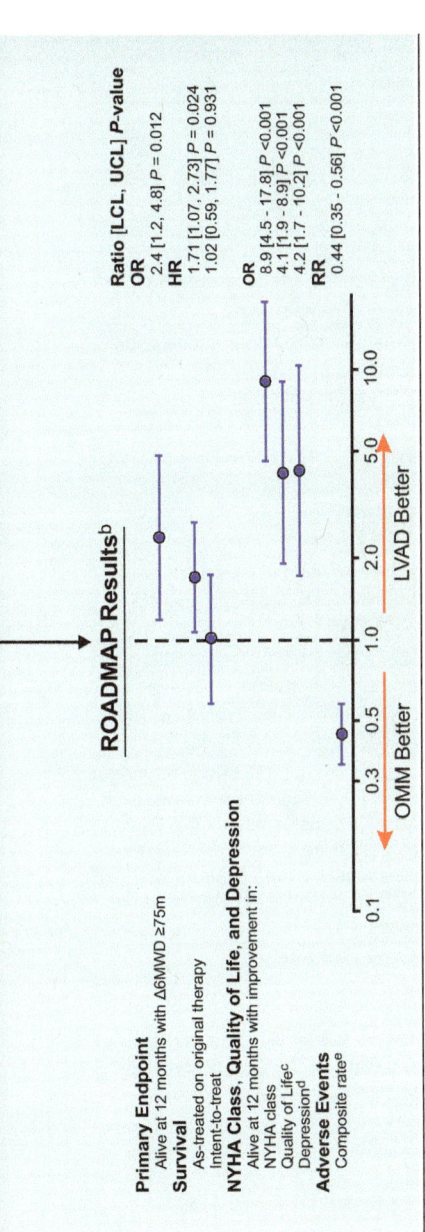

	Ratio [LCL, UCL] *P*-value
Primary Endpoint	OR
Alive at 12 months with Δ6MWD ≥75m	2.4 [1.2, 4.8] *P* = 0.012
Survival	HR
As-treated on original therapy	1.71 [1.07, 2.73] *P* = 0.024
Intent-to-treat	1.02 [0.59, 1.77] *P* = 0.931
NYHA Class, Quality of Life, and Depression	
Alive at 12 months with improvement in:	OR
NYHA class	8.9 [4.5 - 17.8] *P* <0.001
Quality of Life[c]	4.1 [1.9 - 8.9] *P* <0.001
Depression[d]	4.2 [1.7 - 10.2] *P* <0.001
Adverse Events	RR
Composite rate[e]	0.44 [0.35 - 0.56] *P* <0.001

OMM Better ← | → LVAD Better

[a] US Food and Drug Administration (FDA) destination therapy indication includes: New York Heart Association (NYHA) functional class IIIB or IV, left ventricular ejection fraction ≤25%, not listed (or planned) for heart transplantation, and on optimal medical management (OMM).
[b] The ROADMAP (Risk Assessment and Comparative Effectiveness of Left Ventricular Assist Device [LVAD] and Medical Management) trial results.
[c] EuroQol visual analog scale improvement >20 points in patients with baseline score <68.
[d] Patient Health Questionnaire–9 score improvement ≥5 points in patients with baseline mild or worse depression severity.
[e] Sum of bleeding, infection, thrombus, stroke, arrhythmias, and worsening heart failure.

Estep JD, et al. *J Am Coll Cardiol.* 2015;66(16):1747-1761.

TABLE 8.3 — Terms Describing Various Indications for Mechanical Circulatory Support

BTD/BTB	Use of short-term MCS (eg, ECLS or ECMO) in patients with cardiogenic shock until haemodynamics and end-organ perfusion are stabilized, contraindications for long-term MCS are excluded (brain damage after resuscitation) and additional therapeutic options including long-term VAD therapy or heart transplant can be evaluated.
BTC	Use of MCS (usually LVAD) to improve end-organ function in order to make an ineligible patient eligible for heart transplantation.
BTT	Use of MCS (LVAD or BiVAD) to keep patient alive who is otherwise at high risk of death before transplantation until a donor organ becomes available.
BTR	Use of MCS (typically LVAD) to keep patient alive until cardiac function recovers sufficiently to remove MCS.
DT	Long-term use of MCS (LVAD) as an alternative to transplantation in patient with end-stage HF ineligible for transplantation or long-term waiting for heart transplantation.

Key: BiVAD, biventricular assist device; BTB, bridge to bridge; BTC, bridge to candidacy; BTD, bridge to decision; BTR, bridge to recovery; BTT, bridge to transplantation; DT, destination therapy; ECLS, extracorporeal life support; ECMO, extracorporeal membrane oxygenation; HF, heart failure; LVAD, left ventricular assist device; MCS, mechanical circulatory support; VAD, ventricular assist device.

Ponikowski P, et al. *Eur Heart J.* 2016;37:2129-2200.

---

13. Wan B, Rahnavardi M, Tian DH, et al. A meta-analysis of MitraClip system versus surgery for treatment of severe mitral regurgitation. *Ann Cardiothorac Surg.* 2013;2:683-692.
14. Auricchio A, Schillinger W, Meyer S, et al. Correction of mitral regurgitation in nonresponders to cardiac resynchronization therapy by MitraClip improves symptoms and promotes reverse remodeling. *J Am Coll Cardiol.* 2011;58:2183-2189.

TABLE 8.4 — Patients Potentially Eligible for Implantation of a Left Ventricular Assist Device

Patients with >2 months of severe symptoms despite optimal medical and device therapy and more than one of the following:

- LVEF <25% and, if measured, peak VO_2 <12 mL/kg/min
- ≥3 HF hospitalizations in previous 12 months without an obvious precipitating cause
- Dependence on IV inotropic therapy
- Progressive end-organ dysfunction (worsening renal and/or hepatic function) due to reduced perfusion and not to inadequate ventricular filling pressure (PCWP ≥20 mmHg and SBP ≤80-90 mmHg or CI ≤2 L/min/m^2)
- Absence of severe right ventricular dysfunction together with severe tricuspid regurgitation

Ponikowksi P, et al. *Eur Heart J.* 2016;37:2129-2200.

---

15. Pleger ST, Schulz-Schönhagen M, Geis N, et al. One year clinical efficacy and reverse cardiac remodeling in patients with severe mitral regurgitation and reduced ejection fraction after MitraClip implantation. *Eur J Heart Fail.* 2013;15:919-927.

16. Franzen O, van der Heyden J, Baldus S, et al. MitraClip® therapy in patients with end-stage systolic heart failure. *Eur J Heart Fail.* 2011;13:569-576.

17. Vakil K, Roukoz H, Sarraf M, et al. Safety and efficacy of the MitraClip® system for severe mitral regurgitation: a systematic review. *Catheter Cardiovasc Interv.* 2014;84:129-136.

18. Kowey PR, Mohmand-Borkowski A, Burke JF. *Clinical Management of Atrial Fibrillation*, 2nd ed. West Islip, NY: Professional Communications, Inc. 2015.

19. Wiebe J, Franke J, Lehn K, et al. Percutaneous left atrial appendage closure with the Watchman Device: long-term results up to 5 years. *JACC Cardiovasc Interv.* 2015;8(15):1915-1921.

20. Price MJ, Reddy VY, Valderrabano M, et al. Bleeding outcomes after left atrial appendage closure compared with long-term warfarin. *JACC Cardiovasc Interv.* 2015;8(15):1925-1932.

21. Desai AK. Implantable hemodynamic monitoring in ambulatory heart failure: who, when, why, how? *Curr Cardiol Rep.* 2015;17:113-120.

22. Bourge RC, Abraham WT, Adamson PB, et al. Randomized controlled trial of an implantable continuous hemodynamic monitor in patients with advanced heart failure: the COMPASS-HF study. *J Am Coll Cardiol.* 2008;51:1073-1079.

23. Abraham WT, Adamson PB, Bourge RC, et al. Wireless pulmonary artery haemodynamic monitoring in chronic heart failure: a randomised controlled trial. *Lancet.* 2011;377:658-666.

24. Costanzo MR, Stevenson LW, Adamson PB, et al. Interventions linked to decreased heart failure hospitalizations during ambulatory pulmonary artery pressure monitoring. *JACC Heart Fail.* 2016;4(5):333-344.

25. Rose EA, Gelijns AC, Moskowitz AJ, et al; for the Randomized Evaluation of Mechanical Assistance for the Treatment of Congestive Heart Failure (REMATCH) Study Group. Long-term use of a left ventricular assist device for end-stage heart failure. *N Engl J Med.* 2001;345:1435-1443.

26. Estep JD, Starling RC, Horstmanshof DA, et al. Risk assessment and comparative effectiveness of left ventricular assist device and medical management in ambulatory heart failure patients: results from the ROADMAP study. *J Am Coll Cardiol.* 2015;66:1747-1761.

27. Arnold SV, Jones PG, Allen LA, et al. Frequency of poor outcome (death or poor quality of life) after left ventricular assist device for destination therapy: results from the INTERMACS registry. *Circ Heart Fail.* 2016;9(8). pii: e002800.

28. Sajgalik P, Grupper A, Edwards BS, et al. Current status of left ventricular assist device therapy. *Mayo Clin Proc.* 2016;91:927-940.

9. Acute Heart Failure

Approximately 80% of patients who are hospitalized with the diagnosis of acute decompensated heart failure (ADHF) have, in fact, experienced an episode of decompensation of chronic HF.[1] As noted in the earlier discussion of clinical trials of ambulatory hemodynamic monitoring (see *Chapter 8*), hemodynamic deterioration in these HF patients often precedes the clinical events by 2 to 3 weeks. New-onset HF accounts for some 15% of ADHF admissions, and Stage D patients refractory to standard therapy account for the remaining 5% of admissions. Clinicians must keep this heterogeneity in the ADHF population in mind when addressing interpretation of data from large studies.[2]

The ADHF population is relatively equally divided between those with HF-rEF and HF-pEF. As detailed in earlier chapters, HF-pEF patients tend to be older, are more likely to be female, and more likely to have significant hypertension, but less likely to have CAD.[3]

Even though four out of five patients with acute HF have previously diagnosed chronic HF and are presumably receiving medical care, the prevalence of ADHF continues to increase. In the US, over 1 million patients are hospitalized each year with the primary diagnosis of HF,[4] and 3 million additional hospitalizations list HF as a secondary or tertiary diagnosis.[5]

Most importantly for the patient with HF, an episode of decompensation represents a sentinel prognostic event in the natural history of his or her illness.[6] A hospitalization for HF is associated with a high risk for recurrent hospitalization and/or death. A retrospective analysis of data from the Candesartan in Heart Failure: Assessment of Reduction in Mortality and Morbidity (CHARM) trials included 7572 patients of whom 1455 had at least one hospitalization for HF. The risk of death was greatest early after discharge from a HF hospitalization and was directly related to the number of previous HF hospitalizations and their duration. **Figure 9.1** shows the relationship of the hazard ratio for mortality to time from discharge and numbers of prior HF hospitalizations.[7]

FIGURE 9.1 — Hazard Ratio for Mortality Based on Number of HF Hospitalizations

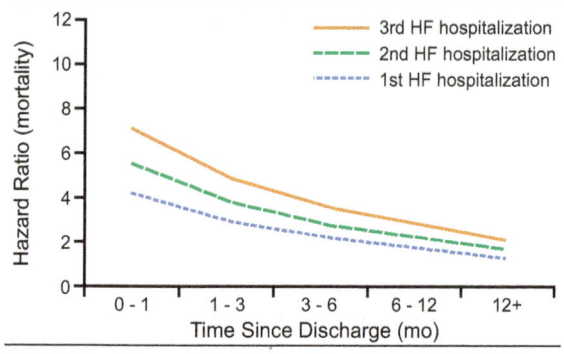

Modified from Solomon SD, et al. *Circulation*. 2007;116:1482-1487.

In an attempt to understand whether hospitalization itself changes the risk profile for individual patients, the EVEREST investigators conducted a post hoc analysis that supported hospitalization-independent and time-independent differences in risk factors as the predominant drivers of post-discharge mortality. In this view, the requirement for repeated hospitalization is a marker for deteriorating pathophysiology, and "although there is transiently elevated individual patient risk in the 90 days before and after discharge, the patient's individual risk profile, rather than temporal change in risk relative to hospitalization, remains the main determinant of mortality."[8]

Table 9.1 details the signs and symptoms of patients presenting with ADHF. The majority of patients present with deterioration of previously known HF, and most have signs and symptoms of increasing fluid retention with peripheral edema, visceral congestion, and some manifestation of difficulty breathing, including dyspnea with exertion or at rest, nocturnal dyspnea, or orthopnea.

The clinical data can be integrated as shown in **Figure 9.2** in a straightforward assessment of the degree of congestion and the degree of hypoperfusion that can help to direct therapeutic intervention. In this scheme, assignment to the "warm and dry" quadrant represents the goal of HF management. Patients who are "wet" will generally benefit from decongestion with diuretics; those who are "cold" may require cautious use of vasodilators or inotropes. The few who are "cold and dry" may require short-term circulatory support with inotropic agents.

The major benefit of this approach is the emphasis placed on careful clinical evaluation of the individual patient's signs and symptoms in directing medical management. There is a wide spectrum of pathophysiology involved in ADHF, and management must be tailored to the individual situation. Although interventions such as invasive hemodynamic monitoring and parenteral vasodilators or inotropic support are not recommended as routine care measures, they may be critically important for selected patients.

The evaluation of patients with suspected acute decompensation includes an investigation of precipitating factors, evaluation of the patient's current cardiovascular status, and assessment of prognosis. **Table 9.2** outlines the initial evaluation of ADHF patients.

A careful search for precipitating factors should always be part of the initial evaluation of a patient with an episode of ADHF. **Table 9.3** outlines common precipitating factors.

Overall goals of therapy in ADHF include:
- Symptomatic relief
- Identification and correction of possible precipitating factors
- Optimization of long-term management.

TABLE 9.1 — Clinical Presentations of Acute Heart Failure

Signs	Symptoms
Pulmonary or Systemic Congestion ("wet")	
<ul><li>Weight gain</li><li>Tachypnea</li><li>Jugular venous distension</li><li>Rales</li><li>S3 or S4 gallop</li><li>Hepatojugular reflux</li><li>Hepatomegaly/splenomegaly</li><li>Peripheral edema</li><li>Ascites</li><li>Anasarca</li><li>Low O_2 saturation</li><li>Chest x-ray findings of congestion, pulmonary edema, pleural effusions</li><li>Increased BNP or NT-proBNP</li></ul>	<ul><li>Dyspnea on exertion</li><li>Dyspnea at rest</li><li>Orthopnea</li><li>Paroxysmal nocturnal dyspnea</li><li>Cough</li><li>Chest pressure</li><li>Abdominal distension bloating</li><li>Early satiety</li><li>Leg edema</li></ul>

Low Cardiac Output ("cold")

- Hypotension
- Narrow pulse pressure
- Tachycardia
- Altered mental status
- Cool extremities
- Worsening renal and/or hepatic function

- Fatigue
- Decreased urine output
- Decreased mental acuity/altered mental status
- Nausea/vomiting

Nonspecific

| Hyponatremia | Cachexia and anorexia |

Cook TD, et al. *Am J Cardiol.* 2016;117:611-616.

FIGURE 9.2 — A Scheme for Integrating Signs and Symptoms of ADHF Into an Overall Circulatory Assessment

Congestion at rest?
(eg, orthopnea, elevated jugular venous pressure, pulmonary rales, S3 gallop, edema)

	NO	**YES**
Low perfusion at rest? (eg, narrow pulse pressure, cool extremities, hypotension) **NO**	Warm and Dry	Warm and Wet
YES	Cold and Dry	Cold and Wet

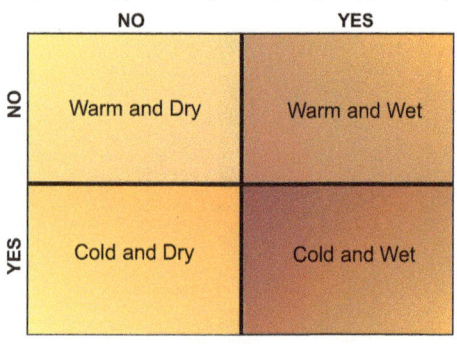

Classification of patients presenting with acutely decompensated heart failure.

Adapted from Thomas SS, Nohria A. *Circ J.* 2012;76:278-286.

TABLE 9.2 — Initial Evaluation of the ADHF Patient

- History and physical examination
- ECG, chest x-ray
- CBC, renal function and electrolytes, metabolic panel
- Biomarkers: natriuretic peptides, troponin
- Imaging: 2D and Doppler echocardiography

Symptomatic Relief

This chapter focuses on agents available for symptomatic relief for the ADHF patient, including diuretics, vasodilators, and inotropes. Although morphine has been included among agents for symptomatic relief in the past, and the ESC guidelines allow for consideration of morphine administration, neither the HFSA nor the ACC/AHA guidelines recommend its use. In an

TABLE 9.3 — Common Precipitating Factors for ADHF

Medications	Non-adherence to prescribed medications
	Adverse effects (diltiazem, verapamil)
	Sodium retention (NSAIDs)
Non-cardiac illness	Infection (pneumonia, UTI)
	Pulmonary emboli
	Worsening CKD
Cardiac events	Atrial fibrillation or other arrhythmia
	Acute ischemia (ACS)
	Worsening mitral regurgitation
Substance abuse	Alcohol
	Cocaine
	Methamphetamine

observational analysis of 147,362 HF admissions from the ADHERE database,[9] administration of morphine was associated with an increased frequency of adverse events including mechanical ventilation, ICU admissions, and mortality.

■ Diuretics, Vasopressin Antagonists and Ultrafiltration

Diuretics remain the most commonly used agents for symptomatic relief in volume overloaded ("wet") ADHF patients, but rigorous clinical data about dose and administration of diuretics are limited. The Diuretic Optimization Strategies Evaluation (DOSE) trial[10] included 308 patients with a mean ejection fraction of 35%; 27% of the patients had an ejection fraction of 50% or greater. Using a 2'2 randomized factorial design, patients were assigned to either a low-dose diuretic strategy (total intravenous furosemide dose equal to their total daily oral loop diuretic dose in furosemide equivalents) or a high-dose strategy (total daily intravenous furosemide dose 2.5 times their total daily oral loop diuretic dose in furosemide equivalents) and also to administration of furosemide either by intravenous bolus every 12 hours or by continuous intravenous infusion.

The patient's global assessment of symptoms, measured with the use of a visual analogue scale and quantified as the area under the curve (AUC) of serial assessments from baseline to 72 hours was the primary endpoint. The investigators found no significant differences in either the global assessment of symptoms or in changes in creatinine levels from baseline to 72 hours when furosemide was administered by boluses compared with continuous infusion or when it was dosed with the low-dose strategy compared with the high-dose strategy (**Figure 9.3**).

The high-dose strategy was associated with greater relief of dyspnea, greater fluid loss and weight loss, and fewer serious adverse events. Although worsening of renal function occurred more frequently with the high-dose strategy in the short term, clinical outcomes at 60 days in the high-dose group were no worse than in the low-dose group.

In summary, a strategy of high-dose intravenous diuretics (total daily intravenous furosemide dose 2.5 times the patients former total daily oral loop diuretic dose in furosemide equivalents) given as bolus doses every 12 hours seems both safe and effective.

Arginine vasopressin is inappropriately elevated in HF, and has an important function in mediating water retention that contributes to congestion and hyponatremia. The Efficacy of Vasopressin Antagonism in Heart Failure Outcome Study With Tolvaptan (EVEREST) was a randomized, double blind, placebo-controlled study with 4133 HF-rEF patients enrolled within 48 hours of an admission and treated with tolvaptan, a V_2-receptor antagonist, or placebo (in addition to standard care) for at least 60 days. The dual primary end points were all-cause mortality and cardiovascular death or hospitalization for HF. Despite a strong pathophysiologic rationale for treatment, and evidence

FIGURE 9.3 — 60-Day Kaplan–Meier Curves for the Clinical Composite End Point of Death, Rehospitalization, or Emergency Department Visit in DOSE

A. Bolus vs Continuous Infusion

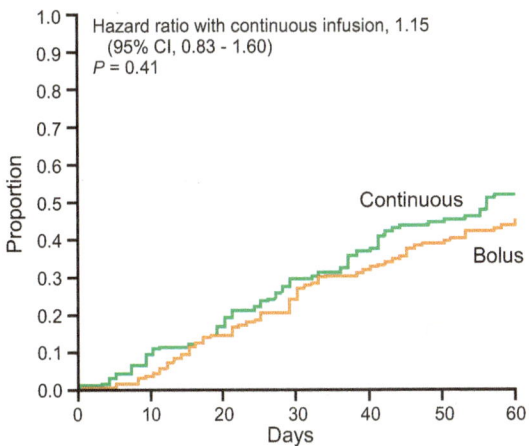

Hazard ratio with continuous infusion, 1.15 (95% CI, 0.83 - 1.60)
$P = 0.41$

B. Low-Dose vs High-Dose Strategy

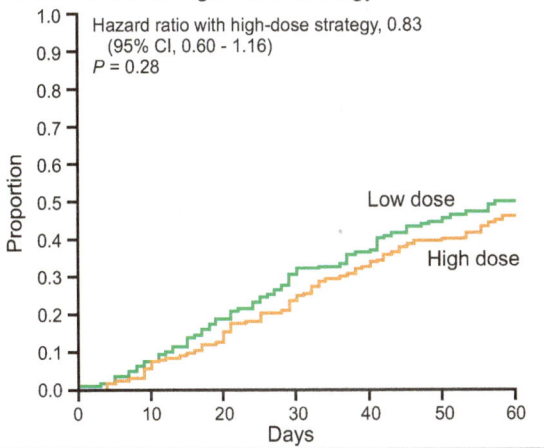

Hazard ratio with high-dose strategy, 0.83 (95% CI, 0.60 - 1.16)
$P = 0.28$

Felker GM, et al. *N Engl J Med*. 2011; 364(9):797-805.

of pharmacologic activity, tolvaptan did not have a demonstrable effect on either of the primary endpoints (**Figure 9.4**).[11]

Tolvaptan (Samsca, Otsuka America Pharmaceutical, Inc) is approved for the treatment of clinically significant hypervolemic and euvolemic hyponatremia (serum sodium <125 mEq/L or less marked hyponatremia that is symptomatic and has resisted correction with fluid restriction), including patients with HF, and Syndrome of Inappropriate Antidiuretic Hormone (SIADH). Nonetheless, it is not currently recommended for routine use.

The Cardiorenal Rescue Study in Acute Decompensated Heart Failure (CARRESS-HF) compared ultrafiltration with stepped pharmacologic therapy on renal function and weight loss in 188 HF volume overloaded patients with worsening renal function and persistent congestion. The primary end point was change in serum creatinine level and change in weight from randomization to 96 hours after randomization considered as a bivariate response. The trial was discontinued because the ultrafiltration group showed both a lack of benefit and excess adverse events. The 96-hour serum creatinine level increased significantly in the ultrafiltration group as compared with the pharmacologic-therapy group, and their weight loss was not significantly greater. The investigators concluded that, "Given the high cost and complexity of ultrafiltration, the use of this technique as performed in the current study does not seem justified for patients hospitalized for ADHF, worsened renal function, and persistent congestion."[12]

■ Vasodilators

Intravenous vasodilators that have been used most commonly in management of ADHF include nitroglycerin, nitroprusside, and nesiritide. The appropriate use of parenteral vasodilators for relief of dyspnea in HF patients remains a topic that generates heated debates with striking differences of opinion. Certain subsets

FIGURE 9.4 — EVEREST: K-M Curves for All-Cause Mortality and Cardiovascular Mortality/Heart Failure Hospitalization for Tolvaptan vs Placebo

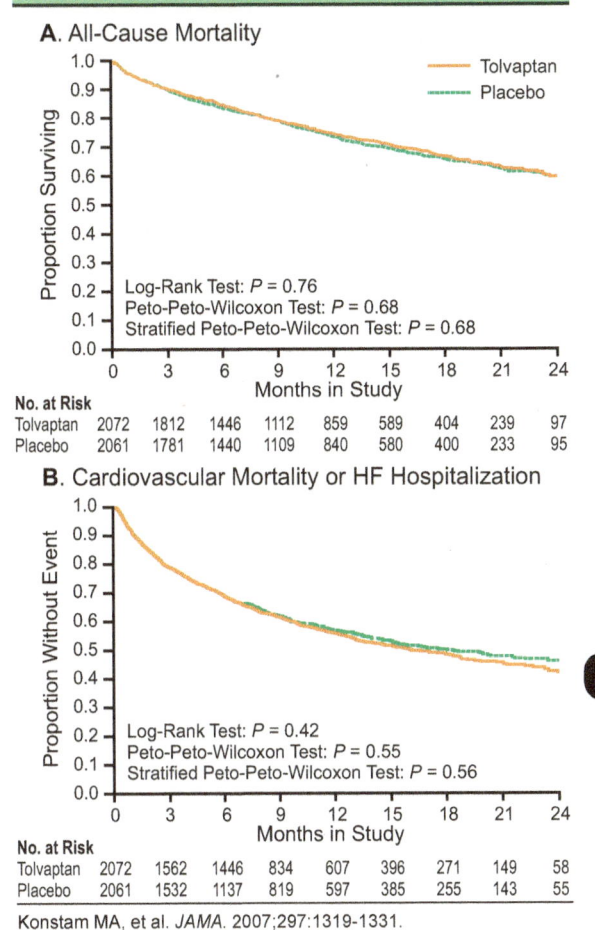

A. All-Cause Mortality

No. at Risk

	0	3	6	9	12	15	18	21	24
Tolvaptan	2072	1812	1446	1112	859	589	404	239	97
Placebo	2061	1781	1440	1109	840	580	400	233	95

Log-Rank Test: $P = 0.76$
Peto-Peto-Wilcoxon Test: $P = 0.68$
Stratified Peto-Peto-Wilcoxon Test: $P = 0.68$

B. Cardiovascular Mortality or HF Hospitalization

No. at Risk

	0	3	6	9	12	15	18	21	24
Tolvaptan	2072	1562	1446	834	607	396	271	149	58
Placebo	2061	1532	1137	819	597	385	255	143	55

Log-Rank Test: $P = 0.42$
Peto-Peto-Wilcoxon Test: $P = 0.55$
Stratified Peto-Peto-Wilcoxon Test: $P = 0.56$

Konstam MA, et al. *JAMA*. 2007;297:1319-1331.

of the ADHF population, including those individuals with significant mitral or aortic regurgitation and those with advanced LV dysfunction (LVEF ≤35%) who have adequate (≥100 mm Hg) systolic blood pressure, may receive substantial short-term symptomatic relief with effective vasodilator management.

If dose titrated to hemodynamic endpoints, there are no objective data to indicate that any single agent is preferable. Both nitroglycerine and nitroprusside require ongoing dose titration and nitroprusside requires invasive arterial pressure monitoring, whereas nesiritide may be given as a fixed dose infusion. As noted in the current ACC/AHA guidelines, "presently there are no data that suggest that intravenous vasodilators improve outcomes in the patient hospitalized with HF; as such, use of intravenous vasodilators is limited to the relief of dyspnea in the hospitalized HF patient with intact blood pressure."[3]

Concerns about blood pressure and possible hypotension are often cited in discussions of the use of vasodilator agents. In a post hoc analysis of the 7141 patient prospective randomized ASCEND-HF trial comparing nesiritide vs placebo, 1555 (21.8%) patients had an episode of hypotension. Of these, 1136 (73.1%) had asymptomatic, 302 (19.4%) had symptomatic, and 117 (7.5%) had both symptomatic and asymptomatic hypotension (**Table 9.4**). In-hospital hypotension was associated with increases in 30-day hospitalization and mortality, *regardless of study drug assignment.* Randomization to nesiritide was associated with hypotension in the trial; however, it had no effect on the association between hypotension and outcomes. These observations suggest that during hospitalization for ADHF, hemodynamic instability itself is a marker for high risk of subsequent adverse outcomes.[13]

These important findings from a large randomized trial suggest two conclusions. First, for patients who are appropriate candidates, careful use of vasodilator agents should not be withheld because of concerns about possible hypotension. Second, hospitalized

TABLE 9.4 — Adjusted Outcomes in Patients With and Without Hypotension[a]

Outcome	Total	No Hypotension	Hypotension	Adjusted HR	95% CI	Cox P Value
30-Day mortality	273/7118 (3.8)	162/5565 (2.9)	111/1553 (7.1)	2.03	1.57-2.61	<0.001
30-Day morality or HF hospitalization	686/6938 (9.9)	455/5422 (8.4)	231/1516 (15.2)	1.58	1.34-1.86	<0.001
30-Day mortality or all-cause hospitalization	1067/6942 (15.4)	747/5424 (13.8)	320/1518 (21.1)	1.40	1.22-1.61	<0.001

Values presented as n/N (%), unless otherwise indicated.

[a] Test for interaction of nesiritide on relationship of in-hospital hypotension and 30-day outcomes: 30-day mortality, $P = 0.874$; 30-day mortality/HF hospitalization, $P = 0.908$; 30-day mortality/all-cause hospitalization, $P = 0.238$.

Patel PA, et al. *Circ Heart Fail.* 2014;7:918-925.

ADHF patients who have episodes of hemodynamic instability should be regarded as at high-risk for short-term adverse outcomes, regardless of their pharmacologic management at the time.

■ Inotropes

Table 9.5 shows the currently available inotropes for management of ADHF. The Outcomes of a Prospective Trial of Intravenous Milrinone for Exacerbations of Chronic Heart Failure (OPTIME-CHF) study, a 951-patient randomized double-blind placebo-controlled prospective trial of routine use of milrinone in HF-rEF patients who had been hospitalized for exacerbation of chronic HF, showed no benefit in outcomes with routine use of milrinone in ADHF and a significant increase in adverse events, particularly arrhythmia[14] (**Table 9.6**) Based largely on the OPTIME findings, the routine use of inotropes for ADHF patients with HF-rEF is no longer recommended.

Nonetheless, observational data have indicated that many physicians managing ADHF routinely employed low-dose ("renal-dose") dopamine or low-dose nesiritide infusion in an effort to enhance the effects of IV diuretics. The 360 patient Renal Optimization Strategies Evaluation (ROSE) trial compared low-dose dopamine (2 µg/kg/min) vs placebo or low-dose nesiritide (0.005 µg/kg/min) vs placebo added to diuretic therapy; the co-primary endpoints were cumulative 72-hour urine volume and the change in cystatin-C from randomization to 72 hours. **Figure 9.5** shows Forest plots of the differences in urine volume across multiple subsets for each active agent compared to placebo.

There was no significant difference between low-dose dopamine vs placebo or between low-dose nesiritide vs placebo in the 72-hour cumulative urine volume, and there was no significant difference in the change in cystatin-C from baseline to 72 hours vs placebo for either active agent. Overall, the ROSE data do not support the routine use of low-dose dopamine

TABLE 9.5 — Intravenous Inotropic Agents Used in Management of HF

Inotropic Agent	Dose (mcg/kg) Bolus	Infusion (/min)	Drug Kinetics and Metabolism	Effects CO	HR	SVR	PVR	Adverse Effects	Special Considerations
Adrenergic Agonists									
Dopamine	N/A	5-10	$t_{1/2}$: 2-20 min R, H, P	↑	↑	↕	↕	T, HA, N, tissue necrosis	Caution: MAO-I
	N/A	10-15		↑	↑	↑	↕		
Dobutamine	N/A	2.5-5	$t_{1/2}$: 2-3 min H	↑	↑	→	↕	↑/↓ BP, HA, T, N, F, hypersensitivity	Caution: MAO-I; CI: sulfite allergy
	N/A	5-20		↑	↑	↕	↕		
PDE Inhibitor									
Milrinone	N/R	0.125-0.75	$t_{1/2}$: 2.5 h H	↑	↑	→	→	T, ↓BP	Renal dosing, monitor LFTs

Key: BP, blood pressure; CI, contraindication; CO, cardiac output; F, fever; H, hepatic; HA, headache; HF, heart failure; HR, heart rate; LFT, liver function test; MAO-I, monoamine oxidase inhibitor; N, nausea; N/A, not applicable; N/R, not recommended; P, plasma; PDE, phosphodiesterase; PVR, pulmonary vascular resistance; R, renal; SVR, systemic vascular resistance; and T, tachyarrhythmias; $t_{1/2}$, elimination half-life.

Yancy CW, et al. *J Am Coll Cardiol.* 2013;62(16)e147-e239.

TABLE 9.6 — OPTIME: Adverse Effects in the Placebo and Milrinone Groups[a]

Adverse Event, No. (%)	Placebo (n = 472)	Milrinone (n = 477)	P Value
Treatment Failure Cause at 48 Hours	43/466 (9.2)	97/470 (20.6)	<0.001
Progression of heart failure	6.8	7.9	0.54
Adverse event	2.1	12.6	<0.001
Events During Index Hospitalization			
Mycardial infarction	2 (0.4)	7 (1.5)	0.18
New atrial fibrillation or flutter	7 (1.5)	22 (4.6)	0.004
Ventricular tachycardia or fibrillation[b]	7 (1.5)	16 (3.4)	0.06
Sustained hypotension[c]	15 (3.2)	51 (10.7)	<0.001
Death	11 (2.3)	18 (3.8)	0.19

Events Within 60 Days			
Myocardial infarction	5/448 (1.1)	10/462 (2.2)	0.21
New atrial fibrillation or flutter	16/446 (3.6)	26/462 (5.6)	0.14
Ventricular tachycardia or fibrillation	20/446 (4.5)	23/461 (5.0)	0.72
Death	41/463 (8.9)	49/474 (10.3)	0.41

[a] Total number of patients listed only when it varies from number randomized as shown.
[b] Reported by the investigator.
[c] Defined as a systolic blood pressure <80 mm Hg for >30 minutes, requiring intervention.

Cuffe MS, et al. *JAMA.* 2002;287(12):1541-1547.

FIGURE 9.5 — ROSE Trial: Differences in Urine Volumes With Nesiritide and Dopamine as Compared With Placebo

A. Nesiritide Strategy Subgroup Analysis: Cumulative Urinary Volume Over 72 Hours

Baseline Characteristics	No. of Patients Placebo	No. of Patients Nesiritide	72-Hour Urinary Volume L; mean (95% CI) Placebo	72-Hour Urinary Volume L; mean (95% CI) Nesiritide	Treatment Difference L; mean (95% CI)	P value
Age						0.92
≤70 y	59	61	8.84 (8.06 - 9.62)	9.30 (8.50 - 10.10)	0.46 (-0.67 - 1.59)	
>70 y	53	48	7.76 (7.03 - 8.49)	8.14 (7.37 - 8.91)	0.38 (-0.68 - 1.45)	
BUN						0.24
≤37 mg/dL	60	51	8.72 (8.00 - 9.44)	8.75 (7.85 - 9.65)	0.02 (-1.13 - 1.18)	
>37 mg/dL	51	57	7.91 (7.09 - 8.73)	8.88 (8.14 - 9.62)	0.97 (-0.15 - 2.08)	
Cystatin-C						0.10
≤1.71 mg/L	54	54	9.03 (8.19 - 9.87)	8.77 (7.97 - 9.57)	-0.27 (-1.44 - 0.90)	
>1.71 mg/L	56	51	7.73 (7.05 - 8.41)	8.83 (7.95 - 9.71)	1.10 (-0.01 - 2.21)	
GFR						0.76
≤44 mL/min	58	57	8.14 (7.45 - 8.83)	8.49 (7.71 - 9.27)	0.35 (-0.71 - 1.40)	
>44 mL/min	54	52	8.54 (7.69 - 9.39)	9.13 (8.30 - 9.96)	0.59 (-0.61 - 1.79)	
Ejection Fraction						0.06
≤50%	89	76	8.13 (7.51 - 8.75)	9.03 (8.31 - 9.75)	0.90 (-0.05 - 1.90)	
>50%	23	33	9.1 (8.01 - 10.19)	8.24 (7.37 - 9.11)	-0.86 (-2.23 - 0.56)	

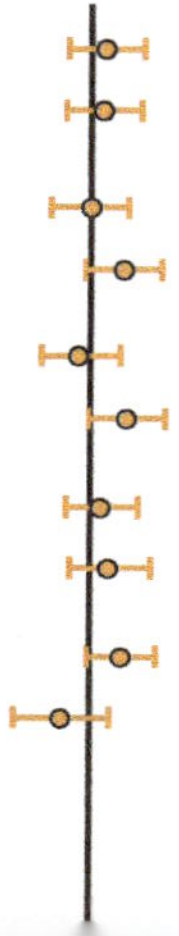

Systolic BP

≤114 mm Hg	57	59	7.87 (7.18 - 8.56)	9.14 (8.44 - 9.84)	1.27 (0.28 - 2.26)
>114 mm Hg	55	50	8.81 (7.98 - 9.64)	8.38 (7.45 - 9.31)	-0.43 (-1.68 - 0.83)

0.04

Difference in Urine Volume (95% CI)

Continued

FIGURE 9.5 — Continued

B. Dopamine Strategy Subgroup Analysis: Cumulative Urinary Volume Over 72 Hours

Baseline Characteristics	No. of Patients Placebo	No. of Patients Dopamine	72-Hour Urinary Volume L; mean (95% CI) Placebo	72-Hour Urinary Volume L; mean (95% CI) Dopamine	Treatment Difference L; mean (95% CI)	P value
Age						0.68
≤70 y	59	55	8.84 (8.07 - 9.62)	9.30 (8.24 - 10.35)	0.45 (-0.86 - 1.77)	
>70 y	53	61	7.76 (7.03 - 8.49)	7.86 (7.18 - 8.55)	0.10 (-0.91 - 1.13)	
BUN						0.71
≤37 mg/dL	60	61	8.72 (8.00 - 9.44)	8.78 (7.90 - 9.65)	0.06 (-1.09 - 1.20)	
>37 mg/dL	51	55	7.91 (7.08 - 8.73)	8.28 (7.37 - 9.19)	0.37 (-0.88 - 1.62)	
Cystatin-C						0.93
≤1.71 mg/L	54	55	9.03 (8.20 - 9.87)	9.18 (8.27 - 10.08)	0.14 (-1.10 - 1.39)	
>1.71 mg/L	56	53	7.73 (7.06 - 8.41)	7.80 (7.00 - 8.61)	0.07 (-0.99 - 1.13)	
GFR						0.49
≤44 mL/min	58	53	8.14 (7.45 - 8.83)	8.00 (7.03 - 8.98)	-0.14 (-1.33 - 1.06)	
>44 mL/min	54	63	8.54 (7.69 - 9.39)	9.00 (8.20 - 9.79)	0.46 (-0.73 - 1.64)	
Ejection Fraction						0.01
≤50%	89	86	8.13 (7.51 - 8.75)	8.82 (8.08 - 9.56)	0.69 (-0.28 - 1.66)	
>50%	23	28	9.10 (8.01 - 10.19)	7.26 (6.44 - 8.08)	-1.84 (-3.21 to -0.47)	

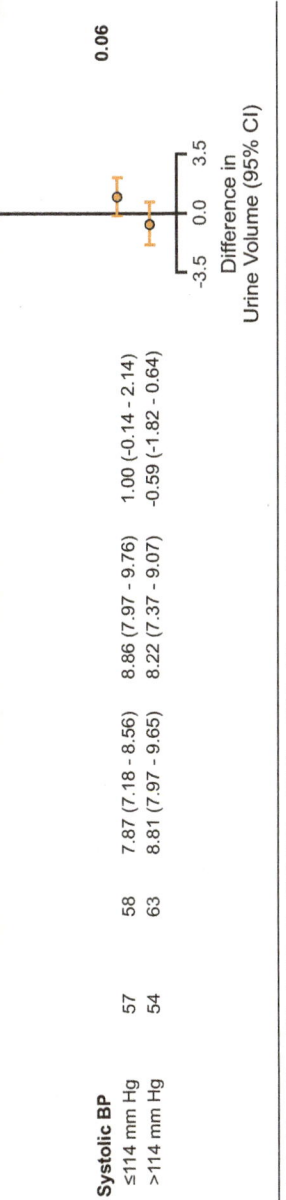

Systolic BP						
≤114 mm Hg	57	58	7.87 (7.18 - 8.56)	8.86 (7.97 - 9.76)	1.00 (-0.14 - 2.14)	
>114 mm Hg	54	63	8.81 (7.97 - 9.65)	8.22 (7.37 - 9.07)	-0.59 (-1.82 - 0.64)	0.06

Adapted from Chen HH, et al; for the NHLBI Heart Failure Clinical Research Network. *JAMA*. 2013;310(23):2533-2543.

or low-dose nesiritide as renal adjuvant therapies in ADHF patients.[15]

Currently, the most common use of inotropes currently is among hospitalized patients with acute decompensated HF-rEF with signs of end-organ dysfunction in the setting of a low cardiac output.[16] Current guideline recommendations support the use of inotropes in the setting of cardiogenic shock and in addition, "Short-term, continuous intravenous inotropic support may be reasonable in those hospitalized patients presenting with documented severe systolic dysfunction who present with low blood pressure and significantly depressed cardiac output to maintain systemic perfusion and preserve end-organ performance."[3] Overall, the current role for inotrope infusion in ADHF is very limited.

Summary

Clinical investigators in recent trials such as ASCEND-HF, CARESS, DOSE, EVEREST, OPTIME, and ROSE have carefully studied the *routine* use of interventions such as inotropes, vasodilators, continuous diuretic infusion, and ultra-filtration in large randomized controlled trials. The data from these trials have generally not provided support for the added complexity, risk, and cost of these approaches in the routine care of ADHF.

Importantly, this lack of efficacy in routine care does not mean that these approaches have no value in the management of selected individuals. From the cumulative efforts of hundreds of clinical researchers studying thousands of patients, we have learned that close to 60% of patients presenting with ADHF respond satisfactorily to intravenous diuretics and supportive care.[17] Nonetheless, we continue to recruit these patients into clinical trials. When this population of standard care-responders are recruited into large "study drug added to standard care" clinical trials, they represent a subset that will do well with placebo. At the same time, they are unlikely to have a significantly enhanced response to a novel agent while remaining vulnerable to its adverse effects. The end result of their inclusion is that trials for novel ADHF agents must be much larger and more costly than truly necessary. Clinicians and guideline writers must recognize the ongoing problem that heterogeneity in the ADHF population poses for interpretation of large studies.[2]

Those patients who do not respond to increased intravenous doses of diuretics represent an ongoing challenge not only for clinicians but also for drug development and clinical researchers. In-hospital optimization of their medical, electrophysiologic, and interventional management may improve outcomes for some of this group, and with the rapidly expanding indications for ventricular support devices, others may have new options in the near future.

REFERENCES

1. Gheorghiade M, Vaduganathan M, Fonarow GC, Bonow RO. Rehospitalization for heart failure problems and perspectives. *J Am Coll Cardiol.* 2013;61(4):391-403.

2. Felker GM, Adams KF Jr, Konstam MA, O'Connor CM, Gheorghiade M. The problem of decompensated heart failure: nomenclature, classification, and risk stratification. *Am Heart J.* 2003;145(2 suppl):S18-S25.

3. Yancy CW, Jessup M, Bozkurt B, et al; American College of Cardiology Foundation; American Heart Association Task Force on Practice Guidelines. 2013 ACCF/AHA guideline for the management of heart failure: a report of the American College of Cardiology Foundation/American Heart Association Task Force on Practice Guidelines. *J Am Coll Cardiol.* 2013;62(16):e147-e239.

4. Lloyd-Jones D, Adams R, Carnethon M, et al; American Heart Association Statistics Committee and Stroke Statistics Subcommittee. Heart disease and stroke statistics—2009 update: a report from the American Heart Association Statistics Committee and Stroke Statistics Subcommittee. *Circulation.* 2009;119(3):e21-e181.

5. Gheorghiade M, Vaduganathan M, Fonarow GC, Bonow RO. Rehospitalization for heart failure: problems and perspectives. *J Am Coll Cardiol.* 2013;61(4):391-403.

6. Mills RM. The heart failure frequent flyer: an urban legend. *Clin Cardiol.* 2009;32(2):67-68.

7. Solomon SD, Dobson J, Pocock S, et al; Candesartan in Heart failure: Assessment of Reduction in Mortality and morbidity (CHARM) Investigators. Influence of nonfatal hospitalization for heart failure on subsequent mortality in patients with chronic heart failure. *Circulation.* 2007;116(13):1482-1487.

8. Cook TD, Greene SJ, Kalogeropoulos AP, et al. Temporal changes in postdischarge mortality risk after hospitalization for heart failure (from the EVEREST Trial). *Am J Cardiol.* 2016;117(4):611-616.

9. Peacock WF, Hollander JE, Diercks DB, Lopatin M, Fonarow G, Emerman CL. Morphine and outcomes in acute decompensated heart failure: an ADHERE analysis. *Emerg Med J.* 2008;25(4):205-209.

10. Felker GM, Lee KL, Bull DA, et al; NHLBI Heart Failure Clinical Research Network. Diuretic strategies in patients with acute decompensated heart failure. *N Engl J Med.* 2011;364(9):797-805.

11. Konstam MA, Gheorghiade M, Burnett JC Jr, et al; Efficacy of Vasopressin Antagonism in Heart Failure Outcome Study With Tolvaptan (EVEREST) Investigators. Effects of oral tolvaptan in patients hospitalized for worsening heart failure: the EVEREST Outcome Trial. *JAMA*. 2007;297(12):1319-1331.

12. Bart BA, Goldsmith SR, Lee KL, et al; Heart Failure Clinical Research Network. Ultrafiltration in decompensated heart failure with cardiorenal syndrome. *N Engl J Med*. 2012;367(24):2296-2304.

13. Patel PA, Heizer G, O'Connor CM, et al. Hypotension during hospitalization for acute heart failure is independently associated with 30-day mortality: findings from ASCENT-HF. *Circ Heart Fail*. 2014;7:917-925.

14. Cuffe MS, Califf RM, Adams KF Jr, et al; Outcomes of a Prospective Trial of Intravenous Milrinone for Exacerbations of Chronic Heart Failure (OPTIME-CHF) Investigators. Short-term intravenous milrinone for acute exacerbation of chronic heart failure: a randomized controlled trial. *JAMA*. 2002;287(12):1541-1547.

15. Chen HH, Anstrom KJ, Givertz MM, et al; NHLBI Heart Failure Clinical Research Network. Low-dose dopamine or low-dose nesiritide in acute heart failure with renal dysfunction: the ROSE acute heart failure randomized trial. *JAMA*. 2013;310(23):2533-2543.

16. Tariq S, Aronow WS. Use of Inotropic Agents in Treatment of Systolic Heart Failure. *Int J Mol Sci*. 2015;16(12):29060-29068.

17. Collins SP, Lindsell CJ, Storrow AB, et al. Early changes in clinical characteristics after emergency department therapy for acute heart failure syndromes: identifying patients who do not respond to standard therapy. *Heart Fail Rev*. 2012;17(3):387-394.

10 Psychosocial Issues in Heart Failure Management

Complete assessment of the HF patient includes more than a correct diagnosis and functional assessment of his or her cardiovascular disease. Success in patient management requires that the team of health care professionals understands the patient's psychosocial environment as well. Frailty, cognitive impairment, and depression are common problems for HF patients and their families. The 2016 European guidelines specifically address these issues, as shown in **Table 10.1** and **Table 10.2**.

None of the conditions require special expertise, complex equipment, or special training to assess. All that is required is attention to the patient.

Frailty

Frailty is defined as a state of increased vulnerability to stressors, independent of any specific disease or disability. It is common in older people and predisposes them to adverse health outcomes. In a review of simple instruments for the diagnosis of frailty,[1] slow gait speed, the PRISMA 7 instrument, and the timed get-up-and-go test all had high sensitivity for identifying frailty.

Gait speed, expressed in meters per second, is measured as the time required to walk either 3 meters or 4 meters at a customary pace without turning.[2] The timed-up-and-go test (TUGT) measures the time taken to rise from a standard chair (with armrests, seat height 46 cm), walk 3 m, turn, walk back to the chair, and sit down.[3] PRISMA-7 is a survey instrument that contains seven simple self-reported components to identify frailty: older than 85 years; male; health prob-

TABLE 10.1 — 2016 ESC Guideline Recommendations on Frailty

- Monitor frailty and seek and address reversible causes (cardiovascular and non-cardiovascular) of deterioration in frailty score
- Medication review:
  - Optimize doses of heart failure medication slowly and with frequent monitoring of clinical status
  - Reduce polypharmacy; number, doses, and complexity of regimen
  - Consider stopping medication without an immediate effect on symptom relief or quality of life (such as statin)
  - Review the timing and dose of diuretic therapy to reduce risk of incontinence
- Consider need to refer to specialist care of the elderly team and to general practitioner and social worker, etc for follow-up and support for the patient and his/her family

Modified from Ponikowski P, et al. *Eur J Heart Fail.* 2016;18(8):891-975.

lems which limit activities; support of another person needed; health problems requiring staying at home; social support; and use of a cane/walker/wheelchair. Each component is scored with a yes/no answer, with a total score ≥3 deemed as indicating frailty.[4]

Because of limited specificity, however, these instruments cannot be used as accurate single tests to identify frailty. Common clinical presentations of frailty (falls, delirium, sudden immobility) can also be used to indicate the possible presence of frailty.

In a comparison of 27 ADHF patients with 197 age-matched stable HF patients, 56% of the ADHF patients met criteria for frailty compared to none of the stable patients.[5] The larger FRAIL-HF prospective cohort study included 450 non-dependent patients ≥70 years old hospitalized for HF; mean age was 80 ± 6 years. Frailty was defined by low physical activity, weight loss, slow walking speed, weak grip

TABLE 10.2 — 2016 ESC Guidelines Recommendations on Cognitive Dysfunction and Depression

Education Topic	Patient Skills	Professional Behaviors
Psychosocial aspects	<ul><li>Understand that depressive symptoms and cognitive dysfunction are found more frequently in people with HF, and that they may affect adherence</li><li>Recognize psychological problems which may occur in the course of disease, in relation to changed lifestyle, pharmacotherapy, implanted devices, and other procedures (including mechanical support and heart transplantation)</li></ul>	<ul><li>Regularly communicate information on disease, treatment options, and self-management</li><li>Involve family and careers in HF management and self-care</li><li>Refer to specialist for psychological suport when necessary</li></ul>

Modified from Ponikowski P, et al. *Eur J Heart Fail.* 2016;18(8):891-975.

strength, and exhaustion. Seventy-six percent of the study patients fulfilled frailty criteria. The frail patients had higher risk for 30-day functional decline, 1-year readmission, and 1-year all-cause mortality.[6] In an outpatient study of 172 cardiac clinic patients over age 65, 40% were classified as frail, and frailty was a strong predictor of disability over the following year.[7]

In summary, frailty is a biologic state, not a disease. Practicing clinicians can use simple and inexpensive methods to assess frailty, and it is common in HF patients.

Cognitive Impairment

Atrial fibrillation, which is highly prevalent in HF, is associated with both silent cerebral ischemia (SCI) and impaired cognitive function. In a meta-analysis of eight prospective observational studies with 77,668 patients (mean age range 61-84 years) who had normal cognitive function at baseline, 11,700 (15%) had AF. After a mean follow-up of 7.7 ± 9.1 years (range 1.8-30 years), 4773 of 73,321 (6.5%) patients had developed dementia. AF was independently associated with increased risk of incident dementia (HR = 1.42 [95% CI 1.17-1.72], $P < 0.001$).[8]

In a detailed study of 270 subjects, 180 patients with AF (90 paroxysmal and 90 persistent) and 90 controls in SR without histories of AF, patients with AF, both paroxysmal and persistent, had a higher prevalence of AF-related SCI on magnetic resonance imaging compared with controls in SR. In addition, the patients with AF also had worse cognitive performance than subjects in SR. **Figure 10.1** shows the results of cognitive testing across five domains.[9]

Clinical observations in HF patients confirm the association between AF and cognitive dysfunction. In a study of 331 stable ambulatory community-living HF patients aged 70 years and older (mean 78 ± 6; range 70-93; 43% women), 30% had atrial fibrillation and 20% had a history of paroxysmal or persistent atrial fibrillation. The atrial fibrillation patients demonstrated a high prevalence of cognitive impairment (corrected Mini Mental State Examination score <24) and frailty (reduced gait speed for 4 m).[10] Similarly, in a study of 188 hospitalized HF patients, 72 had a history of AF. AF was associated with poorer performance on cognitive function, and the association persisted after controlling for confounding cofactors.[11]

In addition to atrial fibrillation and associated silent cerebral ischemia, other pathophysiologic mechanisms for cognitive dysfunction in HF include decreased cardiac output[12] and/or reduction in cerebral blood flow, alterations of cerebrovascular reactivity, and modification of blood pressure levels.[13] Importantly, effective management of HF may be associated with improvement in cognitive function for some patients.[14]

Because patients with significant cognitive impairment may not be able to follow the complex medical programs required for HF management, HF specialty clinics should consider documenting a formal mental status examination as part of the intake process for new patients, and repeating the examination at appropriate intervals.

Depression

The estimated prevalence of clinical depression in HF patients ranges from 24% to 42%, and, after controlling for HF severity, depressive symptoms are associated with an adverse prognosis in patients with HF, as shown in **Figure 10.2**.[15,16]

In a 20-year follow-up study of 662 patients hospitalized with HF in the mid-to-late 1990s,[17] 131 had major depressive disorder at the time of the index hospitalization. Six hundred seventeen (94.1%) patients died during the follow-up period. Major depressive disorder was associated with higher all-cause mortality compared with no depression (adjusted HR = 1.64, 95% CI = 1.27-2.11, $P = 0.0001$). The association

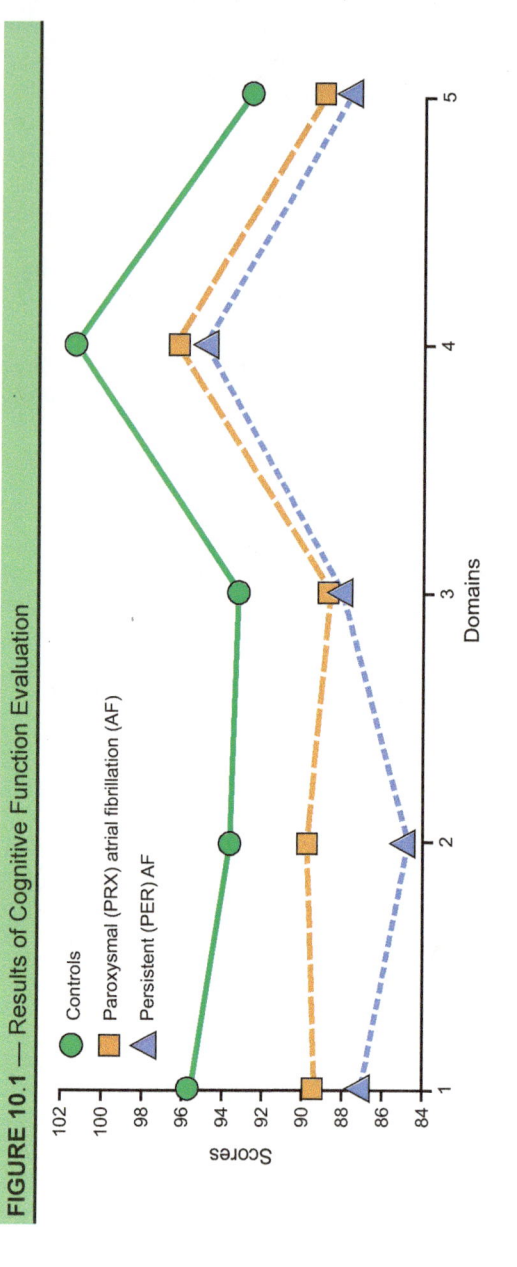

FIGURE 10.1 — Results of Cognitive Function Evaluation

	Controls (N=90)	PRX AF (N=90)	PER AF (N=90)	P Value PRX/Controls	P Value PER/Controls	P Value PRX/PER
Domains						
1 – Immediate Memory	92.4 ± 15.4	86.2 ± 13.8	82.9 ± 11.5	<0.01	<0.01	0.08
2 – Visuo-spatial Abilities	95.6 ± 17.5	89.9 ± 14.7	87.1 ± 16.9	0.02	<0.01	0.24
3 – Language	93.8 ± 16.7	89.9 ± 18.2	84.8 ± 14.8	0.14	<0.01	0.04
4 – Attention	92.9 ± 11.4	88.8 ± 9.1	88.1 ± 8.7	<0.01	<0.01	0.59
5 – Delayed Memory	101.4 ± 21.2	96.6 ± 16.6	94.9 ± 15.6	0.09	0.02	0.47
	93.5 ± 11.7	88.7 ± 14.7	87.7 ± 14	0.02	<0.01	0.64

Graph and results of cognitive function evaluation assessed by Repeatable Battery for the Assessment of Neuropsychological Status (RBANS) score.

Modified from Gaita F, et al. *J Am Coll Cardiol.* 2013;62(21):1990-1997.

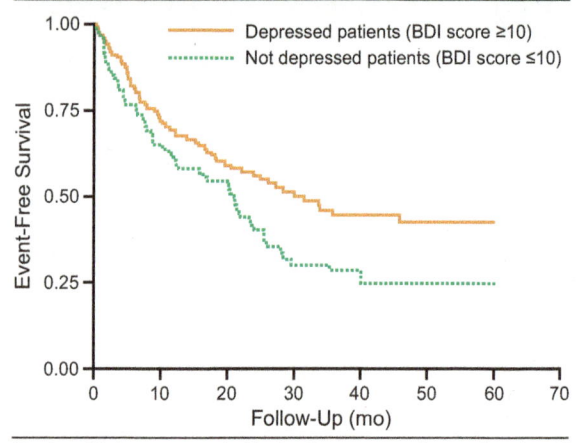

FIGURE 10.2 — Kaplan-Meier Curves Indicate the Composite End Point of Death or Hospitalization Because of Cardiovascular Disease

Kaplan-Meier curves indicate the composite end point of death or hospitalization because of cardiovascular disease in 94 patients with HF with clinically significant symptoms of depression (Beck Depression Inventory [BDI] score ≥10) compared with 110 patients with HF without depression (BDI score <10). Note: $P=0.02$ comparing patients with and without depression, based on proportional hazards models, including adjustment for age, HF etiology, LVEF, N-terminal pro-BNP, and antidepressant medication use.

Sherwood A, et al. *Arch Intern Med*. 2007;167(4):367-373.

with depression was stronger than that of any of the established predictors of mortality included in the fully adjusted model. Patients with persistent or worsening depressive symptoms during the year after discharge were at greatest risk for death. The authors concluded that, "Major depression is an independent risk factor for all-cause mortality in patients with HF. Its effect persists for many years after the diagnosis of depression."

With regard to changes in depression severity during the first year after a hospitalization for HF, worsening of symptoms as indicated by an increasing score on the Beck Depression Inventory (BDI) was associated with increased readmission and mortality compared with patients whose depressive symptoms remained relatively stable over the initial 1-year follow-up period.[18]

In SADHART-CHF, a randomized, double-blind, placebo-controlled trial of sertraline 50 to 200 mg/day vs matching placebo for 12 weeks in 469 HF-rEF patients, all of the participants demonstrated improvements in depression scores from baseline without any additive effect from SSRI treatment.[19] However, among the SADHART patients, those who had greater improvement in Hamilton Depression Rating Scale scores also had significantly greater improvement in physical function, social function, and quality of life.[20]

The MOOD-HF Study (Effects of Selective Serotonin Reuptake Inhibition on Morbidity, Mortality, and Mood in Depressed Heart Failure Patients) enrolled 372 HF-rEF patients with depression who were randomized to escitalopram (10-20 mg daily) or placebo for a median treatment time of slightly over 18 months. The outcomes of death, hospitalization, change in depression score, and safety parameters were all similar for the escitalopram and placebo groups.[21]

In HF-ACTION, 2331 HF-rEF patients were randomized to usual care or aerobic exercise that included three supervised exercise sessions per week for 3 months; patients exercised on a treadmill or stationary cycle ergometer as their primary training mode. Patients were encouraged to begin home-based exercise after 18 supervised sessions and to fully transition to home exercise after 36 supervised sessions. An ancillary study assessed 2322 HF-ACTION participants who also completed the BDI-II at baseline in order to assess the effects of exercise on depressive symptoms and evaluate whether a reduction in depressive symptoms was associated with improved clinical outcomes. Exercise resulted in a significant reduction in depressive symptoms in these HF patients. After 3 months of supervised exercise, patients in the exercise arm achieved a 1.75-point reduction in BDI-II scores compared to 0.98-points in UC controls; differences were even larger for patients with BDI-II scores ≥14.

In summary, the available evidence suggests that HF-rEF patients with depressive symptoms may benefit from an aerobic exercise program, and that the objective benefits are at least as significant, if not more so, than the effects of antidepressant medication. The data from two randomized controlled trials of selective serotonin reuptake inhibition in HF-rEF do not support the routine use of these agents.

End-of-life Planning

Estimates suggest that, at any given time, about 5% of the HF population have Stage D HF. As pointed out in the 2013 ACC/AHA guidelines, formal assessment for frailty and dementia should be part of the palliative care process offered to the patient and family. The 2016 ESC guidelines offer helpful clinical indications for considering end-of-life planning, as shown in **Table 10.3**. One recommended approach to palliative care for advanced HF patients proposes a gradual

TABLE 10.3 — Clinical Indications for End-of-Life Planning

- Progressive functional decline (physical and mental) and dependence in most activities of daily living
- Severe heart failure symptoms with poor quality of life despite optimal pharmacological and non-pharmacological therapies
- Frequent admissions to hospital or other serious episodes of decompensation despite optimal treatment
- Heart transplantation and mechanical circulatory support ruled out
- Cardiac cachexia
- Clinically judged to be close to end of life

Modified from Ponikowski P, et al. *Eur J Heart Fail.* 2016;18(8):891-975.

transition from life-prolonging measures to a focus on palliative care, as shown in **Figure 10.3**.[22]

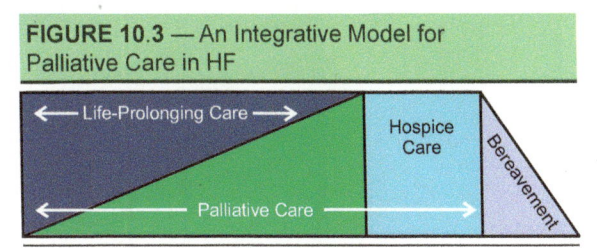

FIGURE 10.3 — An Integrative Model for Palliative Care in HF

Adler ED, et al. *Circulation.* 2009;120(25):2597-2606.

The discussion of prognosis and potential outcomes with HF patients and families is difficult. There are very few data on accuracy of recall in HF patients, although the oncology literature documents that patients' recall of information from "bad news" consultations is poor.[23] Consistent with this, the available data indicate that fewer than 40% of HF patients' family members were aware of a poor prognosis, and only 8% of patients and 44% of family members were told by a physician that the expected duration of life remaining was limited.[22] As compared to oncology patients, HF patients engaged in much less discussion about their condition. Most HF patients did not recall having a specific conversation about prognosis with their doctor.[24] **Table 10.4** outlines some important suggestions for communication with patients and their families.

The 2016 ESC guidelines also suggest that a management plan should be developed through discussion with the patient and his or her family. Such a plan should include:

- A discussion about stopping medication that does not have an immediate effect on symptom management or health-related quality of life, such as agents to lower cholesterol or treat osteoporosis
- Documentation of the patient's decision regarding attempts at resuscitation

TABLE 10.4 — Suggestions for Communication With Patients About HF Prognosis and Care Planning

Assessment	Ask the patient what he or she understands about his or her condition
Prognosis	Be conscious that prognostic uncertainty is no excuse for a failure to communicate about the implications of advanced heart disease
Preparation	Prepare the patient emotionally for what to expect
	Provide approximate time estimates (eg, months or years?)
	Talk about some likely scenarios
Preferences	Discuss healthcare proxy, goals if patient is permanently brain injured, cardiopulmonary resuscitation, ventilators, and location of care
	Discuss deactivation of ICD/cardiac resynchronization therapy/VAD, if applicable
Planning for the worst	Suggest getting financial and emotional affairs in order
	Help to mobilize community and family supports (eg, palliative care, home care, hospice referrals)

Modified from Adler ED, et al. *Circulation*. 2009;120(25):2597-2606.

- Deactivation of an ICD at end-of-life (according to local legal regulations)
- Preferred place for terminal care and death
- Emotional support to the patient and family/caregiver with appropriate referral for psychological and/or spiritual support.

The ESC guidelines manage to convey a critically important sense of the physician's responsibility for the patient dying of HF. In an increasingly data-driven and technologic environment, the recommendations deserve close scrutiny.

REFERENCES

1. Clegg A, Rogers L, Young J. Diagnostic test accuracy of simple instruments for identifying frailty in community-dwelling older people: a systematic review. *Age Ageing* 2015;44(1):148-152.

2. Castell MV, Sánchez M, Julián R, Queipo R, Martín S, Otero Á. Frailty prevalence and slow walking speed in persons age 65 and older: implications for primary care. *BMC Fam Pract.* 2013;14:86.

3. Savva GM, Donoghue OA, Horgan F, O'Regan C, Cronin H, Kenny RA. Using timed up-and-go to identify frail members of the older population. *J Gerontol A Biol Sci Med Sci.* 2013;68(4):441-446.

4. Dent E, Kowal P, Hoogendijk EO. Frailty measurement in research and clinical practice: A review. *Eur J Intern Med.* 2016;31:3-10.

5. Reeves GR, Whellan DJ, Patel MJ, et al. Comparison of frequency of frailty and severely impaired physical function in patients ≥60 years hospitalized with acute decompensated heart failure versus chronic stable heart failure with reduced and preserved left ventricular ejection fraction. *Am J Cardiol.* 2016;117(12):1953-1958.

6. Vidán MT, Blaya-Novakova V, Sánchez E, Ortiz J, Serra-Rexach JA, Bueno H. Prevalence and prognostic impact of frailty and its components in non-dependent elderly patients with heart failure. *Eur J Heart Fail.* 2016;18(7):869-875.

7. Frisoli A Jr, Ingham SJ, Paes ÂT, et al. Frailty predictors and outcomes among older patients with cardiovascular disease: Data from Fragicor. *Arch Gerontol Geriatr.* 2015;61(1):1-7.

8. Santangeli P, Di Biase L, Bai R, et al. Atrial fibrillation and the risk of incident dementia: a meta-analysis. *Heart Rhythm.* 2012;9(11):1761-1768.

9. Gaita F, Corsinovi L, Anselmino M, et al. Prevalence of silent cerebral ischemia in paroxysmal and persistent atrial fibrillation and correlation with cognitive function. *J Am Coll Cardiol.* 2013;62(21):1990-1997.

10. Pulignano G, Del Sindaco D, Tinti MD, et al; IMAGE-HF Study Investigators. Atrial fibrillation, cognitive impairment, frailty and disability in older heart failure patients: In memoriam Giovanni Gaschino. *J Cardiovasc Med (Hagerstown).* 2016;17(8):616-623.

11. Yang H, Niu W, Zang X, Lin M, Zhao Y. The association between atrial fibrillation and cognitive function in patients with heart failure [published online ahead of print April 1, 2016]. *Eur J Cardiovasc Nurs.* doi: 10.1177/1474515116641299.

12. Jefferson AL, Himali JJ, Beiser AS, et al. Cardiac index is associated with brain aging: the Framingham Heart Study. *Circulation.* 2010;122(7):690-697.

13. Leto L, Feola M. Cognitive impairment in heart failure patients. *J Geriatr Cardiol.* 2014;11(4):316-328.

14. Dardiotis E, Giamouzis G, Mastrogiannis D, et al. Cognitive impairment in heart failure. *Cardiol Res Pract.* 2012;2012:595821.

15. Sherwood A, Blumenthal JA, Trivedi R, et al. Relationship of depression to death or hospitalization in patients with heart failure. *Arch Intern Med.* 2007;167(4):367-373.

16. Sherwood A, Blumenthal JA, Hinderliter AL, et al. Worsening depressive symptoms are associated with adverse clinical outcomes in patients with heart failure. *J Am Coll Cardiol.* 2011;57(4):418-423.

17. Freedland KE, Hesseler MJ, Carney RM, et al. Major depression and long-term survival of patients with heart failure. *Psychosom Med.* 2016;78(8):896-903.

18. Sherwood A, Blumenthal JA, Hinderliter AL, et al. Worsening depressive symptoms are associated with adverse clinical outcomes in patients with heart failure. *J Am Coll Cardiol.* 2011;57(4):418-423.

19. O'Connor CM, Jiang W, Kuchibhatla M, et al; SADHART-CHF Investigators. Safety and efficacy of sertraline for depression in patients with heart failure: results of the SADHART-CHF (Sertraline Against Depression and Heart Disease in Chronic Heart Failure) trial. *J Am Coll Cardiol.* 2010;56(9):692-699.

20. Xiong GL, Fiuzat M, Kuchibhatla M, Krishnan R, O'Connor CM, Jiang W; SADHART-CHF Investigators. Health status and depression remission in patients with chronic heart failure: patient-reported outcomes from the SADHART-CHF trial. *Circ Heart Fail.* 2012;5(6):688-692.

21. Angermann CE, Gelbrich G, Stork S, et al. Effect of escitalopram on all-cause mortality and hospitalization in patients with heart failure and depression. *JAMA.* 2016;315:2683-2693.

22. Adler ED, Goldfinger JZ, Kalman J, Park ME, Meier DE. Palliative care in the treatment of advanced heart failure. *Circulation.* 2009;120(25):2597-2606.

23. van Osch M, Sep M, van Vliet LM, van Dulmen S, Bensing JM. Reducing patients' anxiety and uncertainty, and improving recall in bad news consultations. *Health Psychol.* 2014;33(11):1382-1390.
24. Hanratty B, Lowson E, Holmes L, et al. Breaking bad news sensitively: what is important to patients in their last year of life? *BMJ Support Palliat Care.* 2012;2(1):24-28.

11. Resources for Patients

Web-Based Resources

American Heart Association

http://www.heart.org/HEARTORG/Conditions/Heart
Failure/Heart-Failure_UCM_002019_SubHomePage.jsp

Cleveland Clinic

http://my.clevelandclinic.org/services/heart/disorders
/heart-failure-what-is

Heart Failure Society of America

http://www.hfsa.org/patient/

Mayo Clinic

http://www.mayoclinic.org/diseases-conditions/heart
-failure/basics/definition/con-20029801

National Heart, Lung, and Blood Institute

https://www.nhlbi.nih.gov/health/health-topics/topics/hf

National Institutes of Health

http://nihseniorhealth.gov/heartfailure/heartfailure
defined/01.html

National Library of Medicine

https://medlineplus.gov/ency/article/000158.htm

Recommended Books

Success with Heart Failure: Help and Hope for Those with Congestive Heart Failure
    Mark Silver (author)
    Mass Market Paperback
    September 5, 2006

The Cleveland Clinic Guide to Heart Failure
    Randall Starling, MD, MPH (author)
    Paperback
    June 2, 2009

Living Well with Heart Failure, the Misnamed, Misunderstood Condition
    Edward K. Kasper and Mary Knudson (authors)
    Paperback
    May 5, 2010

12 Abbreviations/Acronyms

2D	2-dimensional
6MWT	6-minute walk test
ACC	American College of Cardiology
ACCF	American College of Cardiology Foundation
ACEi	angiotensin-converting enzyme inhibitor
ACS	acute coronary syndrome
ADHERE	Acute Decompensated Heart Failure National Registry
ADHF	acutely decompensated heart failure
AE	adverse event
AF	atrial fibrillation
AHA	American Heart Association
AKI	acute kidney injury
ALLHAT	Antihypertensive and Lipid-Lowering Treatment to Prevent Heart Attack Trial
AMI	acute myocardial infarction
Ang II	angiotensin II
ANP	A-type natriuretic peptide
ARB	angiotensin receptor blocker
ARNI	angiotensin receptor neprilysin inhibitor
ATLAS-2	ATLAS-ACS 2 TIMI 51 (Anti-Xa Therapy to Lower Cardiovascular Events in Addition to Standard Therapy in Subjects With Acute Coronary Syndrome-Thrombolysis in Myocardial Infarction 51) Trial
AVNA	AV nodal ablation
BDI	Beck Depression Inventory [score]
BiVAD	biventricular assist device
BMI	body mass index
BNP	B-type natriuretic peptide
BP	blood pressure
BTB	bridge to bridge
BTC	bridge to candidacy
BTR	bridge to recovery

BTT	bridge to transplantation
BUN	blood urea nitrogen
CAD	coronary artery disease
CHF	congestive heart failure
CHD	coronary heart disease
CI	confidence interval
CIED	cardiovascular implantable electronic device
CKD	chronic kidney disease
CMP	cardiomyopathy
cMRI	cardiac magnetic resonance imaging
CO	cardiac output
COMMANDER-HF	A Randomized, Double-blind, Event-driven, Multicenter Study Comparing the Efficacy and Safety of Rivaroxaban With Placebo for Reducing the Risk of Death, Myocardial Infarction or Stroke in Subjects With Heart Failure and Significant Coronary Artery Disease Following an Episode of Decompensated Heart Failure
CONSENSUS	Cooperative North Scandinavian Enalapril Survival Study
COPD	chronic obstructive kidney disease
CORONA	Controlled Rosuvastatin in Multinational Trial Heart Failure
CPET	cardiopulmonary exercise testing
CRS	cardio-renal syndrome
CRT	cardiac resynchronization therapy
CTEPH	chronic thromboembolic pulmonary hypertension
cTn	cardiac troponin [test]
CV	cardiovascular
CVD	cardiovascular disease
DBP	diastolic blood pressure
DHF	diastolic heart failure
DIG	Digitalis Investigation Group [trial]
DT	destination therapy
dV/dP	change in volume vs change in pressure
ECG	electrocardiogram
ECLS	extracorporeal life support
ECMO	extracorporeal membrane oxygenation

ED	emergency department
EDV	end-diastolic volume
EF	ejection fraction
eGFR	estimated glomerular filtration rate
EMB	endomyocardial biopsy
EKG	electrocardiogram
EPHESUS	Eplerenone Post-Acute Myocardial Infarction Heart Failure Efficacy and Survival Study
EQ-5D	European Quality of Life-5 Dimensions [visual analogue scale]
ERA	endothelin receptor antagonist
ESCAPE	Evaluation Study of Congestive Heart Failure and Pulmonary Artery Catheterization Effectiveness [trial]
ESKD	end-stage kidney disease
EVEREST	Efficacy of Vasopressin Antagonism in Heart Failure Outcome Study With Tolvaptan
FCM	ferric carboxymaltose
FDA	Food and Drug Administration
FEV_1	forced expiratory volume in one second
GDMT	guideline-directed medical therapy
GFR	glomerular filtration rate
GWTG	Get With The Guidelines
HF	heart failure
HF-ACTION	Efficacy of Vasopressin Antagonism in Heart Failure Outcome Study With Tolvaptan
HF-pEF	heart failure with preserved ejection fraction
HF-rEF	heart failure with reduced ejection fraction
HR	hazard ratio
hs-TnT	high-sensitivity troponin T
HTN	hypertension
ICD	implantable cardioverter device
INTERMACS	Interagency Registry for Mechanically Assisted Circulatory Support
IQR	interquartile range
ISDN	isosorbide dinitrate
IV	intravenous

IVC	inferior vena cava
K	potassium
KCCQ	Kansas City Cardiomyopathy Questionnaire
LA	left atrial
LBBB	left bundle branch block
LV	left ventricular
LVAD	left ventricular assist device
LVDD	left ventricular diastolic diameter
LVEF	left ventricular ejection fraction
LVH	left ventricular hypertrophy
LVSD	left ventricular systolic dysfunction
MCS	mechanical circulatory support
MI	myocardial infarction
MR	mineralocorticoid receptor
MR	mitral regurgitation
MRA	mineralocorticoid receptor antagonists
MVO_2	maximal venous oxygen [consumption]
NA	not applicable
NO	nitric oxide
NOAC	new oral anticoagulant
NP	natriuretic peptide
NPM	nonpharmacologic management
NS	not significant
NSAID	nonsteroidal anti-inflammatory drug
NT-pro-BNP	N-terminal pro BNP
NYHA	New York Heart Association
OMM	optical medical management
ONTARGET	Ongoing Telmisartan Along and in combination wtih Ramipril Global Endpoint Trial
OPTIMIZE-HF	Organized Program to Initiate Lifesaving Treatment in Hospitalized Patients with Heart Failure
PA	posteroanterior
PAC	premature atrial contraction
PAH	pulmonary arterial hypertension
PAP	pulmonary artery pressure
PARADIGM-HF	Prospective Comparison of ARNI [Angiotensin Receptor–Neprilysin Inhibitor] with ACEI [Angiotensin-Converting–Enzyme Inhibitor]

	to Determine Impact on Global Mortality and Morbidity in Heart Failure Trial
PARAMOUNT	Prospective Comparison of ARNI with ARB on Management if Heart Failure with Preserved Ejection Fraction
PASP	pulmonary artery systolic pressure
PCP	procollagen type I carboxy-terminal proteinase
PCWP	pulmonary capillary wedge pressure
PDE-5I	phosphodiesterase type 5 inhibitor
PH	pulmonary hypertension
PICP	procollagen type I carboxy-terminal propeptide
PIIINP	peptide of procollagen type III aminoterminal propeptide
PVC	premature ventricular contraction
QOL	quality of life
RAAS	renin-angiotensin-aldosterone system
RALES	Randomized Aldactone Evaluation Study
RAP	right atrial pressure
RBANS	Repeatable Battery for the Assessment of Neuropsychological Status [score]
RNV	radionuclide ventriculography
ROS	reactive oxygen specifies
ROSE	Renal Optimization Strategies Evaluation [trial]
RR	relative risk
RV	right ventricular
RVH	right ventricular hypertrophy
SBP	systolic blood pressure
SCD	sudden cardiac death
SD	standard deviation
SES	socioeconomic status
SERCA2a	sarcoendoplasmic reticulum calcium APTase
sGCS	soluble guanylate cyclase stimulator
SHF	systolic heart failure
SHIFT	Systolic HF Treatment with If Inhibitor Ivabradine
SOLVD	Studies of Left Ventricular Dysfunction

sPRA	selection non-prostanoid prostacyclin receptor
SVO_2	mixed venous oxygen saturation
SVR	systemic vascular resistance
T2D	type 2 diabetes
TKI	tyrosine kinsase inhibitors
TOPCAT	Treatment of Preserved Cardiac Function Heart Failure With an Aldosterone Antagonist
TSAT	tranferrin saturation
TTE	thransthoracic echo
TTR	median time in therapeutic range
VAD	ventricular assist device
val-sac	valsartan-sacubitril
VEGFR	vascular endothelial growth factor receptor
V-HEFT	Vasodilator-Heart Failure Trial
VO_2	volume of oxygen consumption
VSMC	vascular smooth muscle cell
VT/VF	ventricular tachycardia/ventricular fibrillation
VTE	venous thromboembolism

INDEX

Note: HF stands for heart failure.
Page numbers in *italics* indicate figures.
Page numbers followed by a "t" indicate tables.
Clinical trials and studies are indexed under the
acronym of the name.

6-minute walk test, 40, 195, *196*, *200*, 226, 242, *249*

A-type natriuretic peptide (ANP), 51, 88
ACC/AHA
  guidelines for heart failure management, xvi-xviii[t], 258
  stages of heart failure, 40-43, 41t
    relationship to NYHA classification, *42*
ACE inhibitors. See *ACEi-s.*
ACEi-s (angiotensin-converting enzyme (ACE) inhibitors), 83-86
  action mechanisms, 83, *84*
  adverse effects, 86t
  ARBs vs, 83-84, 87-88
  cautions/contraindications, xv, xviii, 86t
  clinical trials, 87-88
    CHARM, 87-88
    CONSENSUS, 84
    ONTARGET, 87
    SOLVD, 84
  efficacy, 84, 87
  indications for
    HF-rEF patients, xviii, 84
    HF with CKD, 194t
  kinins and, 84
  switching to an ARB, 86-87
  switching to sacubitril/valsartan, 91, *94*
Acute coronary syndrome (ACS), 128
Acute decompensated heart failure (ADHF), 253-277
  classification of patients, 255, *258*
    cold and dry, 39t, 255, *258*
    cold and wet, *258*
    cold, cardiac output in, 257t
    cold, treatment decisions for, 255
    hemodynamic patterns, 39t

303

Acute decompensated heart failure (ADHF), classification of patients *(continued)*
    pulmonary congestion ("wet"), 256t
    treatment decisions and, 255
    volume status for "wet" vs "dry", 32t, 259
    warm and dry, 255, *258*
    warm and wet, 39t, *258*
  clinical presentation, 254-255, 256t-257t
    low cardiac output ("cold"), 257t
    overall circulatory assessment, 255, *258*
    pulmonary or systemic congestion ("wet"), 256t
  decompensation as sentinel prognostic event, 253
  goals of therapy, 255
  hemodynamic deterioration
    as marker for high risk of adverse outcomes, 264-266
    number of hospitalizations, mortality risk and, 253-254, *254*
    preceding clinical events, 253
  heterogeneity in ADHF population, 253, 274
  in HF-pEF patients, 253
  in HF-rEF patients, 253
  hospitalization for, 34, *34*, 253-254
    EVEREST study, 254
    mortality risk and, 253-254, *254*
      number of HF hospitalizations and, 254, *254*
  initial evaluation, 255, 258t
  medical management
    challenges in, 274-275
    diuretics, 259-260
    goals of therapy, 255
    heterogeneity in ADHF population, 253, 274
    individualization of, 255, 274
    initial evaluation and, 255, *258*
    summary and evaluation, 274-275
    symptomatic relief, 258-274. See also *specific agents listed under symptomatic relief, below.*
  new-onset, 253
  population characteristics, 253
  precipitating factors, 255, 259t
  prevalence of, 253
  signs and symptoms, 254-255, 256t-257t

Acute decompensated heart failure (ADHF) *(continued)*
  symptomatic relief, agents for, 258-274
    diuretics, 259-260, *261*, 274
    dobutamine, 267t
    dopamine, 266-274, 267t
      vs nesiritide, 266-274, *270-273*
    inotropes, 266-274, 267t
      not recommended for HF-rEF patients with ADHF, 266
    milrinone, 266, 267t
      adverse events with, 266, 268t-269t
    morphine, 258-259
    nesiritide, 264, 265t
      vs dopamine, 266-274, *270-273*
    summary and evaluation of, 274-275
    ultrafiltration, 262, 274
    vasodilators, 262-266, 274
      blood pressure and, 264, 265t
    vasopressin antagonists, 260-262, *263*
Acute heart failure, 22t, 44t. See also *Acute decompensated heart failure (ADHF)*.
Acutely decompensated HF (ADHF), 34, 39-40
ADHF. See *Acute decompensated heart failure*.
Adrenergic agonists, 266-274, 267t
Adrenergic blockers. See *β-blockers*.
Advanced HF, INTERMACS registry of stages for, 242, 244t-245t, *248*
Afterload, 50
Air pollution, 79
Albuminuria, 61, 186
Alcohol intake, 74-76, *75*
Aldactone. See *Spironolactone*.
Aldosterone, 102
Aldosterone antagonists, 102. See also *Eplerenone; Spironolactone*.
  agents, 102
    eplerenone, 102
    spironolactone, 102
Alogliptin, 165t
Alpha glucosidase inhibitors, 165t
Altitude, 78
Alzheimer's disease, comorbid with HF, 160t
American College of Cardiology/American Heart Association. See *ACC/AHA*.

Amiodarone, 143
Anemia, *66*, 193-195
  comorbid with HF, 160t, 162t, 193-195
  iron deficiency, 193, *201, 202*
  iron supplementation treatments, 194-195, *196-200*
Angina, 36t, *46, 171*
Angioedema
  as ACE-i side effect, 86t
  contraindication for sacubitril/valsartan, xv, 89
  minimizing risk for, xviii
  prior, as medication contraindication, 86t
Angiotensin, 50, 183. See also *Renin-angiotensin-aldosterone system.*
Angiotensin I, *85*
  conversion to angiotensin II, *85*
Angiotensin II, *85*
Angiotensin II receptor blockers. See *ARBs.*
Angiotensin-converting enzyme (ACE) inhibitors. See *ACEi-s.*
Angiotensin receptor neprilysin inhibitor (ARNI), xv, 88. See also *Sacubitril/valsartan.*
Anti-platelet agents, 125-127
Anti-thrombotic agents, 125-131
Anti-Xa anticoagulants, 127-128
Antibiotics, *154-155*
Anticoagulants, 127-131
  anti-Xa anticoagulants, 127-128
  clinical trials
    ATLAS-2, 131
    COMMANDER-HF, 130-131
  HF and AF, 127-128
  HF with AF and CAD, 128-130
  HF without AF, 130-131
  implantable devices and, 152, *153*
  indications for, 127-128
  oral, use with clopidogrel, 130
  triple therapy, 129
  warfarin, 127, 128
Antidepressants, xx, 287
  SSRIs, xix-xx, 287
  tricyclic, xx

Aortic stenosis, 217-219, *218*
  approved TAVR systems, 218-219
    decision making for TAVR patients, *224*
    Edwards Sapien transcatheter valve system, 218
    Medtronic Evolut R System, 218
  post-procedure improvements, *220-223*
ARBs (angiotensin II receptor blockers), 83-84, 86-88
  ACEi-s vs, 83-84, 88
  action mechanisms, 83-84
  adverse effects, 86, 86t
  ARBs, 83-84, 86-88
  cautions/contraindications, 86t
    combining sacubitril/valsartan with, xv, xviii
  clinical trials, PARAMOUNT trial, 60-61
  discontinuation of, 87
  dosage of, switching from ACEi to, 86-87
  efficacy, 87-88
  indications for, xix, 86-88
    HF-pEF, 88
    HF-rEF, 88
    HF with CKD, 194t
  switching to sacubitril/valsartan, 91, *94*
  tolerability, 86
Arginine vasopressin, 260
  vasopressin antagonists, 260-262, *263*
ARNI (angiotensin receptor neprilysin inhibitor), xv, 88. See also *Sacubitril/valsartan.*
  PARAMOUNT trial, 60-61
Arrhythmia. See *Atrial fibrillation.*
Arthritis, comorbid with HF, 160t
ASCEND-HF, 264, 265t, 274
Aspirin, 129
Asthma, 160t, 162t
ATLAS-2 trial, 131
Atrial fibrillation (AF), 26t, 127-131
  ADHF precipitated by, 259t
  anticoagulants. See also *Anticoagulants.*
    contraindication for, 228-229, 231
      Watchman Device as alternative, 229-231, *230*
  cardiac resynchronization therapy (CRT) for, 147-151
  cognitive impairment and, 282-283, *284-285*
  heart failure plus CAD with, 128-130

Atrial fibrillation (AF) *(continued)*
  heart failure with, 127-128, 160t
  heart failure without AF, 130-131
  incidence in HF patients, 228
  management of, left atrial appendage (LAA) closure, 228-231, *230*
  prevalence, 127, *128*
  progression of HF and, 35
  stroke risk, 127
Atrium, left. See *Left atrial appendage (LAA) closure.*
AV nodal ablation, 147-151, *151*
Avandia (rosiglitazone)
Azotemia, 86t

B-type natriuretic peptide (BNP), 51, 88
  increased, 256t
  using to evaluate HF with COPD, 169, *179*
β-Blockers, 96-99
  benefits of, xv
  efficacy, 96-98
    comparison of β-blockers, 98t
    differences between β-blockers, 97, 98
    in HF-pEF, 98-99
    vs ivabradine, 99
  indications for, 96, 98-99
    HF patients with COPD, 169-173, 181t, 183t
    in patients with HF-rEF, xviii
  ivabradine and, xv
Bile acid sequestrants, 165t
Biomarkers, 25t
Biopsy, endomyocardial, 31
Bisoprolol
  efficacy, 96
  indications for, HF with CKD, 194t
Blood glucose, 25t
Blood pressure. See also *Hypertension; Hypotension.*
  cognitive dysfunction and, 283
  vasodilators and, 264, 265t
Blood urea nitrogen (BUN), 25t
BMI (body mass index), 23, 73
Body mass index (BMI), 23, 73
Bradykinin, 84

Brain natriuretic peptide, diagnostic importance of, 25t
Brain natriuretic peptide. See *B-type natriuretic peptide (BNP)*.
Bromocriptine mesylate, 165t
Bumetanide, 115
BUN (blood urea nitrogen), 25t

CABG surgery, 159-161
Caloric restriction, 73-74
Canaglifozin, 165t
Cancer, 202-210
  anti-HER2 and VEGF cardiotoxicity, 203, 210t
  anticancer drugs and their CV effects, 206t-207t
  cardiotoxic effects of anticancer agents, 202-203, *204-205*
  CV risk assessment, monitoring, and management recommendations, 212t-213t
  frequency, mechanism, and reversibility of cancer therapies, 208t-209t
  QT-prolongation, 203
  radiation therapy, 203-210
  signaling inhibitor agents, 203, 207t
Candesartan, clinical trials of, 87-88, 186, 190-193, *192*
Canrenone, 106-107
Cardiac catheterization. See *Catheterization*.
Cardiac decompensation. See *Acute decompensated heart failure*.
Cardiac output, 39t, *64*, 111
  assessment of, 31
  in cardiogenic shock, 39t
  decreased, cognitive dysfunction and, 283
  in HF-pEF, 57
  in HF-rEF, 54
  low, 257t
  preload/afterload in, 50
  renal impairment and, 56t
Cardiac resynchronization therapy (CRT), 143, *146, 148-149*. See also *Pacing*.
  in AF patients, 147-151
Cardiac surgery. See *Surgical treatments*.
Cardiac transplantation, 30, 31, 73, 237
Cardio-oncology, 202-210. See also *Cancer*.
Cardio-renal syndrome (CRS), 55, 55t

Cardiogenic shock, 22t, 39t, 244t
  hemodynamic patterns in, 39t, 244t
  inotropes for, 274
CardioMEMS HF System, 236-237
Cardiopulmonary function testing, 29-30, 30t
Cardiovascular history, 23, 23t
Cardiovascular implantable electrophysiologic devices (CIEDs), 141-158. See also *Implantable hemodynamic monitoring.*
  anticoagulation, 152
  cardiac resynchronization therapy (CRT), 143, *146*, *148-149*
    in patients with AF, 147-151, *151*
  CIED therapy and clinical management, 152
  dyssynchrony induced by RV pacing, 147, *150*, 150t
  implantation of a new device, *155*
  importance and summary, 153-156
  infection, 152-153
    treatment of, *154-155*
  QRS widening, 143, *146*
  sudden death, 141-143
Cardioversion defibrillators, implanted, 141-143, *144-145*
  ACC/AHA guidelines, 143
CARESS trial, 262, 274
Carvedilol, 96-97
  efficacy, 96
  indications for, HF with CKD, 194t
Catheterization
  ESCAPE trial, 39
  left heart, for diagnosis, 30-31
  of right heart
    clinical outcomes and, 39
    diagnostic, 31
CHAMPION trial, 236-237, *238-241*
CHARM, 87-88, 186, 190-193, *192*
Chemotherapy, 23t
  cardiotoxic effects, 202-203, *204-205*
Chest X-ray, 27-28
  information from, 27t
Chlorpropamide, 165t
Chlorthalidone, 113-115
  combined with MRA, 115
  compared with hydrochlorothiazide, 114t

Chronic heart failure, 22t, *34*, 44t. See also
  Nonpharmacologic management of chronic heart failure;
  Pharmacologic management of heart failure.
 acute exacerbation of, 35
 acute exacerbation, vs slowly progressing, 35
 nonpharmacologic management of, 71-82
 pharmacologic management of, 83-140
Chronic kidney disease (CKD), 185-193
 ADHF precipitated by, 259t
 comorbid with HF, 159, 160t, 185-193
  impact for HF-pEF, 190-193, *191*, *192*
  impact for HF-rEF, 186, 187t, 189-190, *192*, 193
  Kaplan-Meier plots, 186, *188*, *191*, *192*
  management principles, 193, 194t
  negative feedback cycle in, 186, *189*
  prevalence and severity of hospital admissions, 189, *190*
  prevalence of coexisting CKD in HF population, 186-189, *190*
 definition and pathophysiology, 185-186
 GFR in, 185, 186
 MDRD formula, 185, 186
 prevalence in general population, 187t
 prevalence of in HF population, 186-189, *190*
 in HF-rEF patients, 187t
Chronic obstructive pulmonary disease (COPD), 35, 60, *66*, 169-185
 comorbid with HF, 159, 160t, 162t, 169-185
  β-blockers for, 169-173, 181t, 183t
  ivabradine for heart rate reduction, 173-179, 184t, *185*
  recommended therapies, 173, *180*
  using B-type natriuretic peptide levels to evaluate, 169, *179*
 heart failure and, 37t, 60, 169-185
 HF-pEF and, 60, *66*
 HF-rEF and, 173-179
 prevalence in HF population, 169
 SHIFT trial, 173-175, 182t-184t
Chronic pulmonary hypertension, 60
Chronic thromboembolic pulmonary hypertension (CTEPH), 38
Chronotypic incompetence, 54, 68t, 99
CIEDs. See *Cardiovascular implantable electrophysiologic devices.*

Circulatory support, mechanical, 237-246
Classification of heart failure, 33-47
  ACC/AHA stages of heart failure, 40-43, 41t, *42*
  acute HF, *34*, 44t
    acutely decompensated HF (ADHF), 34, 39-40, 255, *258*
  based on anatomy and function, 35-40, *38*, 44t
    hemodynamic patterns, 39-40, 39t
    HF-rEF, 38-39
    left heart failure, 38-39, *38*
    right ventricular failure, 35-38, *38*
  based on timing of symptoms, *34*, 44t
    acute vs chronic, *34*, 44t
  chronic HF, *34*, 44t
    acute exacerbation, vs slowly progressing, 35
  comorbid processes and, 35
  demographic data, 36t-37t
  heart failure syndromes, classification of, 35-39
  NYHA classification, 40-43, *40*, 41t, *42*
  phenotypes of HF patients, 43, *46-47*
  treatment context provided by, 43, 44t
Clinical syndromes and staging of HF, 33-47. See also *Classification of heart failure.*
Clinical trials. See *specific agents, treatments, and specific trials by name.*
Clopidogrel, 130
Coenzyme Q10, 76
Cognitive impairment, 282-283, *284-285*
  atrial fibrillation and, 282-283, *284-285*
  dementia, 160t, 282
  ESC Guideline recommendations on, 281t
  silent cerebral ischemia (SCI), 282, 283
Colesevelam, 165t
COMMANDER-HF, 130-131
Comorbid conditions, 36t-37t, 49, 159-216. See also *specific conditions, eg, Diabetes mellitus.*
  Alzheimer's disease/dementia, 160t, 282
  anemia, 160t, 162t, 193-195
  arthritis, 160t
  asthma, 160t, 162t
  atrial fibrillation, 127-128, 160t
  cancer, 202-210
  cardiovascular conditions and risk factors, 36t

Comorbid conditions *(continued)*
  challenges to HF management, 159
  chronic kidney disease (CKD), 159, 160t, 185-193
  commonly associated with HF, 159, 160t, 162t-163t
  COPD, 159, 160t, 162t, 169-185
  coronary artery disease (CAD), 159-161
  depression, 160t, 283-288
  diabetes, 159, 160t, 161-169, 162t, 165t
  geriatric conditions, 37t
  HF and atrial fibrillation, 127-128
    with CAD, 128-130
  HF-pEF and, 49, *66-67*
    COPD, 60
  hyperlipidemia, 160t
  hypertension, 36t, 160t
  ischemic heart disease, 160t
  obesity, 162t
  other medical conditions, 37t
  progression of HF and, 35
  psychosocial conditions, 37t
COMPASS-HF trial, 231-236
Computed tomography (CT)
CONFIRM-HF study, 195, *202*
Congestion, pulmonary or systemic, 255, 256t, *258*
CONSENSUS trial, 83
Contrast ventriculography, 30
COPD. See *Chronic obstructive pulmonary disease.*
Cordarone (amiodarone), 143
Corlanor. See *Ivabradine.*
Coronary angiography, 30-31
Coronary artery disease (CAD), 159-161
  CABG surgery, 159-161
  heart failure and, 36t, 159-161
  heart failure and AF with, 129-130
Coronary disease, progression of, 35
Cough, ACE inhibitors and, 86t
CTEPH (chronic thromboembolic pulmonary hypertension), 38

Dapagliflozin, 165t
Decompensated heart failure. See *Acute decompensated heart failure (ADHF).*

313

Decompensation, as sentinel prognostic event, 253
Defibrillators: implantable cardioverter-debfibrillators, 141-143, *144-145*
Depression, xix-xx, 283-288
  adherence to therapy and, xix
  antidepressants, xx, 287
  clinical trials on, 287
  cognitive behavioral therapy, xix
  ESC Guideline recommendations on, 281t
  evaluation instruments, 287
  exercise and, 287-288
  heart failure and, 37t, 160t, 283
  HF-rEF, 287-288
  HF prognosis and, 283, *286*
  hospitalizations and mortality and, 283-287, *286*
  prevalence of, 283
  screening for, xix
  SSRIs for, xix-xx, 287
  worsening of symptoms, 287
Diabetes mellitus, 23t, *66*, 161-169
  comorbid with HF, 159, 160t, 161-169, 162t
    effects of anti-diabetic agents, 161-169
    optimal management strategy, 169
    potential adverse effects of anti-diabetic medications in HF, 161-169, *167, 176-177*
  heart failure and, 36t, 161-169
  heart failure treatment in, 159
  management of, 161-169, 165t
    DPP-4 inhibitors, 165-166, 165t
    efficacy data, review of, *170-172*
    metformin, 165t, 166
    SGLT2 inhibitors, 165t, 167-169, *168*
      adverse effects, 169, *176-177*
      CV outcomes trials, 178t
  type 1 diabetes, 161
  type 2 diabetes, 161-169
    drugs used in treatment of, 161-169, 165t
    efficacy data, review of, *170-172*
Diagnosis of heart failure, 21-32, 32t, 56. See also *Classification of heart failure; Clinical syndromes and staging*
  cardiac imaging studies, 28-29, 29t
    2D and Doppler echochardiography, 28, 28t

Diagnosis of heart failure, cardiac imaging studies *(continued)*
  comorbidities and, 29
  important data from, 28t
 chest X-ray, 27-28, 27t
 electrocardiogram (12-lead resting), 24-27, 26t
 exercise testing in, 30, 30t
 functional studies, 29-30, 30t
 history, 22-23
  cardiovascular history, 23, 23t
 initial evaluation in ADHF patient, 255, 258t
 invasive studies, 30-31
  cardiac catheterization, 30-31
  contrast ventriculography, 30
  coronary angiography, 30-31
  endomyocardial biopsy, 31
  right heart catheterization, 31
 laboratory tests, 23-24, 25t
 natriuretic peptides in, 25t
 outcomes of HF evaluation, 32t
 physical examination, 23, 24t
 presentation, 21, 22t, 43, 256t-257t
 salt and water retention, exercise intolerance, and dyspnea, 21, 22t
Diet, 71-77
 alcohol intake, 74-76, *75*
 caloric restriction, 73-74
 dietary supplements, 76-77
  coenzyme Q10, 76
  nitrate supplementation, 76-77
 fluid restriction, 72
 sodium (salt) limitation, 71-72
  clinical evidence for, 71
  conversion factors, 72t
  RAAS activation associated with, 71
 summary of recommendations, 74t
DIG trial, 116-117, *126*, 190, *191*
Digoxin, 116-117, *126*
 adverse effects, 116
 clinical trials of (DIG trial), 116-117, *126*
 indications for, 117
 monitoring of serum digoxin levels, 117
 risk ratio, 116-117

Diuretics, 113-116. See also *specific agents.*
  adverse effects, 115
  agents
    chlorthalidone, 113-115, 114t
    furosemide, 33, 115, 122t-124t
    hydrochlorothiazide, 113, 114t
    torsemide, 115-116, *118-119, 120-121,* 125t
  clinical trials, 113-115
    ALLHAT, 113
    DOSE, 259-260, *261,* 274
    ROSE trial, 266-274, *270-273,* 274
  combined with MRA, 115
  comparison of, 114t, 122t-124t, 125t
  continuous infusion with, 274
  dosage, low-dose vs. high-dose strategy in ADHF, 259-260, *261*
  efficacy, 113-116
  indications for, 113, 116
    in acute decompensated heart failure, 259-260, *261*
  loop, 115-116
  thiazide, 113-115
Dobutamine, 267t
Dopamine, 266-274, 267t
  low-dose ("renal-dose"), to enhance effects of diuretics, 266-274
  vs nesiritide (ROSE trial), 266-274, *270-273*
Dopamine receptor agonists, 165t
Doppler echochardiography, 28, 28t
DOSE trial, 259-260, *261,* 274
DPP-4 inhibitors, 165-166, 165t
Dyspnea, 21, 22t, 56, 255, 256t
  nocturnal, 255
  vasodilators for, 262-264

Edema, 255, 256t
  acute pulmonary, 39t, 43, 256t
  pulmonary edema, 22t, 43
Ejection fraction. See also *Heart failure with preserved ejection fraction (HF-pEF); Heart failure with reduced ejection fraction (HF-rEF).*
  heart failure with mid-range ejection fraction (HF-mEF), xviii

Ejection fraction *(continued)*
  heart failure with reduced ejection fraction (HF-rEF), xviii, 38-39
    treatment recommendations, xviii
  left ventricular (LVEF), 97, 110, 185
    in HF pathophysiology, *38*
    treatment decisions and, xviii
Elderly patients. See also *Psychosocial issues.*
  atrial fibrillation in, 127, *128*
  cognitive impairment/dementia, 282-283
  frailty, 279-282
  heart failure in, 37t
Electrocardiogram, 24-27, 26t
  12-lead, 24-27, 26t
  common findings in HF, 26t
Electrolytes, 25t
EMPA-REG OUTCOME, *174-175*
Empagliflozin, 165t
Enalapril, *92-93*, 189-190
End-of-life planning, 288-291
  clinical indications for (ESC Guidelines), 288t
  management plan, discussing with patients and families, 289-291, 290t
  palliative care, 288-289, *289*
  suggestions for communication with patients, 289-291, 290t
Endomyocardial biopsy, 31
Endothelin receptor antagonists, 132t
Entresto. See *Sacubitril/valsartan.*
Environmental conditions, 78-79
  altitude, 78
  particulate pollution, 79
  temperature, 78-79
Eplerenone, 102
  clinical trials, 103, 106-107
    EPHESUS, 103
  dosage, 104t-105t
  indications for, 103
ESCAPE trial, 39, 55
Escitalopram, xx
EVEREST trials, 133, 260-262, *263*, 274
  hospitalizations and future risk, 254

317

Exercise, 77, 287-288
   cardiopulmonary exercise evaluation, 30t
   clinical trials of, 287
   depression, reduction in symptoms, 287-288
   in HF-pEF, 77
   in HF-rEF, 77
Exercise intolerance
   in diagnosis, 21, 22t
   onset of, 22-23
Exercise testing, 30, 30t

FAIR-HF study, 193-194, 195, *202*
Familial heart disease, 22, 23t
Fibrillation, atrial. See *Atrial fibrillation.*
Filling pressures, 31, 39t, 50-51, *51*, 57
   in HF-pEF, 68t
Fluid restriction, 72
Fluid retention, 255, 256t. See also *Edema.*
FRAIL-HF study, 280-282
Frailty, 279-282
   ADHF patients, 280-281
   diagnosis of, 279-280
     gait speed, 279-280
     PRISMA-7 survey, 279-280
   ESC guideline recommendations on, 280t
   FRAIL-HF, 280-282
   medication review, 280t
   referral to specialist, 280t
Furosemide, 33, 115
   vs torsemide, 122t-124t

Gender, hospitalization rates for HF and, *34*, 35, 36t
GISSI-HF study, 76
Glimepiride, 165t
Glipizide, 165t
Glitazones, 165t
Glomerular filtration rate (GRF), 25t, 61, 104t-105t
Glyburide, 165t
Guidelines for heart failure management, xiv-xx
   2013 ACCF/AHA Guideline, xiv
   2016 ACC/AHA/HFSA, xiv-xv
   2016 ESC Guidelines, xiv, xv-xx, 258-259

Guidelines for heart failure management *(continued)*
  ACC/AHA recommendation system, xvi-xviii[t], 258
  consensus view in, xx
  critical information on, xiv
  ESC Guidelines, xiv, xv-xx, 258-259
    on psychosocial issues, 280t, 281t
  guideline-directed therapy, xii, xiv
  for ivabradine, xix, xv
  level (quality) of evidence, xvii[t]
  limitations of, xii
  for sacubitril/valsartan, xv
  strength/class of recommendations, xvi[t]
  updates to, xiv-xx

Heart failure. See also *Treatment of heart failure.*
  acute heart failure, 253-277
  classification of, 33-47
  clinical syndromes and staging, 33-47
  comorbidities, 36t-37t, 159-216, 160t, 162t-163t
  diagnosis of, 21-32
  hemodynamic patterns in, 39-40, 39t
  interventions for, 217-252
  pathophysiology of, 49-69
  psychosocial issues, 279-294
  resources for patients, 295-296
  subcategories of, 22t. See also *specific subcategories.*
    heart failure with mid-range ejection fraction (HF-mEF), xviii
    heart failure with preserved ejection fraction (HF-pEF), 56-61
    heart failure with reduced ejection fraction (HF-rEF), xviii, 38-39
    timing of: acute vs chronic, 22t
  symptoms of, 21, 22t, 256t-257t
Heart failure with mid-range ejection fraction (HF-mEF), xviii
Heart failure with preserved ejection fraction (HF-pEF), 44t
  acute decompensated heart failure (ADHF) in, 253
  comorbidities, 49, *66-67*
    chronic kidney disease (CKD), 190-193, *191*, *192*, 193
    COPD, 60
  definition of, 56-57

319

Heart failure with preserved ejection fraction (HF-pEF) *(continued)*
  exercise recommendations, 77
  pathophysiology of, 56-61, *64*
    cardiac changes, 68t
    comorbidities and, 49, 60, *66-67*
    hypertension, 88
    musculoskeletal responses, 61, 68t
    pulmonary responses, 57-60, 68t
    renal responses, 60-61, *67*
  phenotype, 43, 49
  physiology of (LV pressure/volume), 56-57, *62-63*
  precapillary pulmonary hypertension and, 131-132
  treatment
    ACEi-s, 8
    ARBs, 8
    β-blockers, 98-99
    hydralazine/ISDN, 113
    MRAs, 106-109
    sacubitril/valsartan, 91
Heart failure with reduced ejection fraction (HF-rEF), 38-39, 44t
  acute decompensated heart failure (ADHF) in, 253
  comorbidities
    anemia, 195
      treatment algorithms, *201, 202*
    chronic kidney disease (CKD), 186, 187t, 189-190, *192*
    COPD, 173-179
  effectiveness of therapies, xviii, 49
  exercise recommendations, 77, 287-288
  pathophysiology in, 49-56
    CAD and, 161
    cardiovascular responses, 51-54, *52-53*
    hemodynamic congestion, 50-51
    myocardial injury as initiator, 49, *50*
    negative feedback cycles, 49-56, *50*, 83-84
    pulmonary abnormalities, 54-55
    RAAS activation, 50, *50*, 51, *51*
    renal responses, 55-56, 55t, 56t
    salt and water retention, 50, *50*
  treatment
    ACEi-s, xviii, 84-86

Heart failure with reduced ejection fraction (HF-rEF), treatment *(continued)*
    ARBs, 86-88
    β-blockers, xviii, 96
    digoxin, 117
    inotropes, 274
    ivabradine, 99
    MRAs, xviii, 102-106
    sacubitril/valsartan, 91

Heart rate
  CardioMEMS HF System for monitoring, 237
  in diagnosis, 24t, 26t
  elevated, 50
  inotropic agents and, 267t
  ivabradine for heart rate reduction, xix, 101, 173-179, 184t, *185*
  resting, 26t
  sympathetic nervous system and, 50

Heart rhythm, 26t

Heart transplant, 30, 31, 73, 237

HeartMate II device, 242, *243*

Hemodynamics
  in acute decompensated heart failure
    deterioration, as marker for risk of adverse outcomes, 264-266
    deterioration preceding clinical events, 253
  hemodynamic congestion, 50-51
  hemodynamic patterns in HF, 39-40, 39t
    in advanced HF, 244t-245t
    in cardiogenic shock, 39t, 244t
  implantable hemodynamic monitoring, 231-237
  vasodilator use and, 264-266, 265t

Hemoglobin/hematocrit, 25t

HF-ACTION Study, 287
  patient phenotypes ("clusters") in, *46-47*

HF-pEF. See *Heart failure with preserved ejection fraction.*

HF-rEF. See *Heart failure with reduced ejection fraction.*

History, in diagnosis, 22-23
  cardiovascular history, 23, 23t
  familial heart disease, 22, 23t

Hospitalization for heart failure
  for acute decompensated heart failure (ADHF), 253-254, *254*, 264-266, 265t
  demographic data, 36t
  discharges, number of, 34, *34*
  hospitalization rates, trends in, 34-35, *34*, 36t
  hospitalizations for depression, 283-287, *286*
  hypotension and, 264, 265t
  mortality risk and, 253-254, *254*, 264, 265t
    before and after discharge, 254
    number of HF hospitalizations and, 254, *254*
Hydralazine, 109-113
  action mechanism, 109-111
  African Americans and, 111-113, *112*
  clinical trials of
    A-HeFT, 111-113, *112*
    V-HeFT-I and V-HeFT-II, 111
  in combination with ISDN, 111, 112-113
  hemodynamic effects, 110-111
  indications for, 111, 112-113
Hydrochlorothiazide, 113, 114t
Hyperkalemia, 102
  ACE inhibitors and, 86t
  ARBs and, 86t
  CKD patients, 194t
  MRAs and, 106, 109
Hyperlipidemia, 160t
Hypertension, 38, 60, 131-133. See also *Diuretics.*
  alcohol intake and, 74, *75*, 76
  chronic pulmonary, 38, 60
  heart failure and, 36t, 160t
  precapillary pulmonary hypertension, 131-132
  pulmonary, agents targeting, 131-133
Hypokalemia, diuretics and, 115
Hyponatremia, 257t
  diuretics and, 115
  fluid restriction for, 72
Hypotension
  ACE inhibitors and, 86t
  ARBs and, 86t
  hospitalization and, 264, 265t
  vasodilators and, 264, 265t

Imaging studies, in diagnosis of HF, 28-29, 29t
  2D and Doppler echochardiography, 28, 28t
Implantable electrophysiologic devices.
  See *Cardiovascular implantable electrophysiologic devices.*
Implantable hemodynamic monitoring, 231-237
  CardioMEMS HF System, 236-237
    FDA approval of, 237
  CHAMPION trial, 236-237
    changes in medications, 236-237, *240*
    dosage changes in medications, 237, *241*
    management algorithm, 237, *238-239*
  COMPASS-HF trial, 231-236
Individuals
  individualization of therapy, 255, 274
  prognosis, variation in, xiii
Infection
  ADHF precipitated by, 259t
  implanted electrophysiologic devices (CIEDs) and, 152-153, *154-155*
Inotropes, 266-274, 267t
  adverse events, 266, 268t-269t
  agents available, 267t
  indications for, 274
    acute decompensated HF-rEF, 274
    cardiogenic shock, 274
    hospitalized patients with severe systolic dysfunction, 274
  low-dose, 266-274, *270-273*
  not recommended for HF-rEF patients with ADHF, 266
INTERMACS registry of HF stages, 242, 244t-245t, *248*
Interventions for HF, 217-252
  aortic stenosis, 217-219, *218, 220-223*
  implantable hemodynamic monitoring, 231-237
  left atrial appendage (LAA) closure, 228-231
  mechanical circulatory support, 237-246
  mitral regurgitation, surgical repair of, 219-228
  transcatheter aortic valve replacement (TAVR), 217-219
Iron/iron-binding capacity, 25t
Iron deficiency, 193
  algorithm for diagnosis, *201*
  algorithm for treatment, *202*
Iron supplementation, 194-195, *196-200*

Ischemic heart disease, comorbid with HF, 160t
Ivabradine, 99-102
  action mechanism, 99
  β-blockers and, xv
  clinical trials, SHIFT, 99, *100-101*
  dosage, initiation and up-titration of, xv
  efficacy, 99-102, *100-101*
  FDA approval, 99
  guidelines for, xv
  indications for, xix, 99-101
    2016 ACC/AHA/HFSA guidelines, xv
    EMA approved uses, xix
    heart rate reduction in HF-rEF patients with COPD, xix, 101, 173-179, 184t, *185*
  vs β-blockers, 99

Kidney disease. See *Chronic kidney disease (CKD)*.
Kinins, 84

Laboratory tests, 23-24, 25t
LCZ696, xviii, 89. See also *Sacubitril/valsartan*.
Left atrial appendage (LAA) closure, 228-231
  AF patients with contraindication for chronic anticoagulation, 228-229, 231
  Kaplan-Meier curves, 229, *232-233*
  Kaplan-Meier curves for bleeding, *234-235*
  Watchman Device, 229-231, *230*
Left ventricular assist devices (LVADs), 237-242. See also *Mechanical circulatory support*.
  patient eligibility criteria, 246, 251t
Left ventricular ejection fraction (LVEF), xviii, 97, 110, 185
Left ventricular (left heart) failure, 38-39, *38*
  impaired LV systolic function (HF-rEF), 38
Leukocytes/leukocytosis, 25t
Linagliptin, 165t
Loop diuretics, 115-116. See also *Diuretics*.
  torsemide, 115-116, *118-121*
  torsemide vs furosemide, 116, 122t-124t, 125t
LVEF. See *Left ventricular ejection fraction*.

Magnetic resonance imaging (MRI)
Mechanical circulatory support, 237-246
　ECS Guidelines, 246, *248-249*
　　for patient eligibility, 246, 251t
　HeartMate II device, 242, *243*
　INTERMACS registry of advanced HF stages, 242, 244t-245t, *248*
　left ventricular assist devices (LVADs), 237-242, *248-249*
　　patient eligibility criteria, 246, 251t
　REMATCH study, 237
　ROADMAP study, 242-246, *243, 249*
　terms used in indications for, 250t
　treatment algorithm and decision guide, *248-249*
Meglitinides, 165t
Mental status assessment, 281t, 282-283, *284-285*
Metformin, 165t, 166
Metoprolol, 194t
Metoprolol succinate (sustained-release), 96-97
Microalbuminuria, 186
Miglitol, 165t
Milrinone, 266, 267t, 268t-269t
　adverse events, 266, 268t-269t
Mineralcorticoid receptor antagonists (MRAs), 102-109.
　　See also *specific agents*.
　action mechanism, 102
　adverse events, 106
　　hyperkalemia, 106, 109
　　renal dysfunction, 109
　approved agents (eplerone, spironolactone), 102
　clinical trials, 103-109
　　EPHESUS, 103
　　RALES, 103
　　TOPCAT, 107, *108*
　combined with chlorthalidone (diuretic), 115
　discontinuation of, 103
　dosing, 104t-105t
　efficacy, 103-109
　guidelines and recommendations, xviii, 102, 109
　indications for
　　HF-pEF, 106-109
　　HF-rEF, xviii, 102-106
　　HF with CKD, 194t
　monitoring, 103, 109, 110t

Mitral regurgitation (MR), 133, 219-228
  ADHF precipitated by, 259t
  catheter-based approach, 225
  EVEREST II trial, 225-226
  exercise and, 54
  guidelines on repair, 219-228
  in HF-rEF, 54
  incidence of, 219
  MitraClip device, 133, 225-228, *225*
    complications, 228t
    indications for, 226
    meta-analysis of outcomes, 226, *227*
    safety data, 226-228
  surgical repair of, 219-228
Mitral valve regurgitation, 35
MOOD-HF Study, 287
MRAs. See *Mineralcorticoid receptor antagonists.*
Musculoskeletal responses to HF, 56, 60t, 61, 68t
  nitrate supplements and, 76-77
Myocardial fibrosis, torsemide effects, *120-121*
Myocardial infarction, prior, heart failure and, 36t, 38
Myocardial injury, 35
  in HF-rEF pathophysiology, 49, *50*
Myocardial ischemia, stress testing for, 30t
Myocardial remodeling. See *Remodeling.*
Myocardium
  contractility of, *52-53*
  "stretch-squeeze" relationship, *52*, 54

Nateglinide, 165t
Natriuretic peptides, 88
  A-type (ANP), 51, 88
  augmentation of, 88
  B-type (BNP), 51, 88, 169, *179*, 256t
  RAAS activation and, 51, *51*
  using to evaluate HF with COPD, 169, *179*
Negative feedback cycles, 49-56, *50*, 83-84
  in HF and CKD, 186, *189*
Neprilysin enzyme, xv, 88. See also *ARNI (angiotensin receptor neprilysin inhibitor).*

Neprilysin (NEP) inhibitor. See also *Sacubitril/valsartan.*
  angiotensin receptor neprilysin inhibitor (ARNI), xv, 88
  LCZ696 and, xviii, 89
Nesiritide, 264, 265t, 266-274
  low-dose ("renal-dose"), to enhance effects of diuretics, 266-274
  vs dopamine (ROSE trial), 266-274, *270-273*
Neuro-hormonal antagonists (ACEi-s, MRAs, β-blockers), xviii
New York Heart Association (NYHA) classification system, 40-43
  ACC/AHA stages, relationship to, *42*
  maximal oxygen uptake, 40, *40*
Nitrates, 109-113
  action mechanism, 109-111
  dietary supplementation, 76-77
  hemodynamic effects, 110-111
  hydralazine, 109-113
Nitric oxide, 76-77
Nitroglycerine, 264
Nitroprusside, 264
  hemodynamic effects of, 111
Nonpharmacologic management of chronic heart failure, 71-82. See also *Diet.*
  dietary interventions, 71-77
  environmental conditions, 78-79
  physical activity, 77
NSAIDS, ADHF precipitated by, 259t
NYHA classification. See *New York Heart Association (NYHA) classification system.*

Obesity, *67*, 73
  comorbid with HF, 162t
ONTARGET, 87
OPTIME-CHF, 266, 268t-269t, 274
Orthopnea, 255, *258*
Oxygen, maximal consumption of, in HF-pEF, 57
Oxygen saturation, low, 256t

Pacing
  cardiac resynchronization therapy, 143, *146*, *148-149*
    in AF patients, 147-151
  dyssynchrony induced by RV pacing, 147, *150*, 150t
  right-ventricular, 150t
Palliative care, 288-289, *289*
PARADIGM-HF, 89, *92-93*
PARAMOUNT trial, 60-61, 91-96, *96*
Particulate pollution, 79
Pathophysiology of heart failure, 49-69
  in HF-pEF, 56-61, *64*
    cardiac changes, 68t
    comorbidities, 49, *66-67*
    musculoskeletal responses, 61, 68t
    physiology: LV volume/pressure, *62-63*
    pulmonary responses, 57-60, 68t
    renal responses, 60-61, *67*
  in HF-rEF, 49-56, *50*
    cardiac performance and end diastolic volume, *52-53*
    cardiovascular responses, 51-54, *52-53*
    hemodynamic congestion, 50-51
    musculoskeletal responses, 56, 60t
    negative feedback cycles, 49-56, *50*, 83-84
    pulmonary abnormalities, 54-55
    RAAS activation, 50, *50*, 51, *51*
    renal responses, 55-56, 55t, 56t
    salt and water retention, 50, *50*
    self-perpetuating process, 51
Patient phenotypes ("clusters") in HF, 43, *46-47*
Patient questions, information needed to address, 33
Patients and families
  discussions about prognoses, 289, 290t
  end-of-life planning, 288-291
  management plan, discussing with, 289-291, 290t
Peripheral perfusion, assessment of, 23, 24t, *258*
Peripheral vascular disease, heart failure and, 36t
Pharmacologic management of heart failure, 83-140,
    258-274. See also *specific drugs and drug types.*
  acute decompensated heart failure (ADHF), 255, 258-274
  agents, 84t
    ACEi-s, 83-86
    agents targeting pulmonary hypertension, 131-133, 132t

Pharmacologic management of heart failure, agents *(continued)*
  anti-platelet agents, 125-127
  anti-thrombotic agents, 125-131
  anticoagulants, 127-131
  ARBs, 86-88
  β-blockers, 96-99
  digoxin, 116-117, *126*
  diuretics, 113-116, 259-260
  dobutamine, 267t
  dopamine, 266-274, 267t
  hydralazine/nitrates, 109-113
  inotropes, 266-274, 267t
  ivabradine, 99-102
  milrinone, 266, 267t
  morphine, 258-259
  MRAs (mineralcorticoid receptor antagonists), 102-109
  sacubitril/valsartan, 88-96
  vasodilators, 109-113, 262-266, 274
  vasopressin antagonists, 260-262, *263*
 of chronic heart failure, 83-140
 classes of agents, 84t
Phenotypes of HF patients, 43, *46-47*
Phosphodiesterase inhibitors
 indications for, 132t
 milrinone, 266, 267t
Physical activity, 77. See also *Exercise.*
Physical examination, 23, 24t
Pioglitazone, 165t
Prazosin (Minipress), 111
Prognosis
 depression and, 283, *286*
 discussions with patients and families about, 289, 290t
 individual variation in, xiii
Prostanoids, 132t
Psychosocial issues, 37t, 279-294
 cognitive impairment, 281t, 282-283, *284-285*
 depression, xix-xx, 283-288
 end-of-life planning, 288-291, 288t
 ESC guidelines on, 280t, 281t
 frailty, 279-282, 280t
Pulmonary abnormalities, in HF-rEF, 54-55

Pulmonary congestion, 256t
Pulmonary edema, 22t
  acute, patient phenotype, 43
  hemodynamic patterns in, 39t
Pulmonary examination, 23, 24t
Pulmonary function testing, 29-30, 30t
Pulmonary hypertension
  agents targeting, 131-133, 132t
  referral to a HF center, 132
Pulmonary responses
  in HF-pEF, 57-60, 68t
  in HF-rEF, 54-55

QRS widening, 143, *146*
QT-prolongation, anticancer drugs and, 203

RAAS. See *Renin-angiotensin-aldosterone system.*
Race
  hospitalization rates for HF and, 35, 36t
  hydralazine, African Americans and, 111-113, *112*
RALES trial, 103
Ramipril, clinical trials of, 87
RED-HF trial, 193
Regurgitation. See *Mitral valve regurgitation.*
REMATCH study, 237
Remodeling, 35
  electrical, 54
  in HF-rEF, *50*, 54
  negative feedback cycle, *50*
  structural, 54
Renal dysfunction, *67*
  cardio-renal syndrome, 55, 55t
  heart failure and, 37t
  in HF-pEF, 60-61, *67*
  in HF-rEF, 55-56, 55t, 56t
  mechanisms of, 55-56, 56t
  pathophysiology of, 55-56, 56t, *58-59*
  renal congestion, 55-56, *58*
  renal inflammation, *58-59*
Renal function
  glomerular filtration rate, 25t, 104t-105t
  monitoring with MRAs, 109
  testing for, 25t

Renin, increased levels of, 50
Renin-angiotensin-aldosterone system (RAAS), 50, *50*
  activation of, 50, *50*
    cascade of effects, *85*
    sodium (salt) limitation and, 71
  activation of natriuretic peptides, 51, *51*
  aldosterone in, 102
  renin-angiotensin cascade, *85*
  torsemide effects on, *118-119*
Repaglinide, 165t
Resources for patients, 295-296
Right heart (Swan-Ganz) catheterization, 31, 39
Right ventricular failure, 35-38, *38*
Right-ventricular pacing, cardiac effects of, 150t
Riociguat, 132t
Rivaroxaban, 130-131
ROADMAP study, 242-246, *243, 249*
ROSE trial, 266-274, *270-273,* 274
Rosiglitazone, 165t

Sacubitril
  action mechanism, 89
  as LCZ696, xviii, 89
Sacubitril/valsartan (Entresto), 88-96
  action mechanism, xv, 89
  adverse reactions, xv
    angioedema, xv, 89
      minimizing risk for, xviii
    hypotension, xv
  cautions and contraindications, xv, 89
    combining with ACEi or ARB, xviii
  clinical trials, 89-96
    PARADIGM-HF, 89, *92-93*
    PARAMOUNT, 91-96, *96*
  dosing
    initiation of therapy, 91, *94-95*
    switching from ACEi-s or ARBs to, 91, *94-95*
  efficacy, 89-96
  FDA approval, 89
  guidelines for, xv, 91
  indications for, xv
    2016 ACC/AHA/HFSA guidelines, xv, 91

Sacubitril/valsartan (Entresto), indications for *(continued)*
   HF-pEF, 91
   HF-rEF, 91
   to replace ACEi in HF-rEF patients, xviii, 91, *94*
   initiation of, withholding ACEi prior to, xviii
   LCZ696, xviii, 89
   molecular structure, *90*
   troponin T-sensitivity, 92, *96*
SADHART-CHF, 287
Salt limitation (in diet), 71-72, 72t
Salt retention, 21, 22t, 50, *50*
Saxagliptin, 165t
Selixigap, 132t
Sertraline, 287
SGLT2 inhibitors, 165t, 167-169, *168*
  adverse effects of, 169, *176-177*
  CV outcomes trials, 178t
SHIFT trial, 99, *100-101*
Shock
  cardiogenic, 22t, 39t
  hemodynamic patterns in, 39t
Sildenafil, 132t
Silent cerebral ischemia (SCI), 282, 283
Sitagliptin, 165t
Sleep-related breathing disorders, 23t, *67*
Sodium limitation, 71-72
  conversion factors, 72t
Sodium retention, ADHF precipitated by, 259t
SOLVD, 84
  renal function in, 189-190
Spironolactone, 102
  clinical trials, 103, 106-107
    RALES, 103
    TOPCAT, 107, *108*
  dosage, 104t-105t
  indications for, 103, 106, 109
ST-T waves, 26t
Staging of heart failure, 33-47. See also *Classification of heart failure.*
  ACC/AHA stages, 40-43, 41t
  INTERMACS registry of stages for advanced HF, 242, 244t-245t
  NYHA classification system, 40-43, *40*, 41t, *42*

Statistically significant P-values, xii
STICHES, 159-161, *164*
"Stretch-squeeze" relationship, *52*, 54
Stroke, heart failure and, 36t, 127
Substance abuse, 23t, 43
  ADHF precipitated by, 259t
Sudden cardiac death, 141-143
  incidence of, *142*
Sulfonylureas, 165t
Surgical treatments. See also *Interventions for HF.*
  aortic stenosis, 217-219, *218*, *220-223*
  cardiac transplantation, 30, 31, 73, 237
  cardiovascular implantable electrophysiologic devices
      (CIEDs), 141-158
  implantable hemodynamic monitoring, 231-237
  left atrial appendage (LAA) closure, 228-231
  mechanical circulatory support, 237-246
  mitral regurgitation, surgical repair of, 219-228
Sympathetic nervous system, 50
Symptoms of heart failure, 21, 22t, 254-255, 256t-257t

T waves, 26t
Tachycardia, 26t, *50*
  low cardiac output and, 257t
  milrinone, 268t
  sudden cardiac death and, 141, *142*
Tamponade, MitraClip and, 228t
Telmisartan (Micardis), 87
Temperature extremes (environmental), 78-79
Thiazide diuretics, 113-115
Thiazolidinediones
  adverse effects of, 161
  in diabetes, 161
Thromboses: anti-thrombotic agents, 125-131
Thyroid function tests, 25t
Tolvaptan, 260-262, *263*
  approved uses, 262
TOPCAT, 107, *108*
Torsemide, 115-116
  effects on myocardial fibrosis, *120-121*
  effects on RAAS, *118-119*
  potential benefits of, 125t
  vs furosemide, 122t-124t, 125t

Transcatheter aortic valve replacement (TAVR), 217-219
Treatment of heart failure. See also *specific subjects.*
  in acute decompensated heart failure (ADHF), 255, 258-274
  AV nodal ablation, 147-151, *151*
  cardiac resynchronization therapy, 143, *146, 148-149*
  cardiovascular implantable electrophysiologic devices, 141-158
  classification and staging systems and, 33-47
    patient phenotypes, 43, *46-47*
    treatment context provided, 43, 44t
  goals of, xviii, 255
  guidelines for, xiv-xx, 258-259. See also *Guidelines for heart failure management.*
    2016 ESC Guidelines, xiv, xv-xx, 258-259
      on psychosocial issues, 280t, 281t
    ACC/AHA guidelines, xvi-xviii[t], 258
    guideline-directed therapy, xii, xiv
    limitations of, xii
    neuro-hormonal antagonists (ACEi-s, MRAs, β-blockers), xviii
    statistical P-values, xii
    strength of recommendations and level of evidence, xvi-xviii[t]
    updated guidelines, xiv-xx
  interventions for HF, 217-252
    aortic stenosis, 217-219
    implantable hemodynamic monitoring, 231-237
    mechanical circulatory support, 237-246
  nonpharmacologic management, 71-82
    dietary interventions, 71-77
    environmental conditions, 78-79
    physical activity, 77
  palliative care, 288-289, *289*
  pharmacologic management, 83-140, 84t
    ACEi-s, 84-86
    agents targeting pulmonary hypertension, 131-133, 132t
    anti-platelet agents, 125-127
    anti-thrombotic agents, 125-131
    anticoagulants, 127-131
    ARBs, 86-88
    β-blockers, 96-99
    of chronic heart failure, 83-140

Treatment of heart failure, pharmacologic management *(continued)*
    digoxin, 116-117, *126*
    diuretics, 113-116, 259-260
    dobutamine, 267t
    dopamine, 266-274, 267t
    hydralazine/nitrates, 109-113
    inotropes, 266-274, 267t
    ivabradine, 99-102
    milrinone, 266, 267t
    mineralcorticoid receptor antagonists (MRAs), 102-109
    morphine, 258-259
    sacubitril/valsartan, 88-96
    vasodilators, 109-113, 262-266, 274
    vasopressin antagonists, 260-262, *263*
  psychosocial issues, 279-294
    cognitive impairment, 282-283
    depression, 283-288
    end-of-life planning, 288-291
    frailty, 279-282
  QRS widening, 143, *146*
Tricyclic antidepressants, xx
Troponin T, 92, *96*
Two-dimensional echocardiography, 28, 28t
Type 2 diabetes, 161-169, 165t, *170-172*

U waves, 26t
Ultrafiltration, 262, 274

Valsartan. See also *Sacubitril/valsartan.*
  molecular structure, *90*
Vascular resistance, systemic, 50
Vasodilators, 109-113, 262-266, 274. See also *specific drugs.*
  ACC/AHA guidelines, 264
  blood pressure, concerns about, 264, 265t
  choice of agent, 264
  hypotension and, 264, 265t
  nesiritide, 264, 265t
  nitroglycerine, 264
  nitroprusside, 264
  parenteral, 262-264
  use in acute decompensated heart failure, 262-266

Vasopressin antagonists, 260-262, *263*
  tolvaptan, 260-262, *263*
Ventricle
 left
   left ventricular assist devices (LVADs), 237-242
   left ventricular ejection fraction (LVEF), xviii, 97, 110, 185
   left ventricular failure, 38-39, *38*
   physiology in HF-pEF: LV pressure/volume, *62-63*
 right
   right ventricular failure, 35-38, *38*
   right-ventricular pacing, 150t
Ventricular dysfunction, in heart failure, *52-53*, 54
Ventricular remodeling. See *Remodeling.*
Volume overload, 22t, 50
  causes of, 50, *50*
Volume status assessment, 23, 24t

Warfarin, 127, 128. See also *Anticoagulants.*
  use with clopidogrel, 130
  Watchman Device as alternative to, 229
Watchman Device, 229-231, *230*
Water restriction. See *Fluid restriction.*
Water retention, 50, *50*
Weight gain, 23t
Weight loss, recommendation for, 73-74
White blood cell count, 25t